To be, happier and more effective in your body, in your head, and in your actions. Therefore, to better contribute to the construction of the New World.
And to justify being here.

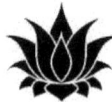

**Bonus :**

**TRAVELER'S ANECDOTES**

**160  INSPIRING QUOTES**

**32  POETRIES FROM THE AUTHOR**

### 101 Guides and 129 Exercises

# To enabled Happiness

**Stéphane Bonduelle**

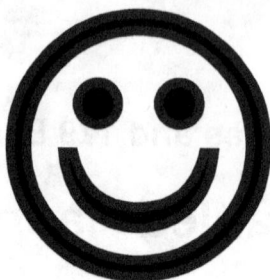

© Stéphane Bonduelle

*To everyone,*

# Summary

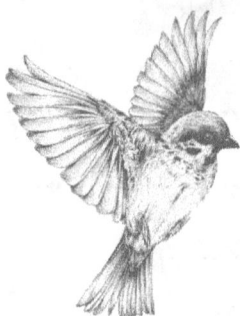

*Happiness is a quest,*

*continually requiring*

*A happy practice.*

Guides and exercises are simple and easy. All are like games. You will want to renew each game. And so, the pleasurable sensations will be refined, amplified and they will settle as your new habits.

Whatever your beliefs, your preconceived ideas, your professional situation, your social situation, your ambitions or your limitations, you will be happy to see improvements in all areas of your life: your health, your thoughts, your emotions, your love your relationships, your performances and your horizons.

All the techniques shared here with you, I practice them, and they bring me much happiness.

# 1. Introduction

My intention, in writing this manual, is to contribute to building a better world by sharing with you, techniques, exercises and feelings, each of which is a new opportunity to cultivate your happiness. You will be more and more happy because, like everything, happiness is addictive. With pleasure, you will raise your consciousness and increase your abilities. It will then be easier for us, and we will take a greater pleasure, together, in building this greater happiness and this better world that we all desire.

The guides and exercises that are offered to you, will bring you a new vitality. They'll make you think differently. They will create in you a desire to act. And they will make of you, another you, happy to be.

A first group of guides will make you happier in your body. A second, will make you happier in your head. And a third, will make you happier in your actions. These three pleasures are complementary, and they are generating a mutual inertia.

You can, if you wish, practice an exercise for several days before moving on to another, and thus, use this manual for a very long time, perhaps forgetting it for a while and then returning to it, always with pleasure. What will be important, in any way, is that you maintain a regular practice. This manual, and the new sensations of well-being that it gives you, will give you the desire, the opportunity, the pleasure and the benefits of practicing regularly.

We all live more or less unconsciously. We are unaware of breathing, hearing, seeing, touching, tasting, feeling, walking, talking, listening, thinking, feeling emotions; we are unconscious in our actions and unaware of our vital energy. We go like zombies. This unconsciousness affects our physical and mental health. We make mistakes. We are subject to forgetfulness. The results of our actions are not as good as they could be. And we miss many opportunities to be alive, to be healthy, to love, to be loved, to be effective and to succeed.

We are not conscious of experiencing these moments of unconsciousness. And maybe even, we have the impression that these moments, when we play possum, correspond to moments of rest; we are mistaken then seriously (out of innocent ignorance), because in these moments our breath is stifling, our body is stressed, we are in fact becoming more tired, and that hurts us a lot, in all aspects of our life (health, happiness, stress, relationship, efficiency, etc.). While a conscious intention to take rest or to conduct any activity, in these precise moments, allows to meet the expectations.

This manual will allow you to perceive, then to correct these trends and to seize new opportunities.

The fourth part of this manual is devoted to the Common Denominator, which is the practice of meditation. Because meditation brings many benefits, including those to feel, to appreciate and to maintain the happiness of living consciously, and, to improve the well-being and performances of the body, thought and actions. Meditation thus catalyzes the dynamics and synergies between body-thought-action.

These benefits and improvements are detailed in this manual, and 100 meditation techniques are explained. Most of these techniques are simple, and all are attractive.

In addition, practicing meditation exercises can be done in seconds, minutes or hours depending on your tastes; so, lack of time cannot be an excuse. It will be easy for you to include the practice of meditation in your daily habits, and you will be very happy with the results.

For millennia we have lived obscurantism; knowledge was reserved for an elite. In the West, in the 70s, we experienced this great movement of peace and love that had a global influence. From these times, meditation has kept the false, repellent and prejudicial images of being reserved for enlightened, privileged, dreamy, idealistic or even drug users. The knowledge revolution has allowed us to understand that these images were false and that the practice of meditation had many and great benefits accessible to all. The evolution of our societies leads us to a natural integration of meditation into our daily lives.
Now is the time for you to get into this dynamic, already very vibrant (in schools, businesses, on U-Tube, etc.).

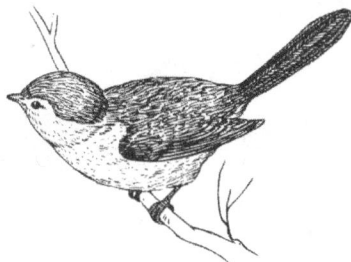

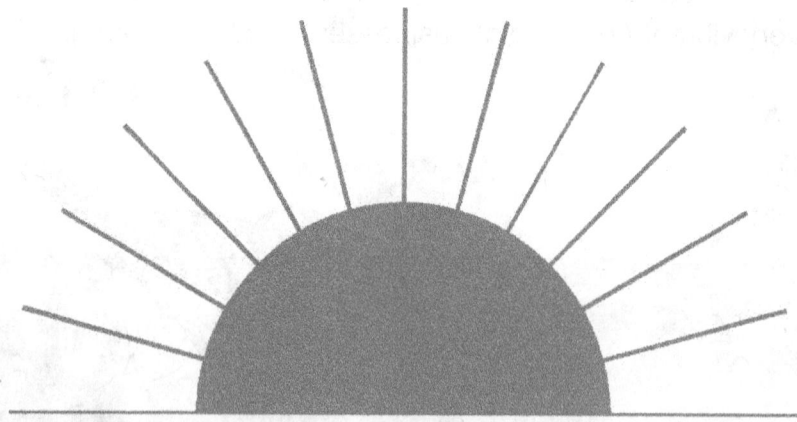

## 2. Preface

We live in a fantastic time; a lot of things is now happening. We have made enormous progress, over the last few decades. We have increased our capabilities and our opportunities.

Naturally, the abilities driven by opposite morals have also benefited. And today we have many insane sources of concern, such as the pollution of the oceans, our air and our soils, the explosion risks of our last world war, Nuclear disasters, etc.

When one observes the history of our civilization, one realizes that similar sources of anxiety have always existed. There has been plague, incessant wars and human rights violations. At the time of the Cold War, students were doing nuclear preparatory exercises, in schools. At that time, millions of children, despite their innocence and the playfulness of the exercise that interrupted classes, together with their parents, felt deep fears, facing the risk of dying in a flash, like did before them the inhabitants of Hiroshima.[1]
We realized that, whatever the circumstances are, even the best that can be, one finds easily 'reasons' to complain, to be sad and to be afraid. Because it easily gives us the feeling to exist.

---

[1] We were then gullible, because he disaster preparedness exercise to take refuge under the school tables is useful in the event of an earthquake, but very futile in the event of a nuclear explosion.

But, complaining and being sad are contrary to happiness. And, it is also regrettable to be afraid. Because fear is disabling. It disrupts our physical, physiological, and intellectual activities. And in doing so, it limits our potential. Fear wins the iron arm against love and against happiness.

Nowadays we realize many other things, for until the end of the 17th century (only a dozen generations[2] ago), our lives were monotonous, and our horizons were narrow. From the age of seven, we began, barefoot, to work very hard. And so, we went on, every day, until we died. When we were injured by a simple scratch, it became infected and we would die from it. In any case we would die young, our life expectancy was only 26 years, (A short time[3] only to learn how to survive). The level of knowledge was very low for most of us and was limited to satisfying our agricultural and domestic activities. Only a very small number of us were scholars, yet with a succinct and often incorrect knowledge.

Then we began to have access to knowledge. In the 18th century, values and humanistic and pacifist ideas, which had developed in a sparse and modest way in previous centuries, have begun to become values and ideas available to the mass of our ancestors.

It was a "knowledge revolution[4]".

---

[2] One generation corresponding to 25 years.
[3] Although high infant mortality contributed to reduce this average.
[4] This denomination, as we shall see, will be used, at the end of the 20th century, to define the computer revolution.

Naturally, as more and more people had access to knowledge, reflection, cooperation and organization, the number of our discoveries and our ways of life have begun to grow exponentially. As a result, our life expectancy has steadily increased[5], allowing us to have more diverse experiences and the opportunity to ask ourselves questions that until then we had not had time to ask, too busy satisfying only our need to eat[6] throughout our short lives.

After a steady progression for 200 years, the curve of evolution of our mass consciousness accelerates in the 20th century. Then, we discovered the theory of quanta, plane, car, galaxy, television, radio, space travel, psychology, woman's liberation, reduction of racial hatred, reduction of domestic violence, relativity theory, vaccines, hygiene, pasteurization, antibiotics, leisure time, holidays and recreation, electronic chip, robotics, computer (whose computing power Double every 18 months), the infinite fractal structure of the elementary particles, the optical fiber, the mobile phone (which appears in 1983), the Internet (which becomes accessible in the 1990s).

The information flow is not anymore limited to printing, radio and television; internet is a new great revolution in our history. With the emergence of social media, our discussion circles have gone from restricted or non-existent to planetary; We find with happiness and facility, people who have similar experiences and interests to ours;

---

[5] Today's life expectancy is more than 80 years.
[6] Survival mode.

While we were isolated and restricted, now we share; This new cooperation is very dynamic and productive. Quantum physics, propelled by Albert Einstein, brought us out of materialism, scientifically unveiling that matter is energy. Transport and access to knowledge have broadened our horizons. And we have expanded the framework of our morality beyond the limits of our villages and finally become global.

In the coming days, we will be experiencing further fantastic accelerations. With soon, the super-internet, already available, that is going to be hundreds of times faster than today. Also, with the ever-increasing capabilities of computers (computing speed, memory, search engine's performance from growing databases allowing more and more accurate responses to precise questions); In the richest countries in the world, research teams are even working on the development of the quantum computer (processing speed superior to that of light). Renewable energy production costs less than nuclear energy production, and we are currently in a period of energy transition. Thanks to global research efforts, renewable energy production, transport and technologies will make enormous progress, in the coming years. And soon all our energy needs will be provided free of cost and clean.

In all areas, the number of innovations continues to accelerate exponentially. To these technologies are added artificial intelligence, new technologies (including nanotechnology) and new discoveries, which will appear and that will amaze us.

While in recent times the variations we were experiencing over a lifetime were minimal, ten years ago no one was able to imagine the world today. The way the world will be in ten years, is even a much greater mystery. We will be essentially the same, but our environment, the way we live and our thoughts will be very different. We will make enormous progress in our ideologies, in respecting the environment, in pedagogies, technologies, sciences, arts, psychology, relational, nutrition, cosmology, sociology and philosophy. In a word, we are going to make enormous progress in the knowledge of ourselves and of everything. We cannot be bored, there are many things to do and to discover. The growing quantities and synergies of each person's thoughts, inspirations and positive innovations lead us to a wonderful evolution.

This better future is confirmed with my 'root cause theory': the study of the 'root causes' of a problem is the study of the causes for which a problem exists. In doing this study, we realize that ignorance is one of the root causes of all problems. Moreover, ignorance is also found to be a root cause of all other root causes. The cognitive evolution we are experiencing now, is named 'The Revolution of Knowledge'. This revolution is characterized by an exponential increase in the flow of information and in our ability to access, filter, process and store information. With the reduction of ignorance, the root cause of all problems, with a better knowledge of the origins of problems, we will find the solutions. We will also find solutions to the neglected human and environmental parameters that currently make us suffer. We will find our ethics. Already, we can see (assuming we watch) a profusion of good wills, inventions, new and promising ideas. We can achieve great things with good and strong intentions, desire, energy, and being active to make them progress, step by step.

We will travel far and fast, perhaps even in an instantaneous way (our advances and our curiosity allow us to remain open to any eventuality). All our cars will be smart, there will be no more accidents and no need for insurance. Our working methods will be radically changed. We will work fewer hours and on short projects. We will have the time and the means to cultivate our curiosity. Our health will also greatly improve, thanks to the knowledge we gained towards better lifestyles, better nutrition and better care of our bodies. Adapting to new methods of education will allow us to know a great deal about many things including on a large number of new things. Our curiosity will give us a clearer mind and a greater ability to question everything, to experience it, then to reject it or accept it. The capacities of each one will be multiplied tenfold; Their sums and their synergies will multiply their effects. All logistics will be far more efficient and well oiled. With our enhanced curiosity, we will be able to see the opportunities; With our increased capacity, we will be able to grasp them and put them into practice.

We will be happy !

We will reach the maximum of our potential because love, the desire to be happy, the desire to evolve and community morality, are in our nature.

All this can only be done through actions.

*The action,*
*and a healthy mind in a healthy body*
*facilitate the maintenance*
*In the consciousness of the reality*
*And in happiness.*

At certain times in our lives it is easier to be happy. Some lives seem easier than others. However, comfort can corrupt, and difficulties facilitate our evolution.
Whatever your situation, this manual will be a good companion. If, at this moment of your life, you are comfortable, you will stabilize your ease and you will be more effective to face the difficulties. If now you are in great distress, the manual will help you out. In any case, a better knowledge of yourself will be very useful.

♦

You will also have the pleasure to taste in this manual, quotes from writers, scientists, and artists. These are quotes chosen for the beauty of words.

Finally, you will find a collection of my poems, each of which is about ideas found in this manual.

*Enjoy !*

# Action

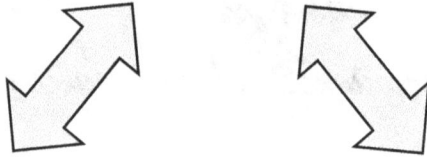

**Body** 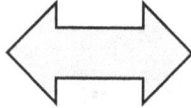 **Mind**

# 3. 101 GUIDES

These guides bring you many opportunities to be happier in your body, in your head and in your actions.

These improvements are individually sources of happiness; Many moments of happiness adding up, to furnish and fill your existence differently.

One in relation to the other, and collectively, these improvements synergize, forming a triangular dynamic. Conversely, weakness or failure in one of the three sectors affects the other two, and this dynamic.

Similarly, if you wish to improve your live in one these three areas (better health, more vitality, more dynamism, better mood, more positiveness, more success, more achievements, etc.), in addition to working on the specific area of your choice, the efforts you will make in the two other areas will greatly contribute to your improvements.

- **3.1. Happy in your body**

- **3.2. Happy in head**

- **3.3. Happy in your actions**

- **3.4. Common denominator : Meditation**

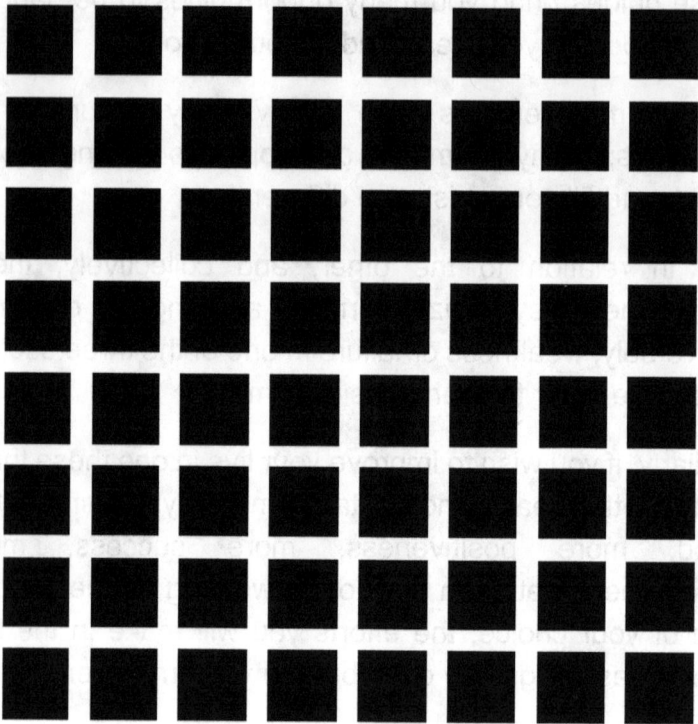

---

[7] To play: observe the optical illusion of the small gray squares, appearing in the drawing above.

## 3.1.  HAPPY IN YOUR BODY

Probably you had the opportunity to see a baby exalted with the joy of laughing. And seeing that it makes his parents laugh, he gets even more exhilarated. We will see, in this manual, the chemical reactions with the hormonal secretions, which participate to this joy. We will also see the importance of re-immersing ourselves, throughout our lives, in the child's happiness and innocence. To find, then, a powerful sensation and a powerful definition of natural happiness.
This happiness is sufficient for the child. He is satisfied, appeased, and satiated.

At each period of life, its specific happiness.
Out of childhood, being happy becomes a quest, or, a treasure hunt. We will play to explore, search, perceive, understand and integrate what makes us happy. We will discover the nature and the amplitude of influences in this triangular body-thought-action dynamic.

We will discover the importance and the existential value of breathing. We will also discover, in this chapter of happiness in his body, the roles of our physiologies in these triangular dynamics.

You will also be surprised to realize how negative stimuli on your body are causing your negative thoughts and failures in your actions. And you can benefit from correcting them.

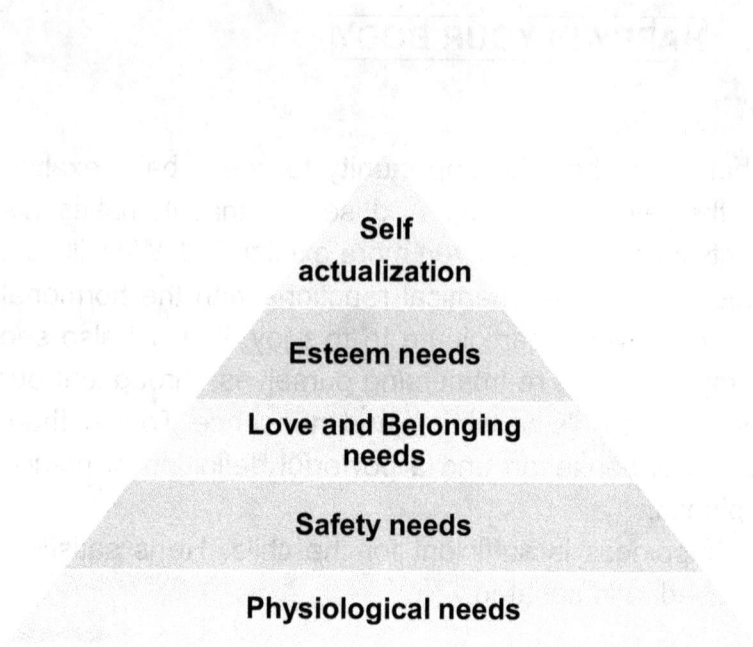

Self
actualization

Esteem needs

Love and Belonging
needs

Safety needs

Physiological needs

[8]

---

[8] Maslow's Pyramid of Needs

# The pyramid of needs

Our physiological needs are at the root of the pyramid of our needs. As with any pyramid, only a solid base can allow a solid, stable and high construction.

To be happy, you must first be alive.

The basic conditions to be alive are: breathing, drinking and eating. One can live for some time without drinking or eating. But if one stops breathing one dies after a few minutes.

In addition, to obtain a better live and to be happier, we will see opportunities to breathe better, to drink better and to eat better.

Our greatest happiness is attained when we fulfill our need of self-actualization. And we can only attain it if our other needs are satisfied beforehand.

The treasure hunt in this chapter will also allow us to play, exploring, searching, perceiving, understanding and integrating, better uses of our five senses, our energy and our emotions, to become happier along the way.

And finally, we will see how essential it is to regularly place our bodies in a natural environment.

## 001 - GUIDE to learn how to breathe

We do not breathe well for three main reasons: we do not breathe well through the nose; we use very little of the diaphragm muscle and we are not conscious of breathing.

Even very often, especially in times of stress, when we face a challenge, or when we are surprised or upset, unconsciously, our breathing becomes shallow and even we hold our breath. We create a feeling of oppression related to our thoughts. And also in these moments, we preferably breathe with the thorax (faster, less deep breathing and less efficient breathing compare to the breathing activating the diaphragm). In these times of stress, rather than operating our body in the best way with the oxygen that it especially need at these challenging times, we deprive of oxygen and we load of carbon dioxide our brain, our muscles, our digestive system, our cells, etc. But when, in these moments, we start to breathe deeply, we manage to correct this feeling of oppression for a feeling of well-being. Thanks to this close connection between our thoughts, our breathing and our emotions, the improvement of our breathing generates the improvement of our thoughts, emotions and efficiency.

The better we breath, better the apparatus and the systems of our body work, and the better we eliminate waste produced by these apparatus and systems[9].

---

[9]Human anatomy and physiology: respiratory, cardiovascular, cerebral, digestive, muscular, nervous, reproductive, lymphatic, urinary, integumentary (including skin), skeletal, glands, visual and auditory.

Make it a habit to observe during your day the way you breathe, especially in times of stress. And when you realize that you are holding your breath, practice several deep inspirations followed by slow expirations, followed by several regular inspirations-expirations, normal in duration, but always deep. Then, breathes normally.

The best way to inspire is, through the nose, rather than through the mouth. Indeed, only inspiration takes place with a muscular effort (mainly with the muscles of the rib cage and with the diaphragm), while on expiration our lungs drain naturally and effortlessly, like a balloon that deflates. The effort to inspire by the nose is less important than the effort to inspire by the mouth. Moreover, when inhaling through the nose, the temperature of the air is better controlled, which is particularly advantageous when the outside temperature is hot or cold to avoid the risk of dehydration or of a cold stroke.
Finally, thanks to the hair and the mucus, the inspiration through the nose allows to filter a lot of the dust in the ambient air, preventing it to enter our lungs.

Exhalation can be done daily, either through the nose or through the mouth. In some cases, it is preferable to exhale through the nose (e.g. by politeness during a face-to-face discussion, or when you want to get the feeling of exhaled air), or to exhale through the mouth (e.g. during meditation).

The diaphragm is the main inspiratory muscle. It separates the rib cage from the abdomen. It is possible that you have no consciousness of this muscle, that you use it very little and that it is thus little developed. It is a pity, because the breathing using the diaphragm is deeper, more efficient and allows a better functioning of your body and its physical and mental faculties. Moreover, the use of the diaphragm allows a massage of the internal organs which stimulates their proper functioning.

Practicing breathing exercises, makes us discover new sensations. For example, we realize that it is nice to have a more fluid and balanced nasal inspiration, and a diaphragmatic (with the abdomen) breathing that works better. And also, that it is very pleasant to breathe, to feel the air which circulates in our noses, our mouths, our throats; The air that swells our lungs and our belly; To visualize and to feel all the benefits brought by oxygen, and to evacuate our negative energies through expiration.

The following exercises are very effective, in quickly eliminating stress, oxygenating and detoxifying our body, increasing our vitality, improving our sleep, increasing our concentration power, improving our digestion, bringing us well-being and making us happier.

These exercises allow us to correct our habits and to adopt a beneficial better breathing daily.

Their practices are easy to include into your daily habits. You can practice them at any time, and several times a day: in the morning on waking, in the evening at bedtime, during a break at work, etc. You can also practice them very discreetly, even in public (eg in your car on the red light, in the subway or bus, in a waiting room, in an elevator, in your chair waiting to pass Before taking a job interview or making a professional presentation, during your concentration before a sporting competition, before and during any important event, etc.). Practicing will be a pleasure and not a constraint.

♦

*'Breathing is the first act of life and the last. Our very life depends on it. Since we cannot live without breathing it is tragically deplorable to contemplate the millions and millions who have never mastered the art of correct breathing'*

Joseph Pilates

♦

*'Have fewer fears and more hopes, eat less, chews more, moans less, breaths more, speaks less, says more, hated less, like more; and all the good things are for you.'*

Swedish proverb

♦

*The experience changes the sighing in breaths'*  Beck

♦

*'When you wake up in the morning, remember yourself how much precious the privilege is to live, to breathe and to be happy'*

Marc Aurel

♦

*'We age when we lock ourselves, when we refuse to see, to hear or to breathe'*

Katherine Pancol

## 👀 Exercise 1 : Fluid nostril breathing

Daily, we inspire a lot of dirt, especially after being exposed to a dusty or polluted environment. But it also happens when you walk in nature. The fact of having so much dirt in the nose is a good thing because it shows the effectiveness of the filtering function of the nose (with hair and mucus) and this allows dirt not to reach the lungs. Yet this dirt hinders our breathing.

I discovered this simple technique of cleaning the nose, more than thirty years ago. And since then, it is part of my daily toilet, and I could not do without it. I even practice it several times a day, when I wash my hands. I am always amazed at the amount of dirt that is eliminated. I am very pleased to have a fluid nasal breath. And I cannot wait to find that fluidity, when it is blocked.

This technique involves inhaling water through the nose. This may seem unpleasant or insurmountable at first. But very quickly it will become pleasant. You will enjoy having a smooth nasal breath; and you may also become to feel the need to clean your nose daily.

Again, inspiration through the nose is more effective than inspiration through the mouth. And better breathing will allow you better oxygenation and better functioning of all the cells of your body. (Note: it is really a large amount of dirt that you will eliminate, so think of cleaning your sink).

**Here is the technique step by step:**

o   Take water from the palm of your hand.

o   Inhale this water through the nose.

o   Exhale through the nose to evacuate this water (like when you blow your nose, using your thumb and index).

o   Renew the exercise three to four times, or as long as you still feel dirt that clogs your nose.

♦

*'The nose is made to inhale.*

*The mouth is made to eat'* Proverb

♦

*'As long as we can still breathe, after the rain, under an apple tree, we can still live!'*

Soljenitsyne

## 👁👁 Exercise 2 : Alternate nostril breathing

It is normal, depending on the circumstances, or merely by cycle, that during the day, we should inhale more easily through one nostril or the other. I invite you, now, to realize, that it is easier for you, to inhale through one nostril than through the other.

o   Use your thumb to close a nostril, and your ring finger to close the other.

o   Begin several times to inhale and exhale through the left nostril, while closing the right.

o   Now inhale and exhale several times through the right nostril, while closing the left nostril.

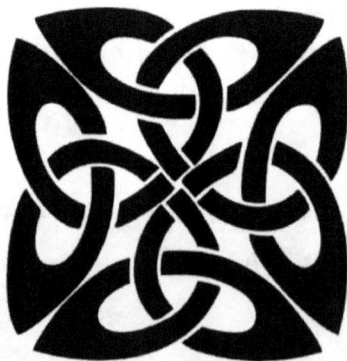

Now practice the following exercise (30 seconds x 3 times):

o With the mouth closed, inhales-exhales through both nostrils several times.

o Inhale-exhale as follows, changing nostrils at the end of each inhale, to a mental count of 5 when inhaling, and to a mental count of 10 when exhaling. Each time clogs the other nostril:

- Inhale with the left nostril.

- Close both nostrils to a count of 3.

- Exhale with the right. Inhale with the right.

- Close both nostrils to a count of 3.

- Exhale with the left. Inhale with the left.

This simple and fast exercise is particularly effective for removing stress. Think of using it, to become more casual and more effective during moments of tension. It can be done discreetly, therefore in all circumstances.

The repeated practice of this exercise will allow you to gain a sustainable balance your breath between the two nostrils. You will experience the great satisfaction of having a more fluid and profound breathing, and, an improvement in your balance, your well-being, your health and your efficiency.

## 👀 Exercise 3 : Diaphragmatic breathing

**In preparation for the exercise**, begins by feeling the movements of your diaphragm:

o When lying down, place your right hand on your stomach to feel it swelling and deflating.

o Place your left hand on your heart to feel your chest cavity swelling and deflating.

o Concentrate on your diaphragm and sense it is going down when inhaling and back up when exhaling.

o Continue this preliminary exercise until you gain a good feeling of the work of your diaphragm.

**Now you can do the actual exercise:**

o Keep your hands on the belly and on the heart as indicated above.

o Counting (1-2-3) deeply inhale through the nose by inflating the belly.

o Counting (4-5) continue your inhale through the nose by now inflating your rib cage.

o Counting (1-2) retain your breath.

o Counting to 10 exhale slowly through the mouth.

o Renew this inhale-exhale cycle at least 10 times, then as many times as you want.

## ◉◉ Exercise 4 : 16 conscious breathing exercises

Usually we are not aware that we breathe. Conscious breathing is very simple to practice. It is closely related to meditation; it is even one of the basic principles. One can even say that practicing conscious breathing is practicing meditation. So, congratulations! What you always wanted to know about meditation, without daring to ask, or without daring to start, now you know, and you do.
Breathing is synonymous with life and existence.

After previous conscious breathing exercises. Here are now sixteen other exercises.
The different techniques and options have each their specific sensory, anatomical, physiological, psychological and psychic qualities.
Some will be more attractive to you than others; seize then the opportunity of this attraction which favors your assiduity of practice. Also be curious and enthusiast to explore other techniques to benefit from their specificities.

## 1.   Exercise: 4 - 4 through the nose

o   Inhale through the nose to a mental count of four.

o   Exhale through the nose to a mental count of four.

o   Continue for at least 2 minutes.

o   After a few days of practice, gradually increase your practice to 6 - 6 then to 8 - 8

## 2. Exercise: Nadi Shodhana breathing

Repeat the Alternate nostril breathing, placing your pointer finger between your eyebrow and focusing on this point.

## 3. Exercise: 10 - 10

o   Inhale through the nose to a mental count of 10.

o   Exhale through the mouth to a mental count of 10.

o   Continue for at least 2 minutes.

## 4. Exercise: Joining breathing in and breathing out

o   Breathing calmly, join breathing in and out.

o   Count "one" to yourself as you exhale. The next time you exhale, count "two".

o   And so on up to "ten", becoming more and more calm each time you exhale.

o   Renew cycle (1 to 10) as many times as you like.

## 5. Exercise: 4 - 4 - 4 - 4     (repeat at least 3 times)

o   Inhale through the nose to a mental count of 4.

o   Retain your breath to a mental count of 4.

o   Exhale through the mouth to a mental count of 4.

o   Retain your breath to a mental count of 4.

## 6. Exercise: 4 - 7 - 8

o   Exhale completely through your mouth emptying your lungs; and making a lion roar with your throat.

o   Closed mouth calmly inhale through the nose, to a mental count of 4.

o   Retain your breath to a mental count of 7.

o   Exhale completely through the nose, making the lion's roar, to a mental count of 8.

o   Repeat the series 3 times, and more if you wish.


## 7. Exercise: Buddha's breathing 8 - 16 (3 times)

o   Slowly inhale with the belly, to a mental count of 8.

o   Slowly exhale with the belly, to a mental count of 16.


## 8. Exercise: Tao breathing 8 - 16 (3 times)

The count is the same as in the previous exercise, but here, the abdominal muscles are contracted on inhales and the chest and lungs are relaxed on exhales.


## 9. Exercise: Muscles of the anus contracted (20 times)

o   Slowly inhale through the nose, contracting the muscles of the anus.

o   Slowly exhale through the mouth, releasing the muscles of the anus.

## 10. Exercise: Even more                    (3 times)

o  Slowly inhale through your nose to fully fill your lungs.

o  Retain your breath to a mental count of 3.

o  Inhale 3 more time.

o  Slowly exhale through your mouth to empty your lungs.

o  Retain your breath to a count of 3.

o  Exhale 3 more time.


## 11.  Exercise: The compressed organs        (3 times)

o  Slowly exhale through your mouth to empty your lungs.

o  Continue to exhale as much as possible, bringing the belly of the spine closer together and contracting the muscles of your anus.

o  You will feel an intense desire to inhale. Remain a short moment feeling this desire.

o  By being relaxed, lower your diaphragm and inhale letting your lungs filling in.


## 12. Exercise: Apnea

Inspire slowly through the nose. Retain your breath to be in apnea. Extends the duration of apneas, as and when practices.

## 13. Exercise: Training the diaphragm

o   Inhale slowly, closing your eyes, and concentrating on the descent of your diaphragm.

o   With a sharp exhaling blow, open your eyes and lift your diaphragm.

o   Do at least 20 inhale-exhale, and more if you wish.


## 14. Exercise: Candles 5 - 15

o   Slowly inhale through the nose, to a mental count of 5.

o   Exhale through the mouth, shaped like you would blow a candle, to a mental count of 15.

o   Do at least 20 inhale-exhale, and more if you wish.


## 15. Exercise: The boxer's breathing

o   Exhale slowly and deeply through your mouth until your lungs are completely empty.

o   Make 4 inhales through the nose, lengthening each time the length of the inhale.

o   Retain your breath to a count of 4.

o   Exhale slowly and deeply through your mouth until your lungs are completely empty.

o   Do at least 20 inhale-exhale, and more if you wish.

## 16. Exercise: Using a Rosary

The rosaries are used in many traditions (for example: mala in Hinduism, Jainism and Buddhism (practice of mantras), tesbih in Islam (for example: practice of dhikr and to recite the 99 names of Allah).

Its use has many advantages:

- Concentration on pearl touch, coupled with concentration on breathing, is an additional opportunity to avoid thinking.

- We are not forced to count; our mind is not busy counting and we avoid getting lost in the count.

- Even if one is aware of the benefits of practicing meditation, and even if one is attracted by the desire to practice, practice regularly (at best daily) and do sessions of several minutes often remain difficulties to overcome.

  Using a rosary, our goal of practicing as many breaths (or mantras) as the number of beads in the rosary is made easy to achieve. More than to bring us discipline, the rosary motivates us and trains us. At the end of a cycle of pearls, one even sees the desire to continue with another cycle.

**Practice example:**

Conscious breathing, by scraping a pearl with each inhale-exhale, until the entire rosary (3x33, 99 or 108 following the rosary used)

## ☻☻ Exercise 5 : The stage breathing

Perform this exercise with the depth of breath that suits you best to feel the best sensations. When you have good sensations, the goal is to look for a natural and relaxed staged breath containing all the following inhaling stages:

o   Start inhaling using the upper part of your lungs.

o   Continue inhaling using the middle part of your lungs.

o   Continue inhaling using the lower part of your lungs.

o   Continue inhaling visualizing that you extend it to your pubis.

o   Expires in a natural way and without forcing, then enchains the following breathing in.

Another stage breathing technic is done in opposite way :

o   Start inhaling at the pubis level.

o   Inhale in the 3 parts of the lungs.

o   Inhale under the clavicles.

o   End at the top of your head.

## ☯☯ Exercise 6 : The energizing breathing

As the name implies, the practice of energizing breathing results in a boost of dynamism and vitality.

o  With your mouth closed, make a series of nasal inspirations-expirations, fast and short.

o  Make 3 breaths-expirations per second.

o  Do these quick cycles for 10 seconds (count on your 10 fingers).

o  After each 10 seconds, breaths calmly for another 10 seconds.

o  Do 3 cycles of 20 seconds.

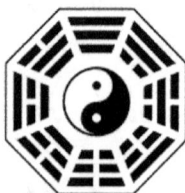

After familiarizing yourself with the previous breathing exercises you can practice the two following techniques.

## Technique 1:

It consists in introducing into your inhale and exhale the sensation of the air passing through the back of the throat. To increase this sensation, you can make a sound with your throat, both when inhaling and when exhaling.

Renew previous breathing exercises by making sure you keep your concentration on this point in your throat. It will certainly happen that at certain moments you lose your concentration on the point, then simply resume.

## Technique 2:

It is to imagine two things when inhaling: that the pores of all the surface of your skin open and that every cell of your body is oxygenated, from the head to the feet. And when exhaling, all the pores on the surface of your skin close again.

You will find this option, for several practices of the manual. It's an interesting option, reflecting reality, that breathing oxygen all the cells in your body. It helps to recognize the value of breathing and optimize its energy intake. It also helps to harmonize the energy throughout your body, rebalancing the areas exhausted.

.

## 002 - GUIDE to ensure sufficient drinking

Majority of us do not drink enough. Strangely, we have a great deal of difficulty correcting this defect. As if we wanted to punish ourselves for something, by refusing to be in good health and a greater well-being. Yet, drinking insufficiently is not a fatality, such as having blue eyes. It can be changed easily and for our greatest benefit.

We need to drink enough so that all the vital processes of our body work well. The amount to be consumed per day varies between 1 and 3 liters depending on the size, weight, activity, more or less warm weather, and the diet more or less rich in fruits and vegetables. For example, for an athlete it is recommended to drink a half liter, two hours before exercise, and then regularly during the effort. (You can lose 1 liter of water in 1 hour of sport).

In fact, one should never feel the feeling of thirst, because then it is a sign of dehydration. We will try to drink regularly so as not to feel thirsty.

Observing the color of your urine will tell you if you drink enough. The optimal color is a barely noticeable yellow. A dark yellow indicates a lack of hydration and the need to remedy it.

**Establish hydration routine :**

Drink a glass of water or fresh fruit or vegetable juice regularly at the same times, such as at sunrise, at bedtime, arriving at work, at break times, at meal times, after each visit to the toilet, at the end of a repetitive task, a glass of water that accompanies each of your coffees of the day, arriving at your place, or at a certain time. Always keep water handy.

Regularly introducing soups into your diet is another good contribution to your hydration. Moreover, their multitude favors the variety of your menus. They are delicious and economical.

By drinking more, you will automatically urinate more. Drink and also urine with pleasure, including that to eliminate waste.

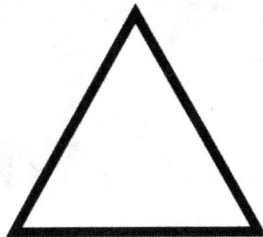

## 👀 Exercise 7 : To drink consciously

We tend to drink, being conscious neither of what we do, nor of what we drink.

o   Fill a glass of water and sit at your table;

o   Give thanks for the chance to be able to drink,

o   Feel the liquid that flows in your body,

o   Be aware of what you drink (the smells, the tastes, the provenances, the well-being that it procures).

You can do this exercise punctually. You can also choose to apply it every time you drink, and so, each time to drink consciously.

You can also practice this exercise by choosing the option to visualize your drink bathing and benefiting each cell of your body, your drink that makes your blood purer and more fluid, water that cleans waste produced by the work of your muscles, the fluid blood that allows your kidneys to do a better job of eliminating toxins from your blood, your body becoming stronger.

*Let's now drink a big glass*

*to our good health !*

## ◉◉ Exercise 8 : The intestinal draining

Intestinal health defines general health.

The length of the intestine is 7 meters; Over the years, waste accumulates on the walls of the intestine, on a layer that can reach a thickness of 1 centimeter. We can thus, accumulate between 5 and 12 kilos of waste in its intestine!

Intestines irrigation is one of the most important health practices, among alternative medicines. For many naturopaths, with fasting, it is key to physical and mental health. This is easy to understand, when one considers the large accumulation of waste, the fact that this waste ferments, putrefies, poison the blood and thus cause many diseases.

Elimination of this waste will directly reduce our overweight. It will allow proper functioning of the intestines, and good nutrients to pass in the bloodstream through the intestinal wall. Thus, we cure, and we avoid many diseases.

Intestines irrigation can be done, thanks to the respectable technique of the enema, which remains a complementary practice. But, it is simpler and easier, to drink, at one time, a large quantity of water in the morning when waking, before breakfast (from 1 to 2 liters). As a result, two minutes after drinking, you will be in a hurry to go to the toilet to eliminate, rectally, this water accompanied by some of the waste. You can use this technique, for example once a month at the weekend, (making sure the toilets are free).

## 003 - GUIDE to change your eating habits

The quality, quantity and cost of what we eat is a concern for all of us. However, the vast majority of us, do not eat optimally to feel at best, and do not use the cost-effective opportunities of healthy eating.

It is observed that the richer a country is, the higher the number of its inhabitants who are overweight. There are also circumstances in life that are conducive to weight gain, due to hormonal upsets, or because of greater temptations to eat (such as, for example, adolescence, pregnancy for women, the first year of marriage for a man, a joyful situation, a sad situation, a depression, a loss of a job, a new job, a move, etc.).

Still, by definition, one feels better when one has his weight form than when one is overweight. If you are overweight and someone says, 'I have a miracle method to make you lose your overweight quickly', do not believe it. Losing your overweight is long (depending on your overweight, a loss of 500 grams to 1 kilo per week is reasonable).

## The only method which works is to change your food habits.

Although it is essential to be active, the overweight is due to 80% to a bad diet and to 20% to a lack of activity.

Without overweight, we move better.

We are less tired.

We protect our heart and our joints.

We have fewer pains.

We avoid medicine.

We make more things.


We are happier !

That being said, if you are currently overweight, it is important that you allow any feeling of exclusion or sadness to pass, and that you replace them by the happiness to breathe, by the desire to observe your behavior, by the integration of the truth that it is advantageous to have better physical condition, and by the energy in motion responding to your intention to change your habits. Indeed, the balance of emotions plays an important part in obtaining the ideal weight.

Clearly the body is resistant, and it appears to be able to function in the worst conditions. The body also demonstrates a formidable capacity to regenerate itself and to compensate. However, the functioning of the body, in these worst conditions, is incomplete, it is missing the advantages of its optimal functioning. The well-being of a person with, for example, a badly functioning liver, bowel, heart or nervous system, is very different from the well-being of another person with these optimal functions. Thus, the decision to change eating habits is obvious. Again, and again: just start, the feeling of the benefits happens quickly, and it is encouraging. One improvement leads to another one, in the trio Body-Head-Action.

◆

*'Physical fitness is not only one of the most important keys to a healthy body, it is the basis of dynamic and creative intellectual activity.'*

John F. Kennedy

Let us see the meaning of changing the eating habits.

This does not necessarily mean becoming fundamentalist on a choice not to eat or to eat such or such thing. It will be advantageous to respect occasional and passing gastronomic conviviality (an evening with friends, an opportunity to appreciate this or that gastronomy, or a punctual desire). Apart from these exceptional events, changing one's eating habits means making life choices, which are followed daily, and over the long term (the short-term causes the effect yo-yo = I lose Weight then I find it back).

We will make the choice to eat what our body needs to feel good. There are foods that should be completely removed (such as sugar, sodas, sweets, industrial foods including fruit juices, refined vegetable oils such as corn, soya and rapeseed, and refined cereals). Also, there are foods that are best avoided, or that you should eaten in moderation (like bread). Finally, there are foods that are beneficial (like fruits and vegetables).

♦

*'Let food be thy medicine and medicine be thy food'.*

Hippocrate

♦

*'Our bodies are our gardens – our wills are our gardeners.'*

Shakespeare

The embryo develops from the primordial intestine. Then along this central trunk are formed all the other organs, which keep nerve connections with the intestines. Because of this, the quality of the diet has great influences, especially on thought, mood, optimal functioning of the body, well-being and action. A good nutrition is a primary condition to a happy life.

For example, such a day, we keep telling ourselves "Oh how unhappy I am! ". It's not that we have new excuses to complain, but because our meal of the day before was too rich.

♦

*'The doctors of the future will no longer treat the human frame with drugs, but rather will cure and prevent disease with nutrition.'*

Thomas Edison

♦

*'We find the proportion not only in measurements and numbers, but also in sounds, weights, time, places, and in every form of energy'*

Léonard de Vinci

♦

*'Don't wait until you've reached your goal to be proud of yourself. Be proud of every step you take toward reaching that goal.'*

unknown

Our digestive system is going from esophagus to anus. It measures about nine meters. It is also named: the enteric nervous system. It is also named the second brain. It contains some 100 million neurons (this is more than the spinal cord). 95% of body's serotonin is found in the bowels.

The second brain is not only involved in the digestion processing, it is also involved in our feeling, emotions, mood and well-being.

Some concepts cannot be understood mentally (like the concept, further developed later in this manual, of "being and not being", the intuition, the inner self, or the "guts feeling"), but they are felt at the level of our second brain independently of the brain, except that these feelings are at the origin of some thoughts in the brain.

The neurogastroenterology is a blossoming field, and we are going to learn interesting facts about the second brain, in the coming years. These facts will allow us to find solutions to many troubles and pathologies; so far, the potential applications already identified are addressing major issue, as: obesity, eating disorders, anxiety, depression and autism.

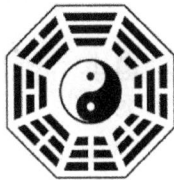

## ◉◉ Exercise 9 : Your ideal body-weight

The Lorentz formula is the most used to calculate the theoretical ideal weight.

This formula is different for the men and for the women as follows:

Women = Height (cm) - 100 - [Height - 150] / 2,5

Men    = Height (cm) - 100 - [Height - 150] / 4

Example: for a woman being 165 cm
Theoretical ideal weight = 165 - 100 - 15/2,5 = 59 kg

Note: there are two conditions of use of this formula:
o   Be of more than 18 years old
o   Measure between 140 and 220 cm

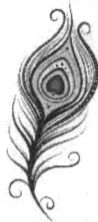

This formula is interesting to set you a goal of loss of weight. However, it is possible that you feel completely dynamic and at ease with yourself with a weight upper or lower than this reference.

## ☻☻ Exercise 10 : Your tailored daily calorie intake

With some variances, depending on gender, age and activity level, the average need of calorie per day is 2200. When the calorie intake is above the calorie consumption, the excess is transformed into fat.

If you wish to lose weight it is recommended to evaluate your daily calorie intake, with data available on packaging or with data found on internet for the food not packed; then, on a long run, to reduce your calorie intake to 2000 calories per day.

Note 1: Physical exercise is important, to not loose muscle from the deficit of calories, but to lose fat. Note that during the physical exercise the consumption of calories is not very high, but the physical exercise increases the speed of the metabolism of your body for many hours after the exercise consequently increasing the number of calories spent.

Note 2: Drinking sufficient quantity of water contributes to the weight loss.

Note 3: Equilibrated intake proportion of carbohydrate, proteins, lipids is 421.

If you wish to gain weight you should increase your calorie intake above 2200 per day.

## 👁👁 Exercise 11 : Eat bananas

One banana contains many of the good things:

o Vitamin C: (11 % GDA[10]) anti-fatigue, resistance to the infections, antioxidant, promotes iron absorption, good for the skin (role in the manufacturing of the collagen), helps to fight against allergies and stress.

o Vitamin B6: (33 % GDA) Good for the nervous system, promotes the production of white blood cell thus favors the immune system, reduces the inflammations in particular at the level of the joints.

o Potassium: (9 % GDA) The lack of potassium is frequent in our nutrition. The potassium is essential to the muscular contraction including in the smooth running of the heart, it is also essential in the transmission of the nervous impulses, promotes the functioning of the kidney, lowers the blood pressure and protects against the heart attack.

o Manganese: (14 % GDA) Essential to the smooth running of the body, essential in the functioning of the brain, vital for the bones growth and for their preservation, activator of enzymes, promotes sexual activity and reproduction, promotes metabolism of fats and carbohydrates, ease premenstrual syndrome, help to the absorption of vitamins.

---

[10] GDA = Guideline Daily Amounts

o Magnesium: (15 % GDA) Essential to the functioning of the muscles including the heart, and the nervous system. Acts in prevention of the diabetes, the atherosclerosis and the high blood pressure.

o Copper: (10 % GDA) Essential to the functioning of the body. It fights against the ageing, promotes the use of the iron, promotes growth, promotes hair growth, reduces arthritis symptoms.

o Calcium: (1 % GDA) The calcium deficiencies are increasing in the modern world. The Calcium is essential to the life. It allows to have good bones and good teeth. It acts in the prevention of the cancer of the colon and the pebbles in loins, it contributes to fight against the obesity.

o Tryptophan: get transformed to serotonin the neurotransmitter which gives us the joy of life and helps us avoid the depression.

o Pectin: help to the digestion.

o Fibers: (23 % GDA) help digestion.

Furthermore, the banana, rich in potassium, stimulates the brain work (it is for example good to eat one before taking an examination or before any other intellectual performances). It also promotes the memory, it relieves the anemia, it protects against the muscular cramp, it is antacid, and it relieves the stomach ulcers.

The banana is very easy to transport, and very easy to eat. You can sometimes, even often, make a meal by eating only bananas.

One banana contains approximately 150 calories, very few proteins and practically no fat. It is however very nourishing, and it calms very well the hunger.
So, to eat bananas is a very good choice for a good nutrition and to allow losing overweight.

The banana is also one of the cheapest food (even organic and in fair trade). Then by eating bananas, you also spend less money to feed.

(Raw carrots bring also many advantages, by their contents, their price and the fact as naturally their chewing is long. And they are so crunchy!)

## *The banana is a tremendous food!*

For my part I eat two bananas at each of the three meals of the day. And I am very satisfied with it.

I am also very satisfied with the menu of my breakfast. And I share it with you below if you want to try:

*Breakfast menu :*

- *Cold drink:*

  - *1 lemon juice*

  - *1/4 teaspoon of turmeric powder*

  - *1 teaspoon of honey*

- *2 Bananas*

- *Hot drink (without sugar)*

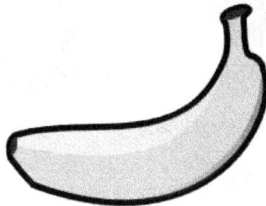

## ◉◉ Exercise 12 : Stop unnecessary food

Industrial food is rich in sugars, oils, salts, colorants, preservatives and other chemicals. It is desirable to avoid it. Sodas, in particular, have no interesting nutritional value. They offer only disadvantages: one bottle of soda (33cl) contains the equivalent of 10 teaspoons of sugar, which corresponds to 160 calories (useless). Very logically, the sodas are very bad to weight-control and fight against overweight. Sodas contribute to the increase in diabetes, increase the risk of heart disease, attack the teeth, promote osteoporosis, are bad for the liver, contain caffeine that promotes dehydration and insomnia, increase risk of kidney stones.

This exercise only concerns you if you drink soft drinks. So, you can now take the decision to stop. According to your past habits, you may feel a strong urge to drink a soda in the following days, you can, then, let yourself go to satisfy this envy; The important thing is your decision for the rest of your life; Little by little, this kind of strong desire will become rarer; Then this desire will be eliminated. If you are parent of a young child, the first thing to do, is never give a soda to your child, then firmly to never have soda at home. In case your child has already tasted the explosive excitement of caffeine and the massive dose of sugar, you can now firmly stop buying sodas, explaining the reasons for your decision.

## ◉◉ Exercise 13 : At every meal

We now know the importance of eating several fruits and vegetables a day.

It is recommended to eat five different ones per meal.
It may seem like a lot to you, it is not. Just start. I sometimes enjoy counting their number in my meal, and the other day the total was 14! (counting different nuts).

However, meals containing little or no fruit and vegetables are not dramatic, when they remain scarce. It is again a matter of changing eating habits.

We love change and diversity. It is therefore normal and desirable that our menus change. We can do this by following the seasons of fruit and vegetable production, enjoying it abundantly, and possibly looking for variants by cooking salads and other dishes.

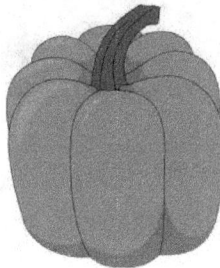

## 👀 Exercise 14 : Risks of deficiency

There are many common misconceptions about deficiencies that a diet favoring fruits and vegetables could generate.

This is the case for calcium. Well this is wrong!
There is enough calcium in fruits and vegetables to satisfy our needs. Moreover, the calcium benefit of dairy products is also a lie, because this calcium is not well assimilated by the body, and even generates calcium deficiencies.

We also hear about a possible protein deficiency that a vegetarian nutrition could generate. Already, these are not proteins we need, but amino acids (the proteins we eat must be destroyed by our digestive system to remove amino acids). And fruits and vegetables (especially green vegetables) are rich in amino acids, simpler, and easier to assimilate.

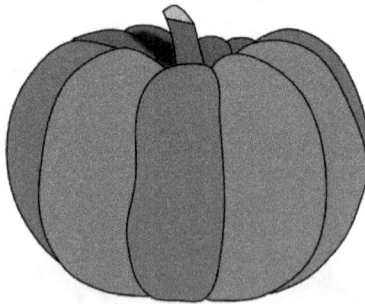

Considers two genuine risks of deficiency:

**Vitamin B12:** We need vitamin B12 to live. Our needs increase with age [0.4 micrograms per day (0.4 mcg / d) in infants up to 3 mcg / d in adults]. Whatever our diet we often see deficiencies. Deficiency causes a risk of anemia over the long term. The problem is less important if you eat animal products (mainly crustaceans and meat). Vitamin B12 is also found in cheese and eggs (about 1.8 mcg / 100 g for both) (the average weight of an egg is 53 g, so the consumption of two eggs satisfies the need for vitamin B12 for an adult - as is the consumption of about 150 g of cheese). On the other hand, for people who choose not to eat any food of animal origin, there is no alternative but to take vitamin B12 dietary supplements (data that show a vitamin intake in certain plants, like Spirulina, appear to be unreliable, Spirulina remaining a food of choice).

**Good cholesterol (HDL):** HDL deficiencies are frequently observed (mainly in smokers, inactive persons and overweight people). They cause cardiac risks. HDL is found in fish (more in fatty fish) and in the following products: nuts, olive oil, avocado, cocoa, onion, beans and lentils, cabbage, etc.

## 👀 Exercise 15 : Eating differently

Use your freedom to eat something else, to eat less, or to experiment with food, here are two examples:

**Experiment eating raw** :

The lovers of raw food diet are becoming more and more numerous, as are vegetarians, vegans, and adepts of fruit and vegetable juices.

Eating raw makes sense, because when you cook the food, 80% of the vitamins, minerals, amino acids and other components are destroyed.

Many properties are attributed to raw vegetarian diets ('living food'), such as the elimination of wastes accumulated in the body, the prevention and cure of diseases such as cardiovascular diseases, cancers, diabetes, digestive disorders, Arthritis, etc. This diet has the advantage of being rich in antioxidant.
This diet is also very effective at losing excess weight and maintaining its weight form.
Eating raw, vegetarian or other, are, with the exploration of subtle tastes, gastronomic experiences. To offer variety, intensity of tastes and to satisfy the pleasure of cooking, seasonings offer many possibilities. In addition, the countless spices, herbs, plants (especially garlic), and oils have other powerful virtues at our disposal.

Begin by gradually adding raw food to your diet, more salads, more fruits and more vegetables.

Out of curiosity, you can, for one or more days eating exclusively raw, including avoiding the bread. And observe these your sensations. Do you feel more dynamic, less tired, lighter, less depressed?

Then, change your diet habits, according to the preferred sensations.


**Eating less meat** :

There is at least a consideration of the management of our planetary resources. Indeed, it is observed that the more the population of a country becomes rich, the more the consumption of meat, dairy and fish is high. There is a growing consumption among the Chinese, the Indians (yet reputed to be vegetarians) and in all the many other countries that are developing rapidly. The largest consumers of meat are the inhabitants of the United States of America. Our planet is already devastated by intensive livestock farming, it does not have the capacity to withstand an increase in the meat consumption of other countries to the height of that of the United States. It is therefore vital to make the choice to limit our consumption of meat (by favoring the consumption of quality meat), or simply to suppress it.

As you started making dietary experiments, do that to reduce your consumption of meat, then that to remove it for a period of time; And again, be attentive to the observation, these days, of the feeling of your sensations.

Then adapt your diet according to the feelings that make you happiest.

## 👀 Exercise 16 : Fasting is a treasure.

It is probable that you have never tasted the riches of fasting, and that the assertion 'fasting is a treasure' may seem surreal to you.

If that's your case, I encourage you to put on your explorer's suit, to go on a treasure hunt. You will discover new pleasures, new clarity of mind, a pleasant sensation of lightness, an increase of your optimism and vitality, the disappearance of common health problems and even the solution to the great diseases of the century[11].

It is indeed an exploration in question. It may be an exploration of your repulsion at the idea of fasting, an exploration of an instinctive impulse of the desire to fast, an exploration of a nascent desire to fast, or the exploration of a deep desire to fast. Then come explorations of feelings of hunger and well-being.

When you explore your repulsion, you observe your cultural and behavioral habits. You also observe your curiosity and your relationship with change. Then you observe the light of the desire to fast, and you will cultivate your intention to pursue this desire.

---

[11]Obesity, hypertension, atherosclerosis / circulatory and cardiac pathologies, diabetes and cancer. Fasting has great preventive virtues. The curative properties should be explored sparingly when the body is weakened by the disease.
But, if you are currently under medical treatment, you shall continue it.

Hunger is of course felt. It is a sensation that is interesting to explore. This sensation is transient, and this impermanence is itself a good subject of observation, but in case it is difficult to bear, it is possible to drink a glass of hot water mixed with a spoonful of honey.

Note that stomach pains when fasting are mistakenly identified with a feeling of hunger. These pains are a good sign that corresponds to the purging of the digestive system. They pass.

After your intention is established, several forms of fasting are at your disposal, each one should be accompanied by a good hydration (2 liters / day), except dry fasting :

Dry fasting:

When one begins to experience the practice of fasting, it is easier to maintain hydration. After a few practices you will be able to experience dry fasting.

Dry fasting has also been practiced for millennia. Its followers attribute to it much greater benefits compared to fasting with hydrations (preservation of mineral salts, detoxification of the body, cell regeneration, elimination of fats, elimination of waste, reduction of inflammations, reduction of cholesterol, regulation of the sugar level in blood, slowing down of aging, prevention of osteoporosis and many other benefits of fasting).

The instinctive impulse :

In normal times, or due to excesses in food, we often feel instinctively the desire to fast. So, rather than forgetting this instinctive impulse, it is beneficial to get used to listening and following it.

A parent, responsible for his or her children, can invalidate the instinctive nutritional desires of their children, including that of not eating. The instinctive impulses are powerful in children, they must be respected. It should be noted that fasting stimulates the secretion of growth hormone. Thus, the practice of fasting is perfectly adapted to children, recommended to sportsmen, and recommended to adults to fight against aging.

We will further explore, in the manual, our relations with the instinctive impulses related to diet. Note that, in case you are feeling an instinctive impulse to eat light, you will also benefit from following it, exploring the sensations, including the growing and disappearing sensations of hunger.


The 24H fasting :

The fast of 24H can be punctual. It can also be practiced with intermittence of one or more days per week.

It is not necessary to choose a day of rest to practice fasting, because on the contrary the choice of a day, during which one is very active, the occupation of our mind facilitates the diversion of the obsession of the sensation of hunger.

Intermittent fasting :

This form of fasting is easy. It is much practiced. It can be your initiation to fasting. It can also become a way of life.

The principle is to establish a period of fasting during the day. This period can be 16 hours (e.g. do not eat from 9:00 pm to 1:00 pm the next day). They may be punctually longer periods, from 17 to 20 hours.

A simple, easy and effective practice is to have your breakfast later (which has the benefit of giving your body more time to wake up), and dinner earlier (which allows you to sleep better) and that also influences your mood the next day when you will feel lighter, more dynamic and less moody).

The 72H fasting :

While the fasting practices described above contribute significantly to the detoxification of our body, it is after a 72H fast that our body is well detoxified.

The long duration fasting :

Great benefits are attributed to the practice of fasting for a period of three weeks. I have never done this experiment (which requires programming), so I will not talk about it.

## 👀 Exercise 17 : Freedom out the cafeteria

Many of us, for professional reasons, must eat at the canteen or at the restaurant. And these meals are usually too rich in sugars, salt and refined oils. For these meals, in the middle of your working day, as for the whole of your diet, it will be useful to you to reflect on your habits. It will also be useful for you to experiment with food. And by doing these experiments, you will evaluate the type of nutrition that suits you best. You will evaluate the foods that make it more dynamic, the ones giving you a better digestive comfort, and those that on the contrary weaken you, and negatively influence your state of mind. These experiences will be especially useful if you have preconceived ideas such as 'I need to eat meat to have enough energy', or 'It is necessary to eat large quantities of food'.

For my part, I realized that a simple and light diet suited me better. I also realized that when I had made a larger meal, during a pleasant event, in addition to the discomfort, the following days the induced addiction to excess gastronomy was exciting me further. To choose, I prefer, enjoying the well-being provided by a simple nutrition, and enjoying exceptionally the profusion of gastronomic sensations.

By choosing, sometimes to replace the canteen meals with a meal basket, you will improve your health, you will see your overweight decrease rapidly, and you will save money.

## Example of basket meal :

Brownie balls + 1 apple + 1 orange + 1 banana

*Recipe Brownie balls*   (Ready in 3 mn, no cooking)

*Ingredients:*   1 ½ glass of peeled nuts

1 teaspoon of vanilla extract

¼ cup of cocoa powder

10 peeled dates

*Preparation:*

Pass the nuts to the mixer. Then add the other ingredients and continue to mix until you get a paste. Made balls with dough.

## ☯☯ Exercise 18 : Intuitive food

The practice of intuitive diet consists in developing our ability to perceive the information that our body gives us, on the diet that suits it for its better functioning.

So we will develop, explore and manage our perception of feelings of hunger, satiety, attraction for a particular food, tastes and eating pleasure. If you've never experienced hunger, or if you've forgotten the feeling of hunger, then you will benefit from exploring the deep sensations it gives. On other hand, the sensation of satiety is full of finesse. It is also good to explore and allows you to stop eating at the right time, and not add to the pleasure of eating the discomfort of having eaten too much.

In the practice of intuitive food we pay attention to the use of the five senses: food is observed and touched (sometimes contemplated, if it is for example fruits and vegetables), we take the time to smell the scents, we extend our trips in the tastes, and we listen to the crackling when we eat.
We also cultivate the pleasure of eating.

One technique is to ask you the question, before a meal, or doing your shopping: What will I enjoy eating in what is available? Then, freely, with pleasure and lightness, procrastination, follow the first idea that comes to mind.
Note, that if you include in your shopping practices the observation of the fruits and vegetables quarter, it is likely that you will be attracted by several of them.

If, occasionally, you find yourself eating a food that is outside your eating habits does not consider it as bad (none is), but instead makes an exploration of its taste.

Become aware of the origin of your desire to eat. And if it is not hunger, but an emotional refuge, look for another way to manage your emotions.

Let's make healthier meals become the new standard, individual, family and even festive with friends. That the happiness of feeling good, becomes associated with culinary joys. Let food experiences become themes for parties with friends.

And finally, if you have children, you can accompany them in their learning of tastes, food intuitions and experiences. Giving them, freedom and responsibility.

◆

*'Although outside circumstances often prevented me from observing strictly a vegetarian diet, I adhere for a long time to this cause on principle. Besides the fact that I agree with the purposes of the vegetarianism for esthetic and moral reasons, I consider that the vegetarian lifestyle, by its purely physical effect on the human temperament, would have an influence of the most beneficial the fate of the humanity'*

Albert Einstein

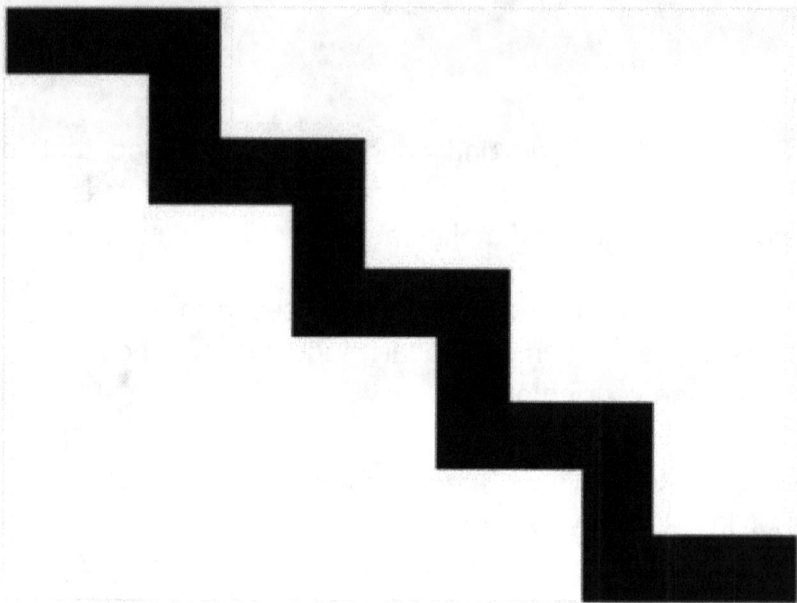

In parenthesis, you will notice that in several places in this manual, you are invited to share the exercises, your sensations and your understandings with your children.

You can make this sharing with generosity, because children will be happy to benefit from your positive discoveries, this will nourish their curiosity and their thirst for learning, and this will enhance the quality of your relationships, as well as the quality of the education you provide.

Keep in mind the importance of this involvement of children in building the better world.

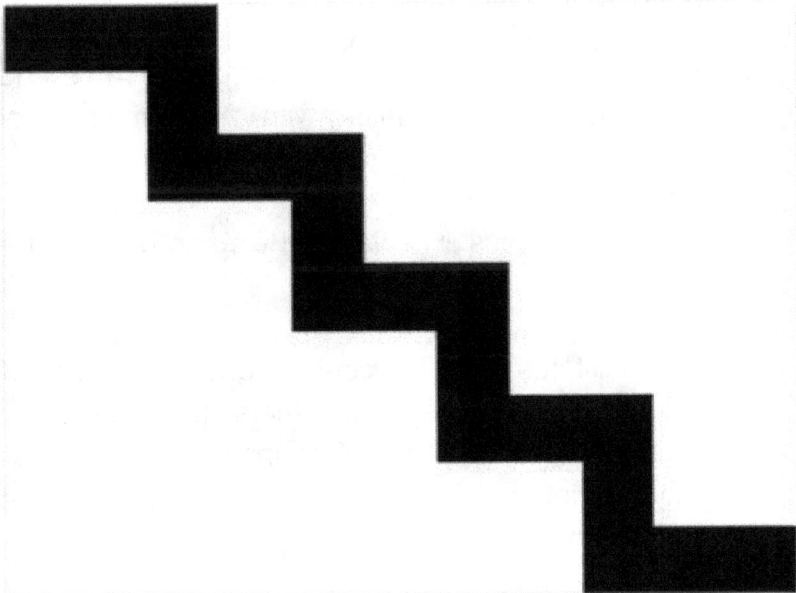

## 004 - GUIDE to sleep better

Getting enough sleep means better mental health, better physical health, a better quality of life, and a reduction of many risks (illnesses, accidents, failures).

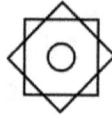

Here are some advantages of getting enough sleep:

○ For the baby, the child and the adolescent, having long sleep times, is important. The production of hormone is promoted by sleep. During growth, the body is subjected to multiple transformations which are favored by a good sleep. Young people need to swallow, process, filter and memorize a lot of information, a good sleep optimizes all this, which is becoming more and more important nowadays with the volume of information increasing exponentially.

○ We are calmer, less irritable. And we can have better relationships with others.

○ Sleep facilitates weight control and the loss of overweight (lack of sleep slows metabolism, therefore decreases fat consumption.) Knowing that the sugars in the diet turn into fat during the digestion process to be released next needs).

- Many studies show a relationship between lack of sleep and diseases such as depression, obesity, diabetes and heart disease.

- Sleep promotes the proper functioning of the immune system thus reduces the risk of disease.

- Sufficient and regular sleep reduces the risk of breast, colon, or other cancer (study of night workers, in addition to the disruption of the biological clock).

- Sufficient sleep promotes good sexuality.

- Lack of sleep increases the risk of accidents (transport, domestic, or other).

- Lack of sleep increases the risk of making mistakes, making bad decisions and failing.

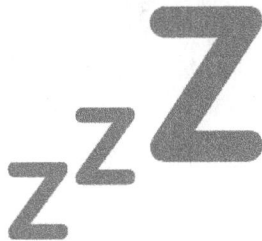

**The need for sleep varies according to age :**

| Age | Hours/day |
|---|---|
| Newborn      (0-3 months) | 16-18 |
| Baby          (4-11 months) | 12-15 |
| Young child    (3-5 years) | 11-12 |
| Child          (6-13 years) | 10-12 |
| Teenager    (14-18 years) | 09-10 |
| Adult         (18-110 years) | 07-08 |

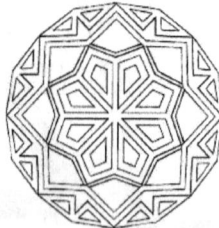

**What is the best position for sleeping?**

The best position is on the side, and more often on the right side (except in the pregnant woman on the left side), with a pillow whose size allows the alignment of the spine.

Sleeping on the stomach is a very bad position. Because, there is then an important pressure on the neck in torsion, which generates chronic pain. If you're used to sleeping on your stomach, you can, and you have to, change it. The position on the back is acceptable without a pillow or a small pillow to avoid twisting of the neck (it nevertheless promotes snoring and sleep apnea).

It is likely that, like many, you suffer from very unpleasant sleep disturbances (need to sleep late, waking up in the middle of the night and insomnia), then experiments to find ways to improve the situation, such as putting you to bed earlier and enjoy reading and doing exercises (sleeping hours before midnight are more restorative than those after midnight).

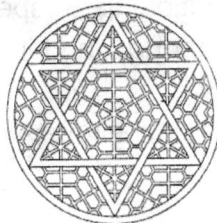

Here are three techniques that will help you sleep well:

## 👀 Exercise 19 : Label the moments

Give labels to the moments of your life. Live fully and exclusively each label, rejecting mix feelings.

o   When you go to bed, you begin your conditioning, to end up with a good night's sleep, by living conscientiously your routine tasks (toilet, preparing the next day's clothes, drinking a glass of water, etc.) And looking forward to being on your way to the next steps.

o   Before you go to bed, you are going to enjoy a routine program that includes exercises, including a review of the good things of the day, and your next day program.

o   The moment to lie down, is a moment, where you prepare for a good rest. This is not a moment to think about anything. For a few minutes, breathe calmly. Immerse, into this calm and sweetness, and in the confidence that you will spend a good night's sleep. Rejoice, and you be safe, thinking, that when you wake up, you will start thinking again, and you will live these 30 seconds of conditioning, to spend a good day. It will be tomorrow, another day, and it is not now.

o   Now, enjoy this exclusive moment, reserved for sleeping.

## ☺☺ Exercise 20 : Wipe out your thoughts

You will soon work in this book at managing your thought.

(You can choose to return to this exercise only after you'll have done this work on your thought.)

The practice of this exercise is exotic, pleasant and effective.

Selected on the Internet (for example on U-Tube), an audio band of the sound of waves. Or of course, take the opportunity to listen to the sound of real waves when you have the chance to be on a beach.

Imagine, with each inspiration, that the waves are passing through your body. And, with each expiration, let preoccupations of the day and your other troubles, leave with the waves. Do this until all your troubles are gone.

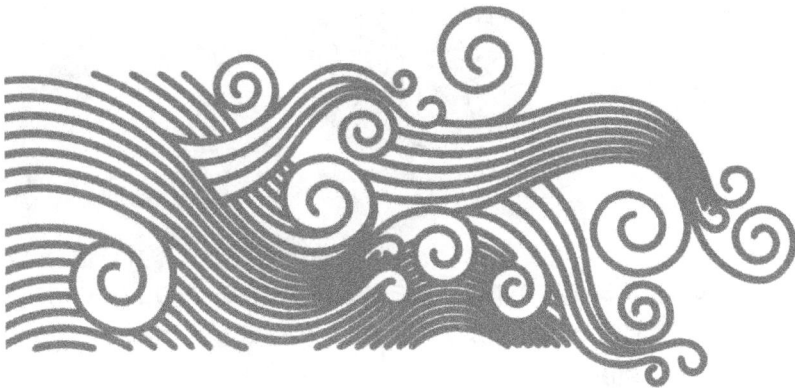

## ☻☻ Exercise 21 : The hyper-relaxation

Relaxing is one of the most important things to have a good life and to be happy ☺ To cultivate your desire to be happier, it is mandatory to learn and practice the technique of hyper-relaxation. Relaxation develops our strengths and blurs our weaknesses. Being relaxed facilitates the success of our actions. Relaxation is fundamental to personal development, because we can then perceive many new and beneficial sensations, that we would miss otherwise.

Some will say 'I am more efficient in times of crisis and when I am tense'. This is also true; however, the tension must then be, the one that allows us to coordinate our multiple actions. It must not be the tension that obscures our mind and makes us make mistakes. For all of us, it is advantageous to practice hyper relaxation.

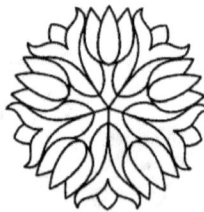

The technique of hyper relaxation described below, is useful to practice regularly (for example every night in your bed, before sleeping):

**Hyper relaxation technique step by step:**

o  Lying on back. Start with a tensioning of your body will allow you a better relaxation: by holding your breath, contract, as long as possible the maximum of muscles of your body (including for example, strongly close your eyes, clench your teeth, tighten your fists, raise your feet, ...).

o  Take long and deep inhale.
   Retain your breath to a count of 3, then exhale by relaxing. Repeat three times (inhale + retain + exhale) by inhaling deeper and deeper, by extending the durations of the exhalations, and by relaxing even more with each exhalation.

o  Now focus your attention on the fingertips of your right foot. And relax each of your toes. Ride along your foot making sure each part becomes very relaxed. Then go to the heel, to the Achilles tendon, and to the ankle.

o  Raise slowly along the leg, focusing on the relaxation of points that you feel tense or painful, to relieve them. The leg is an area that can be particularly tense, especially after walking or practicing a sport, take the time to relax this area to the extent of tension.

o  All along the exercise, when you feel a tense or painful point, focus your attention on it, to get tension or pain. If you feel, at any moment of the exercise, these points in an area that you have already worked in relaxation, then take the time to come back on these points.

o  Then go up to your right knee. Go around the patella. Relaxes tendons all around the knee.

o  Then go back to your thigh, front and back.
   The muscles of the thigh are the biggest muscles of the body, they are frequently tense. Spends enough time to relieve tension and pain.

o  Focus your attention on the fingertips of your left foot. And do the same to the top of your left thigh.

o  Relax now your hips and your genitals.

o  Pay attention to the bottom of your back. It is an area that can be particularly tense and painful. Insists, by pointing accurately and in depth the tense or painful points.

o  Go back slowly along your spine, focusing your attention alternately on the muscles to the right and left of your column.

o  Now go to your right hand. And as you did for your lower limb relaxes well every part: fingers, palm, wrist, forearm, elbow, biceps, triceps, shoulder, and trapezoid.

o   Do the same thing all along your left arm to the trapeze.

o   Now turn your attention to your internal anatomy, starting with the lower abdomen relaxing your anus then slowly ascending, your intestines, your kidneys, your liver, your stomach, your diaphragm, your lungs and your heart.

o   Now go to the relaxation of your neck. Take the necessary time. If you feel the need to move your head lightly, you will get better relaxation.

o   Now go up your face, chin, jaws, teeth, tongue, cheeks, ears, eyes (front and back), forehead, scalp and hair.

If, at any time, you are feeling a tension, somewhere in your body, return to the area to alleviate the tension.

Here you are, you are now hyper relax and you will have a good night.

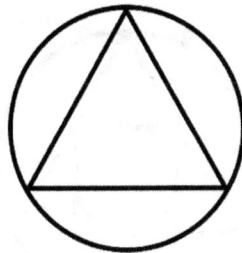

You can also do this exercise at any time of the day. So slowly and deeply if you have the time, or quickly (even a few seconds, when the exercise became familiar to you) when you are on the bus or in the office. However, you may not be able to discreetly (if there are people around) perform the tension of your whole body that is at the beginning of the practice; it does not matter.

Moreover, now that you know the technique of concentration on a tense or painful point, you can also use this technique of relaxation at when and where you feel a point tension, for example, these frequent tensions in the region of the neck.

After some practice, you will be surprised to see, that you are performing, by automatism, a relaxation to feel better, or movements of the head in order to pass a tension at the level of the neck, or Another change of posture to pass a tension in another part of the body.

When practicing meditation exercises, the hyper-relaxation technique is part of the conditioning ritual (with body positioning and staged breathing).

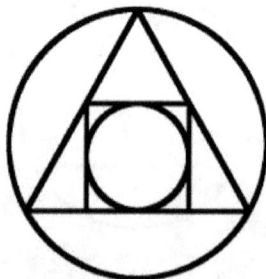

**Realize the tensions :**

Tension can be muscular, after physical activity. Or when you have stayed too long in the same position (for example, tensions in your neck after working long in standing position or seating in front of your computer screen), or after you have made a false move. Or muscular tension can be caused by stress. Or the addition of several of these causes.

Often, we do not realize that we are stressed or tense, but we just feel discomfort. By developing, first, a better consciousness of the tension, then, a better and a more precise feeling of the tension, in is point of origin, it becomes easier, to resorb it, and, at the same time, to absorb the stress, and the discomfort, that accompanies this tension.

Physical tensions, pains, and discomforts are creating negative thoughts. As, negative thoughts are creating tensions pains and discomforts. The relaxation and avoiding negative thoughts (as we will practice later on in the manual), are allowing, both physical and mental comfort.

## 👀 Exercise 22 : Rejuvenate the face

This technique is based on the acupressure of traditional Chinese medicine, and in particular, on the many acupuncture points located on the face.

The exercise is quick to perform (about 2 minutes). It can be done regularly, and even twice a day. It is effective, to relax stress-strained facial muscles, to rejuvenate the face, to delay the appearance of wrinkles on the face, and to reach an immediate state of well-being and general relaxation.

Exercise can be done in both standing and sitting positions.

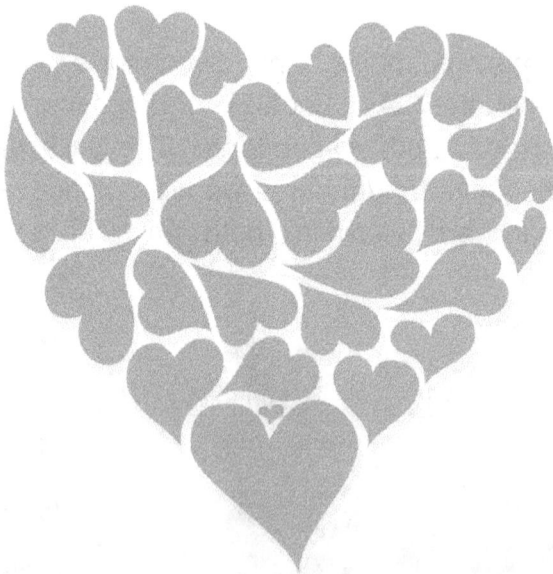

- With the forefinger (right hand for the right-handed, or left hand for the left-handed) make pressure and circular movements, in one direction then in the other, between the two eyebrows. Continue this way, moving the index finger over different points of this area, including the root of the nose.

- With the three fingers of both hands, forefinger, middle finger and ring finger, apply pressure and circular movements, one way then the other, on the eyebrows, moving the fingers on different points of these areas.

  With those same fingers, continue on the forehead, exploring the area generously.

  Continue on the temple, also generously exploring the areas.

  Same thing under the eyes, on the cheeks, on the jaws, in the neck, under the ears and on the ears.

- With the palms and the fingers of both hands, placed flat on the face, move up and down while pressing.

  When going up, pull the skin of the face upwards. And going down pull the skin down. At the passages, press the eyes with the forefingers and middle fingers.

  When going up, make a single long inhale. Ensure the inhale is driving the movement. Similarly exhale when going down.

  Repeat going up and down, 3 times.

## 005 - GUIDE to better see the world

What we look at and what we see defines the world in which we live. We can make choices of quality and quantity of what we look at, which positively influence our definition of the world and our happiness. We can thus choose to look at objects, aesthetic, positive and favorable to our well-being. And not to look at unfavorable objects, while remaining aware of their nature and existence. So, rather than undergo the vision of unfavorable scenes, capable of maintaining our fears, our feelings of persecution or our obsessions, we become masters of our gaze.

There are also techniques, which we are now going to study, that broaden our field of vision, and that result in significant changes in our lives.

We will thus, make the choices, to see a greater number of things, and to see better things.

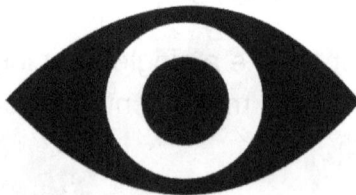

The next three exercises describe very simple and simple techniques that greatly change our awareness of the world we live in, and our awareness of the position of our body in space:

The first two techniques (Exercises 22 and 23: Widen your field of view) develop the muscles of the eyes. They broaden our field of vision in all directions, allowing us to see things that we could not see before, at once. Our world becomes bigger, and more beautiful; These comments are not exaggerated, you will be surprised at the results that the practice of these exercises will bring to you. These exercises are very simple and very fast, you will benefit from practicing them regularly. Note that the amount of mobility of the neck that you will win with the third technique, (Exercise 24: the mobile neck), adds to the gain in magnitude of your vision to give you this more spectacular vision.

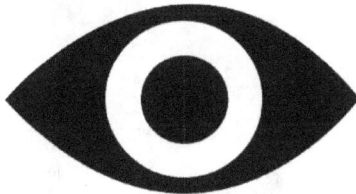

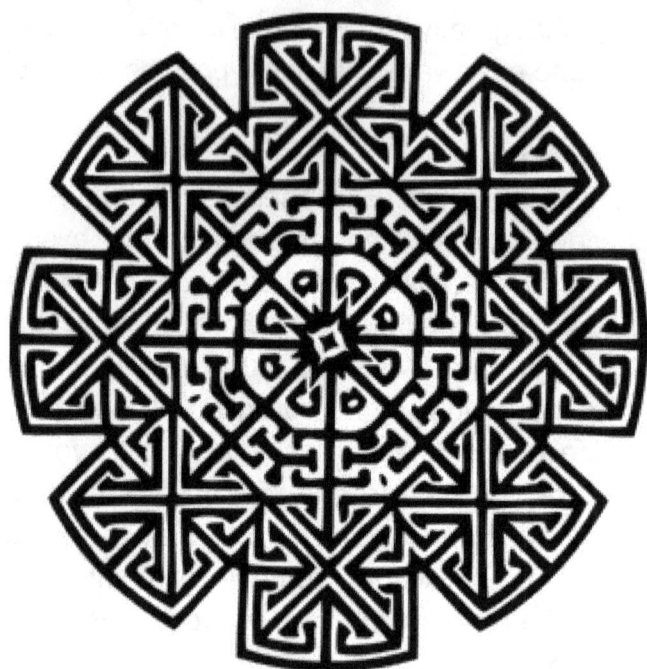

## 👀 Exercise 23 : Widen your field of view 1

Throughout the exercise, you will keep your head still and your gaze fixed. Place yourself in a standing position.

o  Stretch out your arms in front of you, hands clasped in a position of prayer.

o  Extend your arms apart, keeping them taut, and without moving your head or eyes, hold the vision of your hands as long as possible, until your hands come out of your field of vision (once your arms have arrived at the perpendicular of your looks).

   Repeat 5 times. In the beginning, you will tend to move gaze or head, correct this, until performing the technique correctly.

o  Now place your arms stretched out before you, your hands still joined, but this time turn your hands a quarter of a turn to place them flat.
   Spread your hands, lifting one arm and down the other, and hold the vision of your hands for as long as possible, until they come out of your field of vision. Repeat 5 times.

## 👀 Exercise 24 : Widen your field of view 2

Throughout the exercise, you will keep your head still, only your eyes move.

In each direction, you will seek the maximum extent of your gaze by keeping your eyes open.

During the first practices of this exercise, the rotations (directions 9 and 10) will be irregular. After some practices, you will be able to turn your eyes smoothly, faster and drawing ample and regular circles.

Repeat all movements 5 times.

In addition to widening your field of vision, your gaze becomes faster, more vivid and more precise. You will see more things than you had seen before. You'll be more effective. Your capacity for anticipation will be increased, and with it the rapidity of your reactions is also increased.

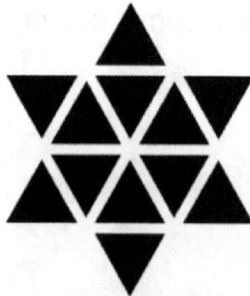

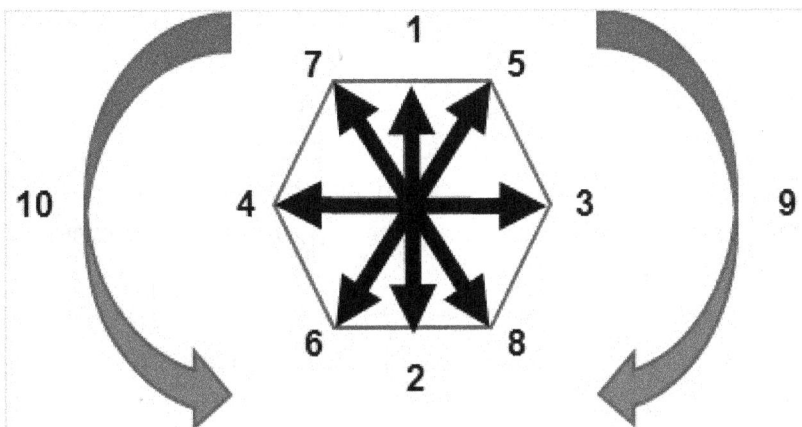

- o Start the exercise by looking straight ahead.
- o Look up                          (direction 1).
- o Look down                      (direction 2).
- o Look to the right             (direction 3).
- o Look to the left              (direction 4).
- o Look diagonally               (direction 5).
- o Look diagonally               (direction 6).
- o Look diagonally               (direction 7).
- o Look diagonally               (direction 8).
- o Turn your eyes clockwise      (direction 9).
- o Turn them counter clockwise   (direction 10).

## ☯☯ Exercise 25 : The mobile neck

The neck is a sensitive area, which is very often, the place, of embarrassing and even disabling pain, in many circumstances (cold stroke, following a false movement, following a bad position during the sleep, as a result of prolonged work positions such as standing or sitting with the gaze fixed on the computer screen, and as a result of long car journeys).

The exercise of the mobile neck contributes, as the previous exercise, increasing the amplitude and the flexibility of the movement of the neck, to a different and broader vision of the world, greater vivacity and responsiveness.

The exercise of the mobile neck also increases, very usefully, the suppleness and power of the muscles which support the head and neck, and the suppleness of the articulations of the cervical vertebrae. This will avoid the pain listed above.

You will do the first time this exercise, by going gently, without forcing on the amplitudes, and with attention to the feeling of, the muscles of the neck and the cervical vertebrae.
Little by little your neck will become more mobile and you will be able to go faster (without going too fast) and with greater amplitudes.
It will be very beneficial for you to get into the habit of practicing this exercise regularly.

**Mobile neck technique step by step:**

o   Start the exercise by looking straight ahead.

o   Toggle your neck back, looking up.

o   Toggle your neck forward, looking down.

o   Turn your head to the right, looking right.

o   Turn your head to the left, looking left.

o   Tilt your head sideways.

o   Toggle your head sideways.

o   Your chin passes from the left clavicle to the right clavicle.

o   Then, from the right clavicle to the left.

o   Form a loose circle with your head in a clockwise direction. Then counterclockwise.

o   Repeat all movements 5 times.

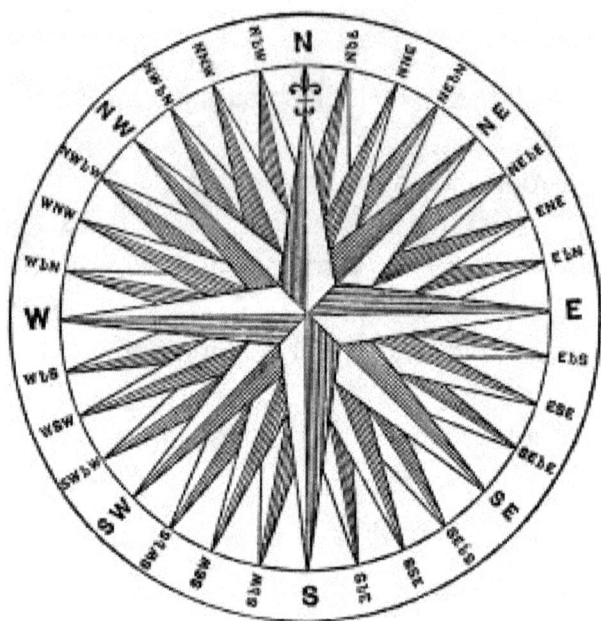

**The eyes precede the movement:**

Practice the exercise of the mobile neck, continuing to concentrate on your muscles and on your vertebrae, and now adding the concentration on, your gaze preceding the movement.

o   To get used to it, start by looking up at the sky before tipping your neck back.

o   From this position, begin by directing your gaze down, before tipping your head down.

Practice several times these two first movements.

o   Now, start looking at the right before turning your head to the right. From this position, start looking to the left, before turning your head, until it is completely left. Do, several times these movements right-left.

o   In the same way, practice several times the three pairs: lateral, from clavicle to clavicle, & whole circles.

o   Now that you are used to this coordination of the movements and the gazes, link up all the movements of the technique of the mobile neck.

**Breathing leads the movements:**

Practice the exercise of the mobile neck, continuing to concentrate on your muscles, on your vertebrae and on your gaze, and now adding the concentration on, your breath leading the movement.

o   To get used to it, start inspiration, with the feeling it is driving the raise of your gaze to the sky, and the rock of your neck to the back. (Here and all along the practice, adapt the speed of the head movements so that your inspirations and expirations are complete, from the beginning to the end of the movement.)

From this position, start your exhalation, direct your gaze and rock your head down.

Do several times these two coordinated movements.

o   Still to get used to the practice, start your inspiration, look right, and turn your head to the right.

From this position, to the right, start your exhalation, look to the left, before turning your head, until completely left.

Done, several times these movements right-left.

o   For the rocking movement of your head on your right shoulder: starts with the inspiration, follow with the gaze, then with the movement of your head. The full inspiration end with the movement of the head.

Feel your exhalation leading your gaze and your return from this position to the straight head position.

Similarly, perform inspirations and expirations driving rocking movements of your head to the left and back.

Do several times these coordinated rocking movements to the right and to the left.

o Place your head in straight position, toppled on the front. From this starting position, beginning with your inspiration, then your gaze looking left, driving the clockwise rotation of your head, end your inspiration when your head is straight. Then link up your expiration, keep your gaze preceding the movement, and end your expiration, when your head is back at the starting point. Do several of such rotation clockwise, by chaining the rotation without interruption, then do several rotations anticlockwise following the same coordination breathing – gaze – rotation. Then, link up all the movements when you are at ease.

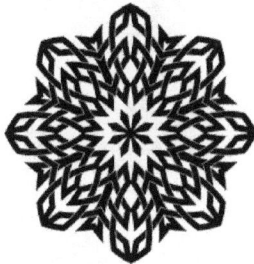

## Feel and remove

Now that you are used to the practice of the mobile neck technique, you will be able to acquire the mastery of the technique of detection and elimination of the emerging tensions, at the level of the neck, before they turn into pain.

o Before practicing the technique, start by doing, very calmly, all the steps of the technique of the mobile neck, described previously (step by step).

o Now, close your eyes, stop concentrating on your breathing, and, by making the ample circular movement of your head clockwise, and / or anticlockwise, concentrate exclusively on the feeling of the muscular envelope of your neck. You are then, learning to feel the painful points and tensions.

o When you feel one of these painful points or tensions, stop the rotation of your head at this point, and stretch the painful muscle by forcing on the maximum amplitude of your head, and exhaling all along stretching. Learns to feel, this type of stretching and the elimination of pain and tension that ensue.

After some time of practicing this technique, you will come, more and more often, and more and more easily, to feel a nascent tension in your neck, and automatically, without even having to think about it, you will make the movement of the neck suitable for stretching muscle and relieving pain and tension.

Note that you may feel, at the beginning, some embarrassment when making automatically these stretching in public. Overcome these embarrassment, because it is obvious, that you are then practicing stretching, making you feeling good.

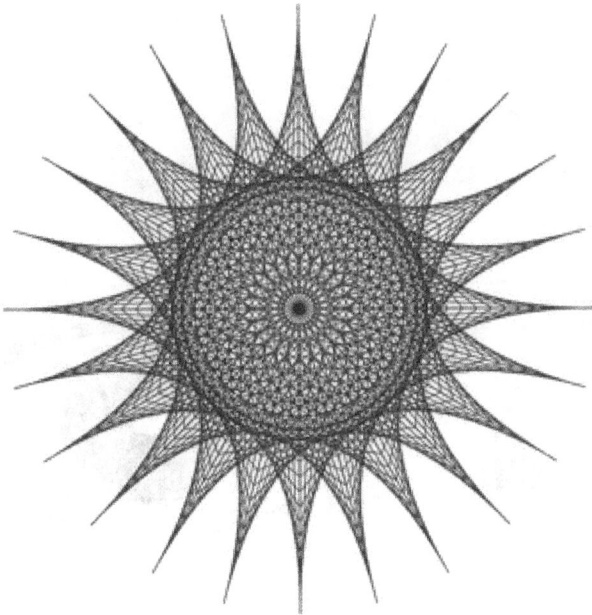

## 👁👁 Exercise 26 : The blind walk

The benefits of this exercise are:

- Increase the notion of your body in space,

- Improve your balance,

- Have a sensation of the seconds passing.

- Gain confidence in yourself and enjoy playing.

The exercise consists in walking with eyes closed.

During the first practices, you will be a little lost, you will lose balance, you will be a little scared, and few seconds will seem very long. But quickly, after two or three practices you will already begin to improve all this.

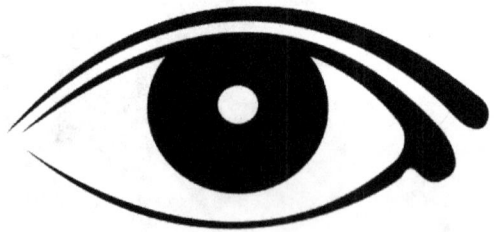

You will do this exercise during a walk on an uncrowded road. Choose a flat path, with no accident and bounded on each side, by a border (like grasses high enough to allow you to feel them with your feet, a barrier or a wall).

o Begin by closing your eyes, only for a short time (two seconds). Continue this preparation until you are comfortable. Then lengthens time, little by little.

o Before closing your eyes, look at the scenery, and position your existing landmarks, in your mind (a tree or a lamppost beside which you are going to pass). Also select one of these markers as the finish line. You will find it very interesting to find yourself closer or further away than you thought you had arrived.

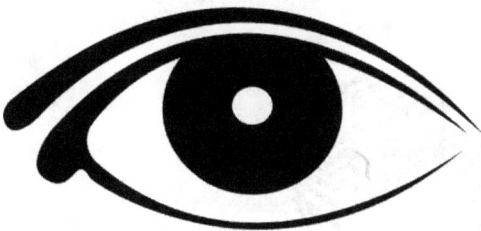

Talking about the big changes in our consciousness of the world, and the consciousness of the position of our body in the space, provided by the three previous exercises made me think of an anecdote:

As I have been travelling a lot, including living in 13 distant countries, for 22 years, I have been moved by the differences when watching the sky, in different parts of the world. Depending on where you are, the aspects of the sky, by day and by night, are significantly different.

By day, different sizes of a different blues sky give different feelings of being on earth.

By night, different brightness and different stars of a bigger sky gives different feeling of being in the universe.

These different feelings contribute, together with the interactions with people, to change the regard on the people living under different skies. It helps understanding that the differences between us are folkloric, historical and sensorial, and that these differences are much minor compare to the similarities of human beings with mostly identical concerns and abilities, and with a common future.

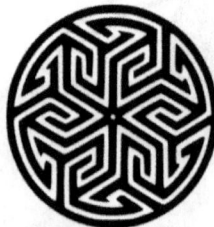

## ☯☯ Exercise 27 : The contemplation

The most wonderful will be found in nature.

A TV reportage highlighted the activities of a charity to teenagers from underprivileged populations, in Harlem to Manhattan. The Association brought a cow that the children saw for the first time. Until then, they thought that the milk they drank was a manufactured product.

Overwhelmed by the pressures of daily life, and sometimes locked up in an urban reality, we forget to see beauty and we lose the sense of reality.

It is very beneficial to take the time to contemplate the beauty of nature.

Thus, to observe the contours of a flower, the veins of a leaf, the meanders of a shell of walnuts, the lamellae of a mushroom, the majesty of motionless trees or dancing with the wind, The spikes of a cactus and sometimes its wonderful flower of a day, the breathing of a frog, the movements of a lizard's head, the flight of a flower butterfly in flower, the path of an insect, the fluffy caterpillar down, a toilet fly, the lace of a dragonfly's wings, an ant carrying a crumb of bread, the movement of waves, the flight of birds, the moon, rising and falling sun, clouds, waterfall, pebble, stars, a drop of water, a snowflake, the fog that rises in the early morning, the dotted skin of a strawberry, the starry heart of a Kiwi, the multicolored wings of ladybug, ...

## 👀 Exercise 28 : Value your gazes

In this exercise you will be following steps to improve the values of your gazes:

o During one week, starting now, you are going to be attentive to the values of your gazes. What thoughts, feelings and emotions are generating the things you are watching. This can be at your accommodation, in the street, in your working place, walking in the nature and any other place you are passing through.

You will then realize that your gazes are generating multiple thoughts, feeling and emotions. Those can be, for instance: sadness, regrets, hatred, jealousy, envy, greed, despair, discouragement, fears, or, joy, love, admiration, satisfaction, encouragement.

This week will be an initiation to this attention given to the values of your gazes. After this week, it will be easier for you to continue giving this attention. And, you can continue to do so for the rest of your life, this will serve you and will give more and better values to your life.

o After this first week, you are going to think how you could correct your gazes or the consequences of your gazes to better serve you.

Can you remove such and such thing from your environment and from your field of view?

Can you stop to include the gaze at this thing from your experience?

Or, on contrary, could you include in your environment and field of view some objects serving you (for instance sacred geometry, as we will see later in the manual)?

Now that you realized seeing this picture or this thing is bringing you undesired thoughts, feeling or emotions, can you modify your reaction? For instance, from sadness or regret to love.

This process can be fast for some things and it will require longer attention and efforts for other things.
Maybe you will desire maintaining some gazing, even if they are generating mix feelings; in that case you can take the necessary time continuing to measure the values of the mix feelings.

○ Doing this training of valuing your gazes, you will also be attentive to realize that repeatedly, by lake of attention, you missed seeing things in your field of view. As result, you lost time, or you missed opportunities. In those cases, take the resolution to become more attentive, more conscient and more alive, in these particular moments.

These invisibilities of things or persons in our fields of view is happening to all of us.

For instance, it happens to hyperactive persons. Theses persons, sometime with a lot of things to do or a lot of responsibilities, are often focusing on the next task to complete. While they desire to be most efficient, these invisibilities consequently affect their efficiencies. This is particularly challenging for these persons as they do not have the feeling to lack presence, consciousness, liveness or consideration for their environments. But these persons would be far more efficient and happier if they could combine their anticipations of events with more presence, rendering invisibilities visible. They would also benefit from the dimension, fulness and relaxation of being in the present moment. And, in the times when they are supposed to relax, they would have more chances of further exploring these qualities of the present moment instead of continuously wondering about the future. These persons will greatly benefit channeling part of their great energy, first to notice that the invisibilities are often occurring, second to correct this deficiency; otherwise, they could spend a lifetime in anticipation of the future and no time in the present.

## 👁👁 Exercise 29 : Bilateral Eye Movements

In addition to be an exercise that improves the mobility and speed of the eyes, and widens the visual field, this is one of the easiest and fastest exercises to improve the consistency between the left and right brains.

This is especially useful for relieving strong and negative emotions.

This technique (also known as: Eye Movement Desensitization and Reprocessing (EMDR)) has proved its effectiveness to unblock and evacuate traumas, fears or negative emotions crystallized in the brain (for example: Post-traumatic stress disorder (PTSD), and disorders related to violence, aggression and other incidents of life).

This technique is also used to improve self-confidence and performance.

o For up to 1 minute, quickly move your eyes back and forth from left to right, without forcing

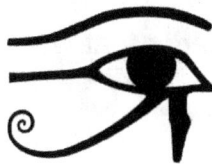

## 006 - GUIDE to tame the television

Probably, you hear more and more people talking about reducing their time watching television, or completely stopping watching it. To get there, it usually does not happen in a day. It is a process.

For 22 years, I lived, for periods ranging from one year to several years, in 13 different countries. I did return regularly to France (about every year), either between two posting or for holidays. At such moments, I was seeing my friends, always with pleasure. And I could see the changes that had taken place. I have been stuck by two things:

- From one year to the next, the general atmosphere was changing in a very significant way. One year my friends were morose and told me that we were on the brink of a civil war. The following year, all this, was out of the question, and all was well.

- On each return, I could hear on television the same speeches, the same problems. As if, not a year but a day had elapsed since the last time I had looked at TV.

Over time, I also realized, that it was useless and harmful to look at the bad news instilled. I also realized that the information and standards that were delivered were often false.

Television and other media have more audiences when they give negative information. These media are above all, merchants, interested in the profit from the sale of their product, whose success is measured by the quantity of the audience and the advertising profits it generates. Thus, it is quite normal that the media prefer to publish bad news, and little good news, however many are. So, if we follow the media diligently, we are overwhelmed with rumors about wars, terrorism, disasters, banditry or crime.

We have every interest in limiting our contact with such bad news. On the one hand, this is depressing, and we are indoctrinated, and on the other hand, we miss the opportunity to be informed about the many positive developments in the same or in other areas, through other sources of information.

In too many homes, watching television is a daily ritual for the whole family (even for children! who are then, unfortunately, exposed to extreme violence). This is most certainly a great source of stress and goes against positive developments and happiness.

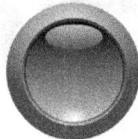

## 👀 Exercise 30 : Watching the news

Choosing our optimal exposure to the quality and quantity of information, is a personal case by case consideration.

Measure your feelings in relation to your own experience, and then experience the changes, and well-being that are right for you.

It is possible that you are interested in this or that "burning" event, perhaps, for now, you feel an obligation, that you will be able to correct, to participate in the social interactions that lament about the new mediatic event of the moment.

However, apart from a case when a catastrophe is close to you and obliges you to keep yourself informed, to make an urgent decision, it will be interesting to you to experience the effects of spacing of exposure to media news as well as to such topics of conversation.

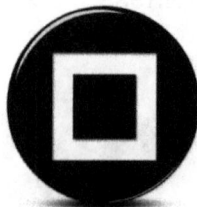

## 👀 Exercise 31 : One week without TV

o   Choose a week, during which you will not watch TV.

o   And use this time saved, to do other things more
    nourishing for your well-being: like walking in nature,
    starting a thing, you always wanted to do, doing
    different things, doing physical activities, reading,
    joining an association, taking classes, spending time
    with family and friends, etc.

o   At the end of this week, when you watch television
    again, judge how far the information differs from last
    week, and what are the consequences of having
    suspended your role spectator.

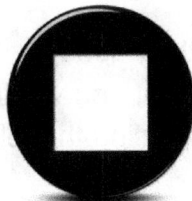

**Stopping TV step by step :**

Stopping watching television can be done, instantly or gradually, and temporarily or permanently. Each improvement in the use of your time is a benefit.

This exercise describes successive and progressive stages:

o At first, rather than being passive about choosing what you are watching, you will make a good selection of programs. This selection must allow you to limit and space your time in front of the screen, and to dedicate it only to interesting programs.

  ▪ Endorse your costume as an explorer, search, and follow the impulses of interest.

o In a second step, you will begin to operate periods of absence of television.

  ▪ Included this second step, in the empty periods of the first; and, to make a pause after busy periods.

  ▪ As you are getting used to, in this manual, to live fully each moment, you will fully live the moments, still unusual, replacing the television periods.

o In a third step, you will feel the urge to totally suppress your TV listening.

The idea of suppressing television may seem sad and reductive. You can satisfy your taste for art and for the show, by watching movies or documentaries, without becoming dependent on the commercial stereotypes. And satisfy your desire to be informed, through use of other media.

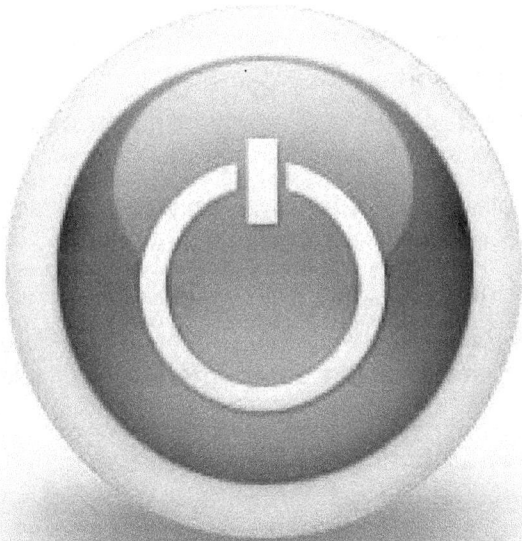

## 007 - GUIDE to listen carefully

As we have recognized the importance of the choice of what we are looking at, the choice of what we listen, also influences our level of happiness, and the definition of the world in which we live.

There are many things to which it will be useful to be more attentive, here are three: listening to others, nature and synchronicities.

○ **Listening to others**

There is a very amusing regional expression to define some of us: 'That one, you say hello to him, he says the rest'. Indeed, some of us, driven by a great need for validation, occupy the entire space of a conversation. They grant themselves the monopoly of speech. They do not allow others to speak, they cannot tolerate an interlude of three seconds of silence, and when the others come to speak they do not listen to them.

Yet when listening to others we can better understand them and, we can better understand ourselves. We can benefit from the contributions or contradictions to improve or to correct our points of view. We have the opportunity to ask questions. Listening and using interludes of silence allow in-depth exploration of ideas. The exchange of ideas allows for synergies. Listening to others, is a respect for them, that is also returned to us. When we listen to others, we encourage and motivate them, rather than frustrate them by locking them in an impossibility of expressing themselves. We may believe that, by maintaining the monopoly of the conversation, we obtain a validation that we need, whereas the opposite is true, we lose the respect and the sympathy of the other one and we miss the chance of enriching our reflection, of possibly receiving advice, finding solutions to problems, and of seeing opportunities. When we increase our listening capacity, we are gaining popularity.

By listening more to others, we are happier.

- ○ **Listening to nature**

The first thing to do, is of course to seek contact with nature, especially when our contacts are non-existent or spaced. Then to listen to the many sounds available. It may also be that we already have the chance to be often in contact with nature, but we do not pay attention to the sounds, so it is now desirable to take the time to listen.

When we listen more to nature, we are happier.

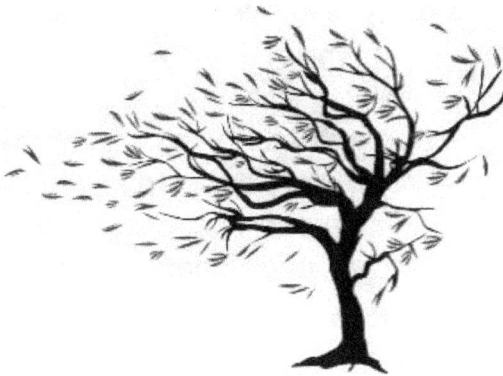

○ **Listening to synchronicities,**

Synchronicities are the pearls of life.

In the analytical psychology developed by Carl Gustav Jung, synchronicity is defined as the simultaneous occurrence of at least two events, that are not causally related, but whose association makes sense for the person perceiving them. Synchronicity is a very rich subject with ramifications in areas like Physics, Metaphysics, romantic relationships, Rock n'roll[12], and so on. In other words, it is these troubling coincidences that defy our understanding of the usual logic, of space and of time. Even if you have a very Cartesian spirit, you certainly have already experienced such events. It can be just a moment when you think of someone you have not seen in a long time, and at the same time, this someone calls you on your phone. Or, it may be a more troubling moment, when you ask yourself a question, and you hear the answer to your question unequivocally, in a conversation on the radio or in a conversation between strangers at the next table, or you see it placarded on a wall in an advertising campaign.

I have had in my life intense, multiple and varied experiences of synchronicity. First, when I was a child, and then knowing nothing about the phenomenon of synchronicity, I was worried and shocked. These worries and shocks continued, until I learned that synchronicity was a normal event. Now, I am very happy every time I see one. Because, it makes me feel the beauty of life.

---

[12]In 1983, the rock band The Police released an album entitled 'Synchronicity'

Synchronicities, can also give us an insight, into the concept of All being a synchronicity.

Visual, auditory or circumstantial synchronicities are always present but rarely noticeable. Naturally, carried away by our desires, ambitions or commitments, we see them without seeing them, we hear them without considering them. Perhaps, for many of us, is it the fear of the unknown, that makes us blind and deaf. Also, some of us, had never seen synchronicity, while others perceive a lot.

It is possible, that you are, like me as a child, frightened by such events that are unknown to you. It is also possible that you are simply surprised. It is also possible that you have never seen synchronicity. In any case, you will find it interesting to begin to be more attentive to the synchronicities.

The synchronicities cannot be understood from a materialistic point of view, even from a quantic point of view. The synchronicities can give us access to the most valuable knowledge : to know that we don't know.

The best way to react when we face a synchronicity can be compared to admiring the beauty of a flower. When we admire this beauty, we are not afraid, we do not attempt to explain or to interpret how a flower can be so beautiful, we simply enjoy this beauty and its reminder of the beauty of life.

## 👀 Exercise 32 : Exercises to listen

○ **Listen to others**

In a first step, measure how much you listen to others, in quantity and quality. And, measure your habit of interrupting others, or even if you tend to cut them to yourself finish their sentences. Then, resolve to improve your listening during your next conversations.

At the beginning of the conversations relax with three deep inspirations and prepare to listen.
Make eye contact calm and relaxed with your interlocutor. Let your interlocutor fully express his idea, by refraining your urge to interrupt him to react. On the contrary, try to understand the ideas and opinions (in particular, the contradictory opinions) expressed, and take the time to refine your interventions. Also, take time to observe and understand the body language of your interlocutor.

◆

*'Listening to the others, it is still my best way to hear what they have to say'*

Pierre Dac

◆

*'When we stop listening to we stop loving'*     M. Bouthot

◆

*'We have two ears and one tongue so that we would listen more and talk less.'*     Diogenes

o **Listen to the nature**

When you are in contact with nature, multiple sounds occur. It will be a song of bird on which you can linger. The breath of wind that you can savor. Or the sound of the wind in the trees, a piece of wood cracking under your feet, the barking of a dog in the distance, an animal that moves or expresses itself, the theft of an insect, the river flowing.

For some time, focus your attention on this specific sound. Listen to its variations, and lets its vibrations passing through you.

♦

*'All the inventions of men are but rude imitations of what nature performs with the last perfection'*

Buffon

♦

*'It is a sad thing to think that nature speaks and that the human race does not listen'*

Victor Hugo

♦

*The nature is full of teachings. Open big eyes. And she will educate you'*

F.R. de Lamennais

♦

*'I remind myself every morning: Nothing I say this day will teach me anything. So if I'm going to learn, I must do it by listening.'*

Larry King

- **Listen to synchronicities**

Be open and attentive to the sound, to the words heard on the radio, on television, or in a neighboring conversation.

Judge if what you hear, is synchronized with a concern you are currently having, and reflect (not much) on the possible meaning of this information. And, just savor the marvelous.

♦

*'In all chaos there is a cosmos, in all disorder a secret order'*

*'Synchronicity is an ever-present reality for those who have eyes to see'*

*'Synchronicity reveals the meaningful connections between the subjective and objective world'*

Carl Jung

♦

*'I am open to the guidance of synchronicity, and do not let expectations hinder my path'*

Dalai Lama

## ☻☻ Exercise 33 : Brainstorming technique

After having discovered this technique with pleasure, I have used it extensively in my job, because it has many merits, such as, using the capacities of each one within the team, developing a project, finding solutions to problems, discovering unknown problems, and greatly promoting the team spirit and the relationship between colleagues.

Using this technique professionally, also allows by extension, and by habit of the process, and of the principles of the technique, to benefit from a very clear improvement of our private communication, and our family, loving, friendly and social relations.

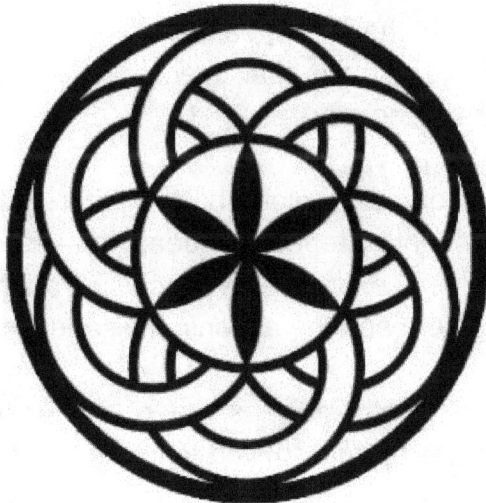

**Here is a step-by-step description of brainstorming technique:**

o A facilitator begins by explaining to the audience the principles of the technique:

  ▪ the expression of idea is free and encouraged.
  ▪ No idea is considered uninteresting, because every idea has a reason to exist. And, it allows to see angles not seen by all alike, making possible to find better solutions to the problem concerned.

o The subject or question that is to be debated is clearly expressed, if possible noted on the wall.

o The facilitator notes all the ideas expressed. He encourages everyone to express themselves, taking particular care to invite people who are shy or lack confidence in them to speak, who certainly have ideas on the subject (ideas that even can turn out to be the best ideas of the day).

o At the end of the session, the facilitator gathers similar ideas, eliminates repetitive ideas, makes an ordered synthesis, and, expresses a conclusion on the solutions of the problem and the actions envisaged.

o When the synthesis has been expressed by the facilitator, the team is invited to correct it or approve it.

## 008 - GUIDE to listen music

Whether one is happier, more relaxed and more efficient in listening to music, is an evidence, which is confirmed by numerous studies (increased secretion of dopamine the neurotransmitter of happiness, decreased secretion of cortisol stress hormone, improved memory, improved athletic performance, decreased depressive states, improved concentration, better performance at school for children who practice a musical instrument. These benefits are certainly due to the mathematical structure of musical notes and musical compositions. We have thus documented the relations of musical notes and musical compositions with the number Pi, the sequence of Fibonacci, and mathematics.

It will be beneficial for you to listen more often to music, whether it is during moments of relaxation, or by studying, working or practicing an activity. It will also be beneficial to explore musical domains that are not familiar to you. And the musical genres are numerous, for example: classical music, rock, jazz, ethnic music, relaxing music, disco, new wave, techno, acid, punk, blues, country, dance, metal, folk, rap, soul.

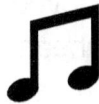

♫

*'The music is, more than any wisdoms and philosophies, the biggest revelation'*

Ludwig van Beethoven

## 009 - GUIDE to sing

Singing has many advantages, it makes us well breathe, relaxes us, gives us emotions.

As for many practices in this manual, singing generates several chemical processes in our body (increased secretion by our brain of the six super-neurotransmitters that bring us happiness, relaxation, activation of memory and libido, better management of our emotions, increasing our creativity and self-esteem, strengthening the immune system, and vivacity).

Singing, laughing, jumping, swimming, dancing, are moments to take full advantage of cultivating freedom, careless and lightness. They satisfy our natural innocence, in which it is good to immerse.

In fact, it will be beneficial for you to seize every possible opportunity to sing. It can be in your car, in your office, in nature or in a choir.

A good opportunity to sing, is when you take your shower.

You can combine listening to music and singing. There are certainly songs you love or loved in your past. And probably you know these songs by heart. So, listen to these songs and sing to heart-joy. Doing so, you can combine a third practice (which will be developed later), that of learning a language other than your mother tongue, then take the words of your favorite songs and sings in that other language.

## 010 - GUIDE to smell fragrances

Smell is the sense, among our five senses, that we use the least. That's why perfumes give us powerful effects. This is also why incense is welcome during our meditation sessions, to provide us with an unusual level of consciousness.

Good perfumes provide intense pleasures, and many other benefits described in aromatherapy (such as: curing a cough, headache, sinusitis, asthma, digestive problems, insomnia, fatigue, anxiety, or antiseptic virtues against bacteria, Viruses, fungi and parasites). Of course, on the contrary, a bad odor produces an unpleasant sensation. And it is desirable to avoid it and eliminate it.

For example, the uses of essential oils are multiple, varied and very positive, it is an area that can be rewarding to study. Essential oils of mint, eucalyptus, pine, grapefruit, lavender, lemongrass, thyme or other.

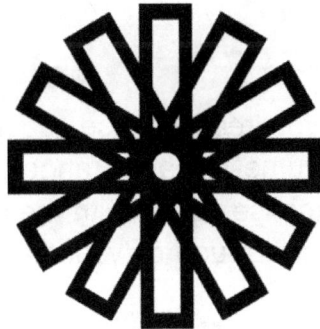

## 👀 Exercise 34 : Six tricks

### A cleaner air in your house :

Opens the windows of your dwelling, 30 minutes a day (even in winter, by closing the heating during ventilation, and vice versa, by closing any air conditioners, in hot weather). Then, the air is purified of allergens, moisture, dust, toxic and polluting gases. Also thanks to ventilation the oxygen level is increased. The best practice is to create a draft by opening several windows.

### Remove bad smells :

Here is a simple trick to get rid of a bad smell in the toilet, the car, or any other place: being careful, burn two or three matches. The sulfur of the match quickly absorbs unpleasant odors.

This exercise is not for young children, because of the risk of fire.

### Smell an orange :

While you work, you read or else, deeply and regularly breathes the perfume of an orange. And sometimes included in this exercise, along with the deep breathing of the perfume, feel the touch of your hand on the orange peel.

## Simple, ornamental, perfumed :

Here is a simple and decorative deodorizer: takes a citrus fruit (orange, grapefruit, lemon, clementine or kumquat) and cloves. Plant the cloves in the citrus by spacing them 0.5cm (the citrus shrunken when drying). Wrap a string or ribbon around, as if to close a package. Then hang the string on a shelf. It will release a pleasant fragrance. This perfume is also anti-mite.

## Pot-pourri :

You can also recover and mix the citrus peels. Dry the peels, by spacing them to obtain bark. Place the bark in a saucer. Then place this saucer, where you want (on a shelf, in a cupboard, ...).

## Three drops of essential oils :

Mint, eucalyptus, pine, grapefruit, lavender, lemongrass, thyme or the like, simply placing three drops in a saucer.

Using incense is also very interesting.

## 011 - GUIDE to touch

Touch is the only one of the five senses, necessary to our survival, and to our development in our environment. Our skin is rich in receptors related to our emotions. Thus, it is desirable to make extensive use of touch in our family relationships (For example, a baby who is not touched by his parents, does not develop normally. While parent's massages are very beneficial), in our friendship, and, in our professional relationships, for example a (very) casual clap on the shoulder (statistical studies show better performances, thanks to this type of use of touch). These contacts bring well-being, reduce stress, and regulate our emotions. Studies also show an improvement in our immune system through touch. Touch reveals us to our humanity, to the reality of our physical consciousness.

For example, we can use a ball, a pebble, Chinese balls (meditation with attention centered on the rotation of the Chinese balls is using the touch), or another object to reduce our stress, to use massages and practice braces and cuddles. And, we will see in the exercise of the multipoint walk, the benefits that one gets, at each step, practicing the touch of the points of the feet's sole.

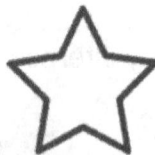

## 012 - GUIDE to take cold shower

I received this teaching of the cold shower, while living in Bangladesh, I went to a week-long retreat, in an ashram in Bangalore, India. There, the charming Guru (Sri Sri Ravi Shankar), who headed this Ashram, had one day given a single recommendation to the large assembly: to take cold showers. I understood then, that this teaching had to be important, and I began to take cold showers. And I have, indeed, found a lot of fun and benefits doing so.
I also later found this teaching of the cold shower, confirmed from several other sources.

Of course, this technique is not easy. It is easier during hot weather, where it also has the advantage (sometimes even the necessity) of lowering body temperature.
It is necessary to start with the feet, then slowly ascend along the body.

Cold showers offer many advantages:

- Increased vitality,
- Increased well-being,
- Improved blood circulation,
- Relief of depressive states,
- Improved skin and hair health.
- By activating the sense of touch, they reinforce our anchoring in the reality.

## 013 - GUIDE to do physical exercise

Physical exercise is important for physical, mental and emotional health. Good health promotes happiness, although one can be happy while being very sick. Regular physical exercise allows the body to work properly, including maintenance of the heart, lungs, muscles, tendons, nervous system, joints and bones. It thus helps to avoid pain and sickness, and the punishments that accompany them.

Physical exercise triggers the secretion of endorphin, the euphoric hormone of happiness, as do smiles, laughter and orgasm. This brings a well-being that you want to renew by doing more physical exercise.

When we do physical exercise, we focus our attention on the management, coordination and precision of movements, and we stop during this time, the convulsive and obsessive thoughts, that one may have facing responsibilities or during depressive states. On the contrary, we have access to new ideas and to new understandings.

Physical exercises should never be excluded, even in tight time management (e.g. coming student exam, domestic or professional responsibilities). The result will be positive, because physical exercise brings greater capacities of concentration, memorization and analysis. Studies show that high school students and students who do physical activity are more successful in their studies.

When talking about time management, the opposite must also be avoided, where time spent in physical activity is too long and to the detriment of other things (studies, family and professional life, or other responsibilities).

Physical exercise allows to have more our feet on the ground. It also makes it possible to know better the position of the body in space, which allows to have more precise gestures, to avoid accidents and to feel better.

From a social point of view, physical exercise, collective or individual, allows to establish relations and to fight the isolation.

It also develops team spirit and leadership. Achievement of a performance (e.g. distance, point gained) increases self-confidence and joie de vivre.

Increasing our mental balance and our desire to feel better, also helps us to better manage and avoid possible excesses (food, cigarettes, alcohol, drugs).

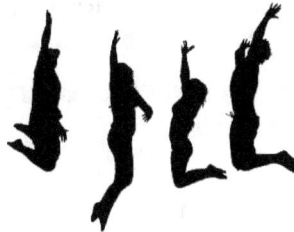

## 👀 Exercise 35 : 30 min. of exercise a day

The resolution to perform a minimum of 30 minutes of exercise each day, will be particularly beneficial if you do not have many opportunities to move in your life, or if you are currently in a difficult period of your life. Respect this minimum, especially on days when you really do not want to move, and even if it rains, take you by the hand and go for a ride; You will finally be very happy; And this routine will become easy and pleasant.

When you feel the disagreeable sensation that accompanies this lack of desire to move, react, with the realization, obviously, that you will be much happier activating and ventilating your head and your body.

Become accustomed to observing yourself, and at times when you understand that you are experiencing feelings of melancholy or sorrow, change your schedule. And replaces these moments with physical exercise.

When you engage in this new occupation, be careful not to feel constraint, but freedom and pleasure. Replace melancholy or disgust to do anything, by the happy feelings of your body, become pleasantly supported by your muscles and more solid. And also, taste the pleasure and the advantage of being able to maintain a straighter posture, for better alignment of the body (prevention of back pain and better circulation of energy).

Enjoy the feeling of your lungs and the contact of your feet with the ground. Find contentment in what you see and in what you feel. Find the happiness to be alive and feeling the energy circulating in your body.

A daily 30 minutes is enough, but short. A longer time is better. You can also, use the technique of adding one more minute each day, and soon the action that seemed insurmountable gives you joy.

Established a routine in your schedule, dedicated to the happy activation of your body. Defends firmly and with a happy conviction the continuity of this routine. Take it back quickly when it is interrupted. And consider these moments as privileged, as a gift that you make to yourself

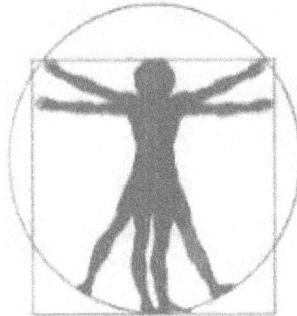

## 014 - GUIDE to stretch without apnea

Apnea is when you stop breathing. Individuals who engage in physical activity, often practice muscle stretching exercises. Yet, most do not know the importance of breathing and its effects, contrary to expectations, when not well used during stretching.

Indeed, for the stretches to be effective, they must be coordinated with the breathing. When stretching is practiced in apnea, as they are often, they on the contrary generate tensions and stiffness.

## Here is the desirable coordination with breathing:

o   Before the stretch takes a deep breath.

o   Then, expires slowly and steadily from the beginning to the end of the stretch. Work the sensation that it is your expiration that drives your movement.

o   When your expiration comes to an end, expire one last time, by emptying your lungs, and at the same time insists on your stretching. Then relax your stretch, while taking the following deep inspiration, and so on. Just as expiration has led the movement, your inspiration must lead it into the phase of relaxation. Thus, at no time, should your breathing be blocked.

It should be noted here, that the inspirations and expirations leading the movements of your body, are desirable to be practiced and adopted in all your gestures. Your gestures will then be more precise and more powerful. You will be more resistant to stress. Your body will be better oxygenated. And your recovery time after exercise will be shortened and less painful.

♦

That being said, the benefits of practicing stretching muscles and tendons are numerous:

- Before physical exercise, the muscles and tendons made more flexible are more effective, and the risk of injury is reduced.

- Stretching helps to correct bad posture and the muscular tension that it has generated.

- They allow a better blood circulation therefore a better feeding of muscles, tendons, cartilages and organs.

- After exercise, stretching reduces risk of muscle pain, and is very useful in maintaining muscle flexibility.

- Stretching is useful to practice daily, even without practicing other physical exercises (e.g. in evening, when simple stretching, in bed, allows better sleep).

- They contribute to stress reduction.

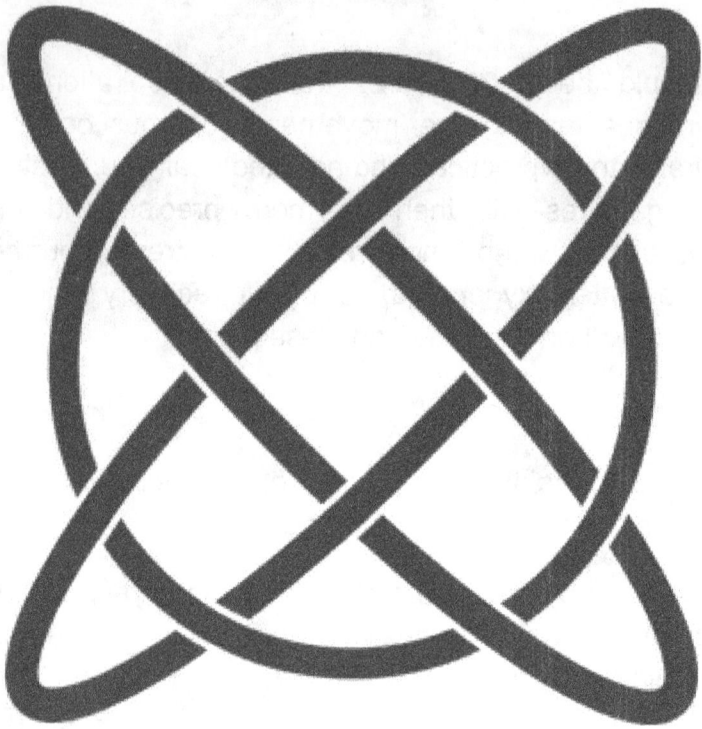

Anecdote: a martial art master told me one day, that he ate his meals on a coffee table, sitting on the floor, as is done in Asia, to maintain the flexibility of his body. The search for longevity, in good health, being a goal of Taoism.

◆

*'To keep the body in good health is a duty, otherwise we shall not be able to keep our mind strong and clear'*

Buddha

◆

'Take care of your body. It's the only place you have to live'

Jim Rohn

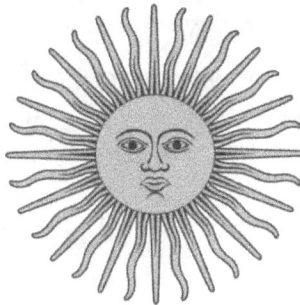

## 015 - GUIDE to merge with nature

With the evolution of our societies, more urbanization, more noise, more technologies, more information, greater horizons, more speed, more activities and more mental work, the contacts and the symbiosis with nature are becoming more and more useful. They are good, to keep us in the reality of life, for our relaxation, our physical and mental health, our ability to concentrate, our effectiveness, our memory, our emotional, psychological and spiritual needs, the quality of our relationships, our joie de vivre, and the reduction of our physical and mental fatigue.

Little is known, about the vegetable, animal and mineral worlds, their medicinal properties, interactions between them and with man. Fascinating things are already known, such as the fact that all the trees in a forest, and logically all the trees in a continent, are connected to, and are interacting with, one another by an enormous entangled network of roots and rootlets (this reality Is also a good subject of meditation in the forest). And we also attribute many properties to crystals (highlights of the evolving branch of minerals) and essential oils of plants (such as essential oils of wood, phytoncides, which you breathe during a walk in the forest).

We are learning and will undoubtedly discover, in our knowledge revolution, fascinating things about these subjects.

Whatever is your life, your job, your family situation, visiting the nature has to be regularly part of your life. This may require an effort to move around to visit nature, to include these tours in your busy schedule, or to go against your preference for urban living. However, you will always be very satisfied with the results.

In any case, contact with nature cannot be excluded from your schedule. Seize any opportunity, and also be enterprising to spend more time with nature and preferably daily. Nature outside cities, or in urban parks, gardens, terraces, etc., there is certainly one place within your reach.

Rather than making excuses to avoid going for a walk (such as rainy or snowy day when smells, sounds, and colors are particular and intense), make the move. In will finally result in bringing you great satisfaction.

Builds a strong conviction of your desire and pleasure to visit nature regularly, based on the memory of well-being provided by each visit.

When you are in nature, merge with it, be completely present, free and happy. Do not ruin this moment by ruminating your thoughts, with shortness of breath. Breathe and be alive.

## 👀 Exercise 38 : Embrace a big tree

This practice is unfortunately ridiculed.

Even if this exercise seems odd or if a preconceived idea makes you feel uncomfortable, do it, then see what you feel.

o  Choose a big tree, it has more interactions (chemical as far as we know) with its community, lovingly embrace it, put your cheek against its bark and thus remains at least one minute.

o  The experience of your relationship, like all spiritual experience, will be unique and intimately personal; It will be part of your privacy.

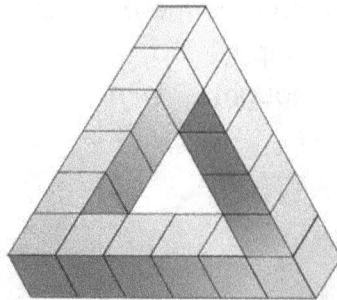

## Grow house plants

Cultivating indoor plants offers several benefits, including: air purification of many toxic polluting gases emitted by furnishings and decoration, carbon dioxide absorption and oxygen production, and the beneficial to health increase in the humidity of the air (whereas the atmosphere of the houses is often too dry).

More and more people are growing indoor vegetable gardens, which, in addition to the joys of gardening, allow them to harvest vegetables. Indoor crops are also fun and educational for children (for example, you can help grow a seed or a core of avocado, orange peels or cuttings). The cultivation of cacti is also very pleasant, there are many varieties, they are very aesthetic, they multiply easily and quickly, and they make very beautiful flowers (one day). The cultivation of wheat grass offers daily harvesting opportunities for making juices or salads.

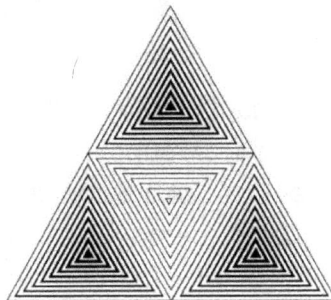

## 016 - GUIDE to sunbathe

Exposure to sunlight, generates an increase in the secretion of the serotonin hormone by the brain. Serotonin makes us calmer, happier, and increases our ability to concentrate. Insufficient exposure to the sun, on the contrary, contributes to depressive states (we tend to have a sad mood in winter). Sunlight in contact with the skin also generates the creation of vitamin D which strengthens our bones. While insufficient exposure induces vitamin D deficiency, the discomforts and pains of lack of bone matter known as osteoporosis (insufficient density and alteration of the microarchitecture of the bones). Also, when our bone density is insufficient our risk of fracture is high. Vitamin D also makes our immune system stronger and reduces our risk of disease.

We can be reassured about our need for vitamin D because short and regular exposures to the sun are sufficient. On the other hand, interpretations of blood tests often give a vitamin D deficiency, but the reference rate used is too high. Note that the best dietary sources of vitamin D are dairy products, eggs, fatty fish and mushrooms.

However, we must remain cautious and follow the medical prescriptions of vitamin D supplements (this is a very inexpensive and easy to take supplement), as opinions differ about vitamin D; some say it is a miracle hormone-like substance that prevents many of the symptoms and conditions (including cancer, type 1 and type 2 diabetes, dental caries, fatigue, muscle weakness, cramps, sometimes dry skin, some other autoimmune diseases (multiple sclerosis, inflammatory bowel diseases, etc.) and cardiovascular disorders with their many consequences)). Some doctors even recommend regular vitamin D supplements for all. The list of symptoms that affect our well-being, and the list of pathologies that can be avoided, are so long that this recommendation appears to be a good idea.

Still, we benefit greatly from bathing regularly in the sunlight (avoiding however the mid-day hours and protecting us during prolonged exposures).

While you are getting used to daily physical exercise outdoor, take few minutes only focusing on benefiting from the energy facing the sun (with your eyes closed).

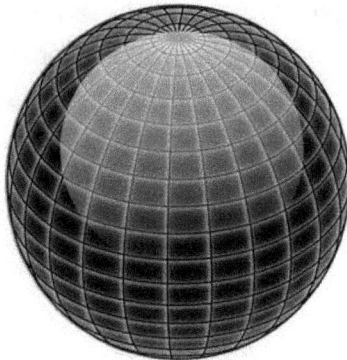

## 017 - GUIDE to respect life

Although progress has been made, we often continue, in the name of short-term profit (return on investment), even if it condemns the long-term, or habit or ignorance, not to include in our activities many essential parameters, especially our physical or mental health, and environmental (environmental impact).

Doing so was a mistake. Continuing to do so is another mistake. To find excuses to justify his error is a third mistake.

The new world will be a world of cooperation, satisfaction and respect for nature and for all. For man cannot live without respecting the logic of a positive environmental impact. When this evidence is our new normality, our super electronic computers will have found the solutions with the new parameters of the equation. Living preferences should be easy. And also, less risky than speculating or going astray by misunderstanding our fundamental interests.

The biggest causes of environmental degradation are industrial, for my part I cannot do very much. But I can make small. And the little streams make the great rivers. And you, if you can make big ones, go! The small gestures, the means, the big ones, the individuals and the collectives, let's go!

*'Success is a lamentable teacher. It seduces intelligent people to think they cannot lose'*

Bill Gates

♦

*'What have they done to the earth?*
*What have they done to our fair sister?*
*Ravaged and plundered and ripped her and bit her*
*Stuck her with knives in the side of the dawn*
*And tied her with fences and dragged her down'*

Jim Morrison

♦

*'It is spring again. The earth is like a child that knows poems by heart'*

R.M. Rilke

♦

*'Our environment and our attitude are the result of our choices'*

Daniel Desbiens

## ◉◉ Exercise 37 : Pick up along the way

When you see a litter thrown on the ground, in a forest or on a street, the exercise consists in collecting this trash, and in bringing it into a garbage can.
It is an exercise whose statement is very simple, and whose prospects are very rich and powerful.

Initially, our frustration to see this trash on the ground is strong. We become Judges and Jurors of the negligence of those guilty of these acts. Perhaps, we have a desire to punish those guilty.

Before knowing the practice of this exercise, the circumstance of the detritus found on the ground, only engendered frustration, disgust and rancor. However, most of the time, we do not react to the reality of this pollution, making the simple to carry it a trash.

It is very common to see a litter on the ground. Individually, we are not going to pick them all up, because they are too many. But their frequency will allow us to often practice the exercise, and to measure the evolution of our feelings. Also, by being more numerous in practicing this exercise, we will be able to change in a very perceptible way the cleanliness of nature and our quality of life.

With the knowledge of this exercise, every time we see a litter on the floor, whether we pick it up or not, we will measure the evolution of our frustration and our resentment in the face of reality.

The most powerful benefit of this exercise is that it allows to cultivate our humility every time we pick up trash on the floor.

We will thus work our balanced position between the negative energies of negligence, disillusionment, frustration and resentment and, on the other hand, the positive energies of respect and love, nature and the environment, as well as the positive energies of humility and our happiness to have carried out this good gesture of picking up the trash.

By measuring and practicing regularly these many variations, we come to benefit from these feeling of pure joys, and from the removal of these negative energies. Then, we also benefit from the dynamics of those.

◆

Another interesting similar behavioral exercise (and simpler because without disgusting, but the only happiness of the gesture well done), is to get into the habit of removing a stone from a road that could cause an accident.

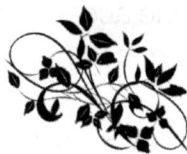

## 👁👁 Exercise 38 : Every drop matters

Look at the list of small streams that follows. And when you see one that corresponds to you, take the resolution to take care of it:

o  I let the tap water flowing continuously, when I wash my teeth, the dishes or my car.
o  I have a leaking tap since a long time.
o  I sometimes produce plastic waste, or other waste, that I could avoid. For instance: I use cutlery and plastic cups.
o  I believe the expiry date relates to safety rather than a quality convention[13].
o  If I leave a room for more than 20 seconds, I leave the light on.
o  I leave my television or my radio on, when I do not watch or listen to it. Or, I leave my computer and my printer on, without using them.
o  I heat more water than I use for my coffee or tea.
o  I leave my charger plugged in.
o  I could avoid using the clothe dryer.
o  My washing machine runs half-full.
o  I still use the old light bulbs.
o  I never check my tire pressure[14].
o  The engine of my car rotates when stopping for more than 20 seconds.
o  I drive my car using the accelerator and the brake rather than anticipating my decelerations.

---

[13] The expiry date relates to quality. Products can be consumed longer
[14] Underinflation results in higher fuel consumption

- I buy this product, while I know the disastrous effects of its production.
- I prefer to fly than the train. I do not use public transport. I could make the journey by bike, on foot, or in car-sharing.
- The cold air, or hot, passes under the door while I could easily stop it.
- I know the carbon and water balance, and the environmental impact of my business. [15] Or I do not even know what it is. Or I know what it is and I do not care.
- I do not use recycled paper. Or, I could avoid printing this document.
- I never cleaned the grills in the back of my fridge[16].
- I throw away the rest of my meal rather than make it with a new good dish.
- I use toxic products to clean.
- I throw away my used batteries instead of placing them in a recycling container[17].
- I do my shopping without sticking to a list.
- I do not eat only the fruits and vegetables of the season.
- I do not carry my bag by going shopping, and have to take new bags every time.
- I leave my refrigerator running when I go on vacation.
- I think of another small stream that is not in this list.
- I could rather buy products in local shops.

---

[15] Carbon weight = tool for calculating the quantity, direct and indirect, of carbon dioxide emissions. Same for water (e.g. 17 liters of water are used to produce a sheet of A4 paper, less for recycled paper).

[16] Should be done once a year. It saves 30% of the energy.

[17] An electric battery thrown into the wild, pollutes, with very toxic materials, 1 cubic meter of earth for many years, as well as the groundwater table.

## 018 - GUIDE to balance your emotional body

Our emotions play an important role in the journey of our lives. During our childhood and adolescence, we discover these unknown emotions, their opposites and their interactions, which are sometimes devastating. Then, our emotions continue to greatly influence our lives.

Let's talk about our emotions as constituting our emotional body. Naturally we want to have a balanced emotional body. We want to feel good in our emotional body. We want it to be useful, rather than to have our emotions harming us, disturbing us or bringing us on destructive paths.

While we are benefiting having a more equilibrated emotional body, we also can use our emotional system to help us in our decisions. This is subtle feeling, which requires attention and practice. A basic functioning of the emotional system is that a thought unfavorable to our evolution, generates a negative emotion. And a thought favorable to our evolution, generates a positive emotion. This emotional system is related to our subconscious intuition. It is therefore, far more reliable than our conscious thinking system, because it is based on wealthier past teaching and on a wider vision.

Yet, our desires and our imagination distort our judgment. Being convinced that such idea or such desire is favorable to our evolution, we ignore the feeling of our emotional system warning us of the contrary. Ignoring this underlying uncomfortable emotion, we risk being carried away by our desires, our joy and our enthusiasm, to later realize that this idea and the choice that followed, were not beneficial to us and drove us to an uncomfortable, even sometime perilous situation.

Therefore, we will look at being attentive to our emotions. We will question arousing thought as being pure emotion of joy and enthusiasm? Or if we fell a subtle uncomfortable emotion together with this thought? We will remain careful in our analysis, because the discomfort can also be part of the normal questioning of the mind evaluating the risks of our choice.

Naturally we have a very large number of thoughts and emotions. In order to make the best choices in this complexity and in this subtlety, it is desirable and beneficial to increase our ability to control the flow of thought and emotion, to take a step back, to be able to shut down and open the tap of the mind. In order to increase our capacity, we have various practices, including meditation. Our consciousness acquires strength drawn from our ability to feel emptiness, in silence and in the present moment. Our thoughts and emotions become more serene and more just. The underlying, false or true and subtle causes emerge. We learn to use our emotional body.

The applications of the technique of understanding our emotions are found in everyday life when we have to make a decision (examples: choice of a romantic or professional relationship, a professional choice, a choice of subject of study, a choice to move to a new place to live, a choice to purchase or sale something, a choice of lifestyle, etc.).

We will see, later in this manual, other benefits of meditation, and a Guide to Meditation. Certainly, the ability to make better choices in our lives, being more comfortable and more stable in our emotional body, is a decisive result in convincing us to practice meditation.

## ◉◉ Exercise 39 : Name your emotions

Observe your emotions and describe them with a word, for example: I am furious. I'm sad. I'm desperate. I'm afraid. I'm disappointed.

Then continue your mental exercise, continuing with:

I am ... because.

And details the reasons for your emotion.

Your emotion then moves from your emotional body to your mental body, and it becomes less intense and easier to manage.

## 019 - GUIDE to merge with animal

People living with a pet, know some aspects of the singular nature of animals and of our relationships with them, especially their constant and generous elk in love when they celebrate with us or ask for caresses.

Beneficial interaction initiatives with animals are increasing, such as in hospitals, prisons and support to autistics. Many scientific studies measure the positive variations in hormone and neurotransmitter secretions, blood pressure, immune system, decreased risk of allergies, numerous therapies, decreased stress and feeling of loneliness, and also greater ability to learn for children.

We talk about a particular healing power of cats, that would be even closer to their masters to treat them when they are sick. We now recognize morally, and even legally, the suffering and the right to the existence of animals. Adopting an animal develops a sense of responsibility to care for and care for a period of up to fifteen years.

We savor even more with a pet the pleasure of walking in nature and being active. Tasting the company of an animal, even a goldfish in an aquarium can reduce our stress levels.

There are also great advantages in observing wild animals, contemplating their beauty, their colors, their shapes or their agility, whether birds, insects or any other animal that one may have the chance to encounter.

## ◉◉ Exercise 40 : Pet healer

This exercise is only for people living with a cat or a dog.

It consists in observing when the animal is particularly cuddly, and then to let you go completely, without even imagining anything other than the value of sharing. The massage, carried out by the mainly by the cat (but also dog), the sound made by the animal and this gift of love which could well be aimed at the care of a physical or psychic disorder, whose healing will be facilitated by your participation and your confidence in the process.

◆

*'We do not have two hearts, the one for the man, the other one for the animal … We are good-hearted or we don't.'*

A de Lamartine

◆

*'The best remedy for those who are afraid, feel alone or unfortunate, is to go to a quiet place, alone in the paradises, nature and God. It is in these moments when we perceive that everything is as he has to be'.*

Anne. Frank

◆

*'For my part I know nothing with any certainty, but the sight of the stars makes me dream'.*

Vincent Van Gogh

## Wild only with eyes

Apart from animal protection programs carried out by professionals, it is necessary to refrain from having interactions with wild animal, other than observing them. Animal skin, coat, plumage or carapace contains oils and bacteria that protect the animal. Touching the animal may damage this protection and make the animal vulnerable to disease. These oils and bacteria can also be causes of diseases for humans. Just as oils and bacteria on our skin can cause diseases to the animal. A wild animal, as beautiful as it may be, and as gentle as it may seem, can easily have sudden aggressive reactions, as an expression of its survival instinct. Feeding a wild animal can also be disastrous for its health. And finally, any interaction produces a modification of the animal behavior that can be fatal to him.

Corrects your possible tendency to interfere with the wild animal. If you are a parent, teach this behavior to your child.

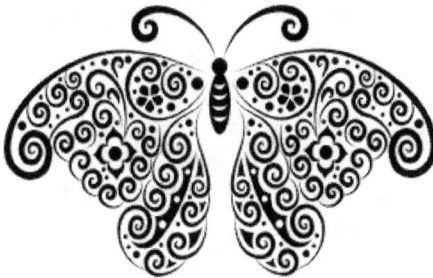

## ◉◉ Exercise 41 : Birds and bugs

Some of us are passionate about bird watching. On the other hand, this activity seems too passive, uninteresting and overly requiring patience, for many of us. I was one of those, and I did not imagine that one day I might be interested. Yet, I found myself living, for a year, in an oasis of an Iranian desert, where there was no opportunity for leisure during free time. I then had a colleague and friend, who was a bird watching enthusiast. So, I accompanied him. And we were lucky enough to be able to observe many birds, big ones, small ones, flamboyant colors or multicolored. So, I started to enjoy this activity. Since then, I have enjoyed every opportunity to observe the birds. And this is an activity I recommend, at least during walks.

Make this experience.

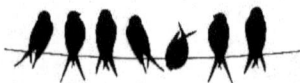

♦

'Storms and darkness scared me, but somehow it encouraged me to learn about nature and I think nothing's dark, dark is beautiful too'.

Bai Ling

It is also beneficial to take every opportunity to observe, even for a long time, the life of the insects, while exercising your patience at the same time. It can be a fly, a beetle, an ant, a spider, a butterfly, or any other. If you are one of those who has a repulsion for insects, it will be similarly beneficial, and will allow you to overcome your phobia.

On your next visit to nature, focus your attention on the discovery of insects, you will certainly have the pleasant surprise to be able to observe a very beautiful one.

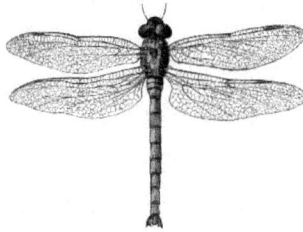

*'The earth laughs in flowers'.*                    R.W. Emerson

♦

*'Some people walk in the rain, others just get wet'*

Henry Miller

♦

*There are always flowers for those who want to see them'*

Henri Matisse

## 020 - GUIDE to balance your chakras

Knowledge, practice and writings about chakras, circuits and currents of energy, is rich and ancient. This richness includes simple and tangible benefits of body perception in space, from the best circulations of energy in the body, to cosmological concepts. This initiation to the knowledge and practice of the chakras, will allow you to feel better in your body and to improve your self-confidence.

If you are impervious to considerations that are not, so called, down to earth, you will still be able to do the first exercise, of body perception, whose practice will still benefit you. If your curiosity allows you to observe the practices of billions of humans since thousands of years, with repertoires of sophisticated points and circuits of energies of the human body, Ayurvedic, Chinese, Hindu or Inca medicines, martial arts, sophrology, osteotherapy, energy medicine and physiotherapy, qi gong, yoga, spirituality, esotericism and meditation, you will have many opportunities to deepen your knowledge.

We also can find the chakras in sacred geometry, in numerous symbols (eg the caduceus of Hermes) and on numerous archaeological remains found on all continents.

The texts of Ayurvedic medicine describe tens of thousands of chakras distributed in the human body. More simply, everyone agrees with the description of seven main chakras with which are associated colors, organs and functions of the body, qualities and emotions. Knowledge about the chakras describes an optimal functioning of the body and the psyche, when energy flows freely. And describes physical diseases and psychic disorders, when the energy circulates with difficulty in one or the other of the centers of energy. Thus, when one wishes to work on an organ, a function, a quality or an emotion one will work by insisting on a specific chakra.

The most important in this chapter is, as always in this manual, the practice of exercises, which engenders perceptions. But before that, here is some information about the chakras that will be useful in the exercises that follow: locations, colors and specificities of the chakras will be used and recalled

The energetic circulation networks of the body are constituted of many ramifications listed. There are two directions of energy flow, one from the bottom to the top, for which we see a column of energy starting from the center of the earth, which enters the body mainly through the root chakra that is located on Lower in the body, which then ascends from chakra to chakra, circulating by the meridians and mainly by the meridian located in the spine, which emerges through the chakra of the crown at the top of the skull to join the cosmos. The second direction of energy flow is from top to bottom, for which we visualize a column of energy, entering through the crown chakra, flowing along this sophisticated arborescent array of channels of energy, meridians and chakras distributed throughout the body, to come out through the root chakra and join the center of the earth. It will be interesting to see simultaneously these two directions of energy circulation (bottom up and top down), however this double viewing is, in my experience, a bit tricky, because we are not used to nature of these energies free from directions. In order to make it easier, we can start by visualizing one direction and then the other. And in a second step, we will consider our body as an antenna crossed by a column of energy, with the confidence that this energy flows naturally from bottom to top and from top to bottom.

There are many applications using the characteristics of the chakras. We will do at the end of this chapter, only a few of the possible exercises. It should be noted in the case of the chakras that, as always in this manual, priority will be given (above all other considerations) to stability, balance, efficiency, comfortable acceptance of our specific and circumstantial human conditions.

The chakra energy system must be conceived as a whole, with links and interactions between the chakras. We begin with the lower chakras (the first three starting from the bottom), ascending through the central chakra of the heart and ending with the three upper chakras. Even if you want to work a specific chakra (for example, a higher chakra), it is recommended to first work (even fast) on the flow of energy through the 7 chakras. Do not worry, because only with a little habit, you can work on the 7 chakras in seconds.

Let us see, in the following pages, the names, the locations, the anatomical, physiological, pathological and psychic correspondences and the associated colors of the 7 chakras, going from the bottom of the body to the top, going along the central axis:

## ☯ <u>The root chakra</u> :

- Location: between anus and genitals.
- Color: red
- Anatomy: linked to adrenal glands.
- Physiology: stimulates the whole body and acts on the blood circulation.
- Pathology: sciatica, anemia and circulatory problems.
- Psychic: balance, fundamental ground anchoring, stability, self-confidence and courage.
- The root chakra is the one that best captures the energy of the earth.

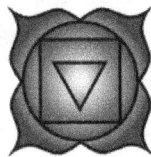

At the time we live, when, we have access to a lot of information; where, spiritual treasures, like the writings of Rumi, have recently become very present in social media; where, the existentialist questions have become popular and shake the egos; where, our horizons have expanded to the dimensions of the infinitely large of the cosmos, as well as to the dimensions of the infinitely small elementary particles constituting the matter, and therefore our bodies; where, we are all concerned with economic and environmental changes; and, where, we engage in the construction of a new world, our terrestrial anchorage is very important. It is the foundation of our being, it ensures our equilibria and our stability. This shall not be neglected. Therefore, while working on the chakra, the work of this first chakra is of the utmost importance.

(Note that if you are not currently interested in exploring the chakras, it is still very important that you strengthen your earthly anchorage, and you shall do so by regularly visiting the nature.)

For, our relationship with the earth, is our only true truth. While, the truths of our faith, our convictions and our ideas are good, and are a joy to explore, but it is our duty to always question them; to admit that we may be mistaken, and to realize that effectively we are often mistaken. These truths, whatever they are, are respectable. They are necessary to our life, for without it would die, having no reason to exist. These truths are also respectable, for we respect them with great enthusiasm, effort and devotion. These truths also always contain their untruths. All in all, these truths are very complicated, it is part of their seductions.

To the complexity of so many truths is added the complexity of the unknown (to which we can however be comfortable, admitting our ignorance).

To best enjoy these complexities, it is necessary that we cultivate a great stability. And this stability is possible only if we have a very close relationship with our only true truth, the earth. That, which is simple, which is not possible to question, and which has no untruth; the one that can be touched; that for whom we cannot lack respect, enthusiasm, effort and devotion, for without it we would not exist and we would die.

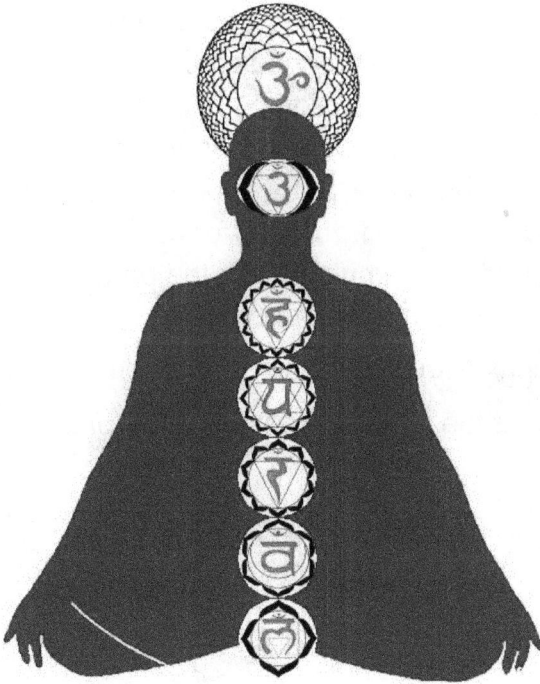

### ☯ **The sacral chakra** :

- Location: point located three fingers (index, major and ring) below the navel.
- Color: orange
- Anatomy: sex glands
- Physiology: sexuality, reproduction.
- Pathology: genital, renal and urinary disorders.
- Psychic: sexuality, emotions, joy, vitality, creativity, enthusiasm and compassion.
- This is the most important point for physical strength, on which it is good to pay attention during a specific or difficult work (like carrying something heavy), as well as during a physical action Simple, like walking. It also corresponds to the center of gravity of the body. We will work on this chakra to improve the quality of our sexuality (not only from a performance point of view, but from greater communion with the partner) and to better manage our emotions and fears.
- This chakra bears the name of sacred, for it is at this point that the soul is localized, when one believes in it.

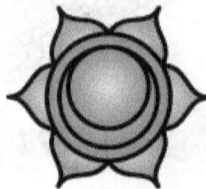

## The Solar plexus chakra :

- Location: at the base of the sternum.
- Color: yellow
- Anatomy: pancreas.
- Physiology: digestion.
- Pathology: digestive disorders, diabetes, obesity (related to satiety).
- Psychic: will, power, balance, spontaneity, self-confidence (one feels this point chakra when after a moment of amazement, one seems to have a heart tight).
- Like all chakras, the solar plexus is a vital point, important in our lives, and on which a violent shock leads to death.

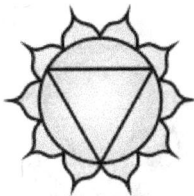

## ☯ <u>The heart chakra</u> :

- Location: point located three fingers (index, major and annular) above the solar plexus.
- Color: Green
- Anatomy: heart and thymus
- Physiology: cardiac function and immune system.
- Pathology: cardiac disorders, tensions and back pain, infections.
- Psychic: love, friendship, sociability or on the contrary coldness, difficulties to establish professional, friendly or loving contacts.
- You can strongly feel this chakra, in moments when you feel light and transported by a feeling of joy or love.
- There are many practices, breathing, meditation, energy and psychic practices (thought, emotions, consciousness, ...) focusing exclusively on this chakra.

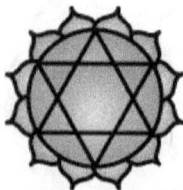

## ☯ <u>The throat chakra</u> :

- Location: point located in the hollow of the throat.
- Color: blue sky
- Anatomy: mouth, tongue, teeth, vocal cords, bronchi, lungs, lymphatic system and thyroid.
- Physiology: speech as well as the functions associated with anatomical correspondences.
- Pathology: sore throat and teeth as well as hearing problems.
- Psychic: communication (even written) and expression, and self-confidence.
- It is good to work this chakra before making a speech, statement or before singing, or when you want to correct a speech disorder or shyness. And before performing a work of written expression.

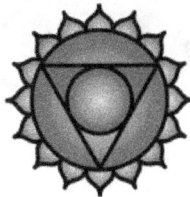

## ☯ <u>The third eye chakra</u> :

- Location: at the top of the nose.
- Color: blue-purple.
- Anatomy: pineal gland.
- Physiology: vision and the nervous system.
- Pathology: headache, eye disorders and nervous diseases.
- Psychic: clarity of ideas, wisdom, intuition, imagination, creativity, self-knowledge and premonition.
- The third eye, and its relationship with the pineal gland are found on all continents and from the time of ancient Egypt. We find this relationship over the centuries and in many practices including martial arts, meditation and yoga.

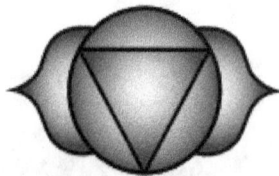

## ☯ <u>The crown chakra</u> :

- Location: at the top of the skull.
- Color: purple and also white
- Anatomy: pituitary gland
- Physiology: immune system, growth.
- Pathology: headaches and immune deficiencies.
- Psychic: decision-making, psychic balance, acceptance of reality, seat of values and beliefs.
- This is the main point of entry of the column of energy going from top to bottom.

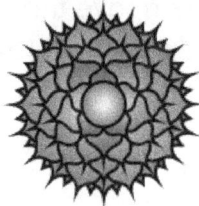

## 👁👁 Exercise 42 : Initiation (1st part)

This first exercise can, therefore be practiced, even by the most skeptical and the most down-to-earth of us, with the advantage of an improvement of the feeling of the body which is always beneficial to improve the knowledge of the localization of the body in space (Allows you to move with greater confidence, greater precision and balance). These physical improvements have their psychic equivalents, all of which equate to an increase in the feeling of well-being and joie de vivre) .

For the less skeptical and the most curious among us, this exercise will be a first contact with the chakras, which will be useful for all other exercises on the chakras (which are very numerous and of which only a few examples are cited here).

The positions of the 7 chakras is recalled here to facilitate the practice of the exercise:

- Root: between the anus and the genitals for the dermal part and at the tip of the sacrum for the precise internal point.
- Sacred: three fingers below the navel
- Solar plexus: at the base of the sternum
- Heart: three fingers above the sternum
- Throat: in the hollow of the throat
- Third eye: above the nose
- Crown: at the top of the skull

The exercise consists in feeling and visualizing the seven chakras. It is done in 2 steps:

- o In a first step, you will touch, with your index finger, the area where each chakra is located. Move your index finger in the specific area of each chakra, making sure to locate exactly the center line of your body, on which the chakra point is located. Then, always with your index finger, massage this point. This massage will allow you a better feeling and memorization of each chakra point that will help you, afterwards to visualize them.

- o A second step is to visualize the 7 points chakra, successively, dwelling at least 30 seconds on each chakra.

If, during the second stage of visualization, you feel the desire to touch any of the chakras, follow your desire without hesitation.

Now that you are initiated into the localization of the chakras, you will sometimes feel again the desire to touch and massage one or other of the chakras. So, let yourself go, to do a massage course (2 to 3 seconds).

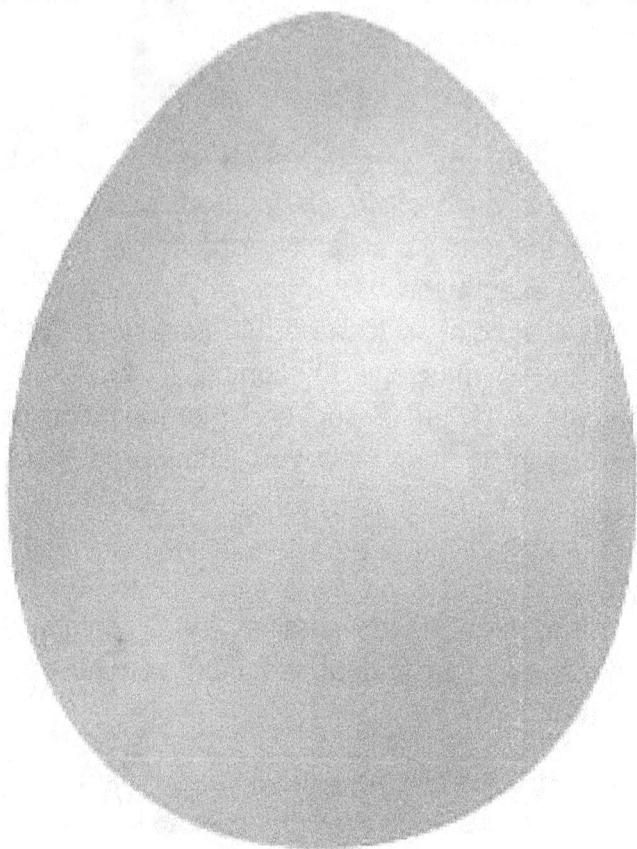

## ◉◉ Exercise 43 : Initiation (2nd part)

This exercise consists in adding to the previous exercise the visualization of the colors associated with each chakra (recalled here to facilitate the practice of the exercise). Moving from one point to the next, imagine the color of the dot mixing with the next.

- Root Chakra: Red
- Sacred Chakra: orange
- Solar plexus chakra: the yellow
- Heart chakra: the green
- Chakra of the throat: the sky blue
- Chakra of the 3rd eye: blue-violet
- Chakra crown: purple or white

After you get used to this localized visualization of the seven colors, you can add, before going from one color to the next, a visualization of each color filling up your entire energetic halo (ovoid shape around your body), as well as the totality of your body to the heart of each cell.. And you can remain for some time in the comfort of this colored egg. And finally, you can stay longer, bathed in the white halo of energy that constitutes your energy envelope.

## ☻☻ Exercise 44 : Cleaning (1st part)

Difficult events, accidents and aggressions of life, leave traces in the chakras, which disrupt the optimal circulation of energy in our body. Traces, good to remove by practicing the cleansing of the chakras.
The ambient energy enters each chakra at a very precise point, at the top of a cone of energy. Around these precise points the energy at the level of the chakras turns clockwise (imagine a clock placed on the body).

In this first part of the chakras cleansing exercise, and in the second part that follows, three steps are described (a total of six steps). These steps may seem complicated. Do not worry, take the time to be comfortable with each step before moving on to the next. You have all your time, do not hurry, enjoy every step. Each step brings its own benefits and satisfactions. Quickly, you will find very simple to practice these techniques.

During the stages, you will visualize each chakra for at least 30 seconds. This minimum time of 30 seconds is necessary for your first practice of cleansing the chakras, as your chakras now need a good cleaning. Later, you can shorten this time, to 10 seconds, if you wish.

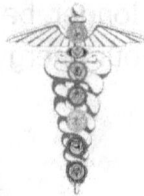

The first step

Visualize, successively for each chakra, this direction of rotation (clockwise direction on the chakra point).

The second step, (is the proper step for cleaning.)

Re-visualize each chakra, but this time by visualizing, a rotation movement in a counterclockwise direction.

The third step,

Visualize for each chakra the rotation restored in a natural clockwise direction and a speed of rotation more and more rapid, even to become very fast.

♦

Once the three steps of this exercise are completed the seven chakras are cleansed.

With a little practice, you can even enjoy a short free time during the day to do quickly (two minutes) these three steps. And you can do this exercise as many times as you want. It is very enjoyable and very beneficial.

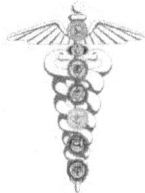

## 👀 Exercise 45 : Cleaning (2nd part)

Apart from the root and crown chakras (which have energy flows in the vertical direction), the other five chakras possess their symmetrical equivalences, at the back of the body. These symmetrical points also have a rotary movement in a clockwise direction (you can visualize a clock placed on the posterior face of your body). The cones of anterior and posterior energies, therefore, turn in the opposite direction.

First step :

○ Visualizes the cone of energy at the top of a column that enters your root chakra, and which rotates clockwise.

○ Visualize a cone of energy penetrating your sacred chakra, on the anterior face of your body, turning clockwise.

○ Visualize a cone of energy penetrating your sacral chakra, on the posterior face of your body, turning clockwise. The tops of two cones meet in the center of your body.

○ Now passes to the solar plexus, and also performs a visualization of the two cones of energy that revolve on the anterior face of your body and then on the posterior face. Do the same for the heart chakra, the throat chakra and the third eye.

○ Complete this first step, by visualizing an energy cone at the base of a column of descending energy that enters your crown chakra crown, with a clockwise rotation.

Second step : (proper cleaning):

Reproduces the first step, with a counterclockwise rotation.

Third step :

Reproduces the first step by visualizing the clockwise rotation going faster and faster, until going very quickly, because the chakras are now well cleaned and function optimally.

Once you are comfortable with this practice, you can add a

Fourth step :

Visualize your whole body, with the flows of energy penetrating the seven chakras; the ascending vertical flow that enters through the first chakra (root), nourished with energy the seven chakras and emerges through the crown chakra; the two horizontal (anterior and posterior) streams of the following five chakras; and the descending vertical flow, penetrating through the crown chakra, nourishing the seven chakras with energy and emerging through the root chakra.

It is good to begin each work session on the chakras, doing a cleansing of the seven chakras.

Then, there are many techniques that consist, depending on the desired effect, to concentrate particularly on one or other of the chakras.

There are also many techniques, with specific goals, working the chakras by different pairs or by different groups.

These techniques may optionally include visualizations of rotations, colors and both at the same time. And as the rotations become faster and faster, the colors become more and more vivid.

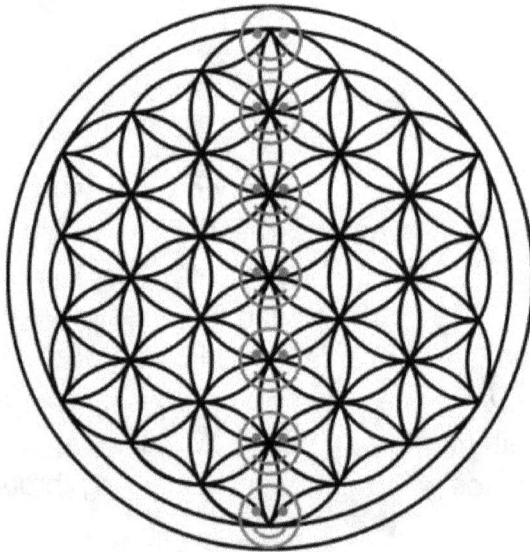

## ◉◉ Exercise 46 : Turning around the body

Now that you have practiced, the locations of the seven main chakras, and the later symmetries of five of them, here is an exercise, that I personally enjoy practicing several times a day (exercise is quick and can be practiced, discretely, everywhere).

It is simply a matter of viewing and concentrating on these 12 points (without colors or rotations), one after the other.

You can start with the crown chakra, follow with the third eye on the anterior face of your face and continue with the next 10 points. You can, after, chain several cycles of these 12 points.

This energy harmonization of your body will be very beneficial to you, at all times and in all circumstances.

You can also use this technique, to relieve specific pain such as a headache, sinusitis, toothache, sore throat, bronchitis, difficult digestion, abdominal pain in the intestines (in particular pains of nervous and psychological origin, which are very common in this region which is much innervated), pre- and post-menstrual pain in women, hemorrhoids, etc. For these pains, first, make several rotations around your body, follow your instinct to linger longer on one or the other of the points chakra, while maintaining the rotation around your body which will make you return on this point, perceive your sensations as well as their evolutions (especially those around the chakra point close to your pain). You can also use this technique to relieve your mind and your body unbalanced by an emotional shock that makes you angry or makes you sad or nervous.

## 021 - GUIDE to know your magnetism

The brain has long been regarded as omnipotent, the only center of our thoughts, memory, sensations and emotions. The heart was given a single role of a blood-pump, and the intestines a single role of digestion. Recently, our certainties have changed. For example, we now give a memory role to each cell of the body; The function of memory and the magnetism of the heart have been discovered; As well as its sophisticated interactions with the brain; And the memory function of the intestine and its primordial role on the nervous system.

The existence of magnetic fields was discovered in the 13th century. But it was not until the 1970s that the biomagnetic function (magnetic fields produced by the electrical activity of living organisms) was scientifically defined. It is already known that the heart has a much more powerful and ample biomagnetism than the brain. And this is an area in which we will make many discoveries. While we discovered the emission of electromagnetic waves from the heart, it is interesting to note, that light is the set of electromagnetic waves visible to the human eye.

The magnetic field of our body has the same structure as the magnetic field of the earth and the magnetic field of the universe (including the same sense of direction of the magnetic lines.) This form is called 'torus'. These magnetic fields are shown on next page:

Human body magnetic field[18] :

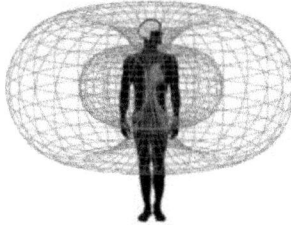

Earth magnetic field :

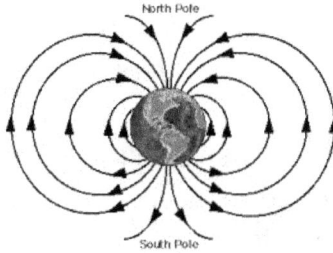

North Pole

South Pole

Universe magnetic field :

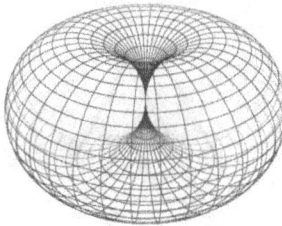

---

[18] Illustration of body magnetic field from Institute of Heartmath Research center.

## 👀 Exercise 47 : The Magnetic walk

In the coming years, we will learn more about the variations of our body's magnetic field. For now, to benefit from a better self-knowledge, it is beneficial to only visualize the existence of our magnetic field.

o   Begin by visualizing the shape of your magnetic field on the charts on the previous page, also its magnitude and the directions and orientations of the magnetic lines.

o   During a walk, preferably in nature, consciously breathe and view all these parameters of your magnetic field.

o   Include a specific visualization of the fluidity of the electromagnetic currents in the region of your heart, which is at the center of your torus.

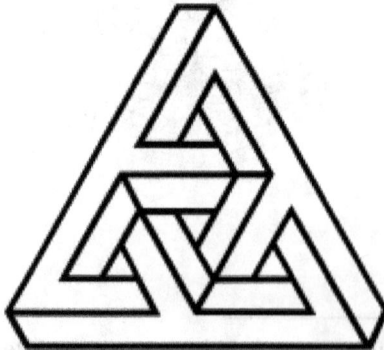

## 👁👁 Exercise 48 : Rewarded heart

Your heart, with its electromagnetic role is the star of this chapter.

This exercise is there to reward it.

Your heart deserves to be rewarded, because he always accompanies you, when you do sports, in your loves, in your fears, in your joys, in your sorrows, in your euphoria and in your anxieties. Your heart is sometimes oppressed, sometimes expanding. You have sometime a 'heavy heart', sometimes a 'light heart'.

This exercise will allow your heart to be, instantly, comfortable, light and happy.

o   The technique is simple. It consists in visualizing, for a few minutes, that you are breathing with the heart, and that the inspiration fills your whole body.

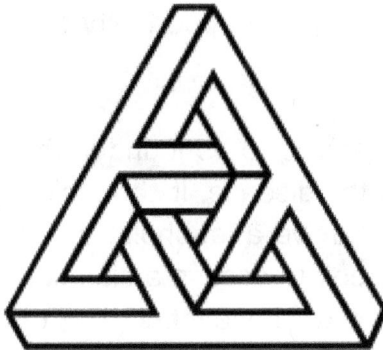

## 022 - GUIDE to appreciate the disease

Becoming happy, in our body, head and actions, very clearly reduces our chances of getting sick.

If you happen to get sick, then, it will be beneficial for you to appreciate the benefits of being sick. This appreciation will enable you, to heal faster, to better live the time of illness and the time that follows. If, on the contrary, you cultivate the sadness and the frustration of being sick, these benefits will escape you.

o   The disease helps to strengthen the body. You can take advantage of the sickness time, to work on feeling your energy and improvement of its circulation.

o   When we focus on our frustration of feeling pain, fever or weakness, or on what the disease prevents us from doing, it creates stress in us. While we can, on the contrary, accept the disease, and take advantage of it to explore, in depth, these unusual sensations. (One more time, taking the opportunity to play the explorer role.)

o   There is a teaching to be found in the introspection of the cause of the disease. It can indicate fatigue due to overwork. It can be a loophole, a call for help, or the need for a break to assess a situation. By discovering this cause, you will have found 50% of its solution.

o  Disease helps cultivate patience and restore humility.

o  It is an opportunity to, take care and to love yourself.

o  It is good to, use the illness period for, reassessing your priorities and finding solutions to the problems you hold dear.

o  This new appreciation of the benefits and opportunities of the disease helps to broaden your horizons and in particular contributes to the appreciation of the benefits of the difficulties encountered in your life and similarly to solve them faster and live better rather than aggravate them.

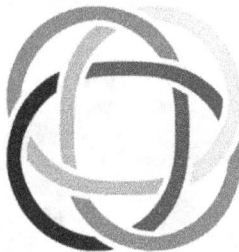

## 👀 Exercise 49 : Take care of your teeth

In many countries, tooth care is traditionally very important. Thus, individuals spend several hours each day, while doing other activities, to clean their teeth with sticks as a toothpick (the first toothpicks appeared in the Bronze Age).

A toothache can be very painful.

In addition, a damaged tooth generates a large production of bacteria that weakens the body and can be the cause of diseases (including heart disease).

Bad dental hygiene gives bad breath, that is harmful for a good social life.

Bad teeth or lack of teeth prevent good nutrition and good digestion and are thus detrimental to a good health.

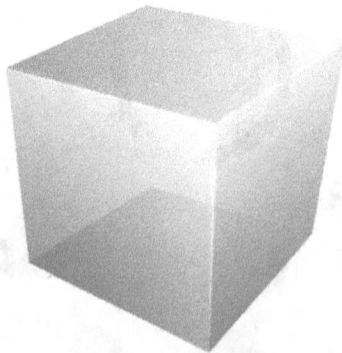

Let's take positive energy from this long list of benefits, to generate the desire and the pleasure of taking good care of our teeth:

o Regular brushing after the three meals;
o Mouth rinsing after a snack and, also <u>before</u> each brushing;
o Sufficient brushing times (at least 2 minutes);
o Refining of brushing technique for optimal efficiency;
o Use of a dental floss daily;
o Banishment of sweets and sugary drinks;
o And, timely care of a damaged tooth.

Start now, according to your needs, to make improvements to the care of your teeth.

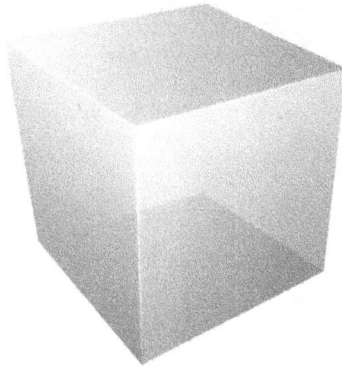

# Acti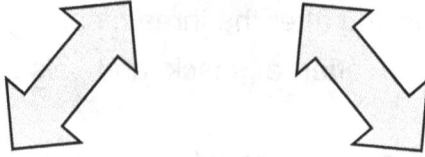n

Body 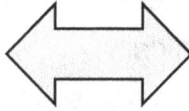 Mind

## 3.2.  HAPPY IN YOUR HEAD

As the happiness of feeling good in our body is powerful, as happiness is above all a state of mind, and as our good actions can fill us with happiness, we may be tempted to make the mistake of believing, that separately this happiness is stable and sufficient.

We discover in this manual, that these three happiness's are optimized and become stable and intense, when they are grown simultaneously.

We also discover how experiences and the practice of happy sensations in one of these three domains generates happy sensations in the other two. And we discover the surprising inertia of these triangular dynamics, which facilitates and multiplies our discoveries.

In this chapter of happiness in our head, we will explore our thinking, our behaviors, stimuli generating cascade effects, and we will discover new treasures.

We will also learn to perceive that, on the contrary, negative stimuli in one or other of the three domains have negative effects in the other two domains. This knowledge will enable us to avoid these negative stimuli, to favor positive stimuli and thus to benefit from positive dynamics.

Here surely, Love with a big 'L' !

Live everything with love.

Love is everything and cannot be defined.

Love is felt.

Love is also more than a feeling.

Love is essence.

Any attempt of description would impose limits.

Love is in the hatred. Hatred is in the fear.

Big love is in the point of balance between love and fear.

No attempt of description could imagine in this point the non-existence of limits.

Nevertheless, it is at this point that it is good to build our stability.

## 024 - GUIDE to measure the belonging

The feeling that the other belongs to us, is a tendency that one often encounters.

In a family, parents easily confuse their responsibilities of education, with a sense of belonging, to the detriment of the integrity of the personality of their children. Such confusion can be seen in other family relationships (brothers-sisters, grandparents-grandchildren, etc.). In a couple, this feeling of ownership, is also often very strong and very devastating. In the same way, one cannot accept that a friend may be different from what one had imagined, or that he may have ideas, tastes and desires different from ours. At work, the demand for productivity, with the feeling that employees belong to the company, is wrong, forgetting the concrete and fundamental human reality, and that better productivity is obtained when this reality is respected.

The correction of this confusion (integrity-belonging), allows us better relations, better cooperation, more efficiency and more happiness.

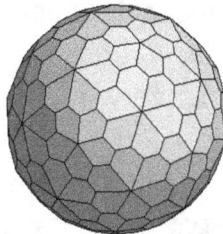

## 025 - GUIDE to adapt to sex equity

The relationships between people of opposite sex are complicated. Because they have a heavy history, and because they evolve quickly and a lot, especially since the end of the last century, and even more so in the West with the women's liberation movement in the 1970s. We progressed from a society, where women were considered inferior, soulless, without the right to express themselves, and without the right to work, to a society where, ideally, there is no such sexist discrimination.

Through this passage, our capabilities are, as it were, doubling. Even in fact, more than doubling, thanks to the synergy of the larger capacities, and thanks to the famous formula of cooperation 1 + 1 = 3.

We shall work to achieve two goals:

o The first, is to continue gender equity efforts, bridging the many remaining cultural gaps, until the moment when iniquity will be for us another of those curiosities of our history

o The second, is for men and women to continue to adapt, to their respective new equitable identities, to their new interactions, cooperation, achievements and independence.

The achievement of these two goals, for which we are currently making great progress, is a very dynamic phenomenon, which is very promising to support the construction of the new world.

The situation being new, our improvised reactions, can be audacious and visionary.

Here is already a good time for you, to observe the Sri Yantra, bellow. The Sri Yantra will be explained in more detail later in the manual. It is a diagram of tantric meditation consisting of nine triangles arranged in duality; One of the meanings of the 4 triangles (on the central axis) pointing upwards is the masculine side, and one of the meanings of the 5 triangles (also on the central axis) pointing downwards is the feminine side.

To the observation of the Sri Yantra is attributed the property of balancing the masculine and feminine sides, right and left-brain hemispheres.
(the kinetic art of graphism may allow this property, You will see, it is amusing, when concentrating on the image (by fixing the central point), one sees the triangles moving).

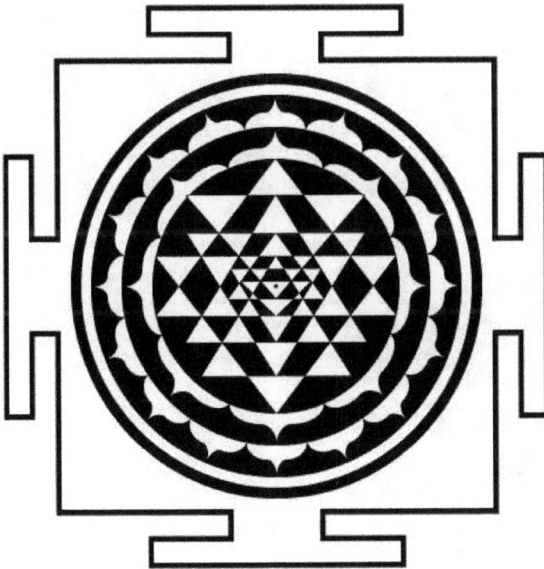

## 026 - GUIDE to develop self-love

The discovery of the concept of 'self-love' was a "key" to me. What is very fun with a key is that, first, and many times, you pass by without seeing it. Then, once the concept has tilt, we see this key everywhere. The principle of a key, is also that it opens doors, makes us progress, and in this case, makes us happier. While the key has opened new horizons, this vision remains ephemeral, it becomes stronger when we use it again, but it fades if we stop watching.

In brackets, this mechanism actually applies to all our thoughts. It explains very well and very easily with the description of our nervous system and its mechanism of memory.

Here is the diagram of a neuron:

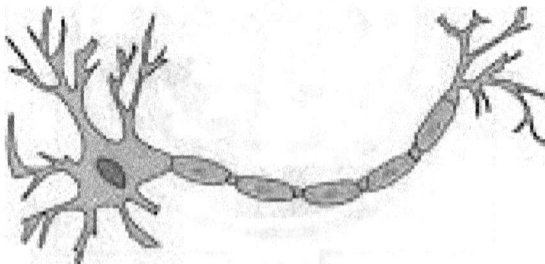

Neurons are the cells that make up our nervous system. They are found throughout the body, mainly in the brain, heart and intestines. As can be seen in this diagram, a neuron has tree structure at its two ends. The neurons bind to each other, in chain, at the levels of these trees, according to mechanical and chemical mechanisms.

When we have a thought, it is printed at the level of neurons by creating a specific link in these trees that constitutes our memory. When we renew this thought, other bonds are created between our neurons, the tree corresponding to this thought becomes more abundant and stronger. When, on the contrary, we cease to have this specific thought, the links and the corresponding tree branches are atrophied, and the influence of this thought diminishes until it disappears.

One thus understands the physiological mechanism of thought, and the interest of making addictive choices in favor of positive thoughts while weaning negative thoughts.

Note that while they atrophied, the tree branch remains, maintaining knowledge of the totality of the life experiments. A mass of enormous knowledge that fuels our subconscious and conscious mind.

We further appreciate here the interconnections between our body, our mind, our emotions, our thoughts and subsequently the interconnections with our actions, which are either enhanced or either enhancing.

Let's go back to the concept of 'self-love'.

He may at first surprise us, for we are not accustomed to speaking of 'self-love' as a positive thing, perhaps even to attribute to it a negative connotation, identified by error to selfishness. On the contrary, it is the lack of self-love, which cultivates egoism, and which is at the origin of all abuses. For it is easier, more direct and more rapid, to define oneself, to define our ego, with suffering rather than with love. And because the impulse of suffering, if it is not stopped, generates a cascade of additional suffering.

Would it be by modesty, humility, impatience, or more simply by habit of self-underestimating, we are not accustomed to delight in the pleasure of the good results of our capabilities. However, it is gentle, beneficial and realistic to feel, in love, beautiful and having great qualities. And when we practice the tasting of the respect and the self-love, the reasons to do so continue to improve. Then, we become accustomed to these changes in our personality, as well as to changes in our relationships with others. This metamorphosis is progressive. It may be challenging to newly situate ourselves, and to situate our new relationships with others. Likewise, the others must re-establish their relations with us. However, we will observe the others, seduced by sharing the real, superficial and deep dimensions of our new personalities.

The stable integration of self-love, generates positive changes in all our relationships, listed here to emphasize their importance: family, loving, friendly, social and professional.

Finally, to love oneself, is also necessary for our survival.

So, if you have a lack in your ability to love yourself, and if you now manage to fulfill it, you will see your life transformed. And it is very probable that this capacity is lacking to you, for it is a weakness that we all have, and that we all are improving, by gaining knowledge. It is quite natural, that at a time when some had no consideration, and even had disgust with respect to others, because of their castes, their sexes, or their colors of skins, it was difficult for these others to love themselves. As these denigrations are now greatly leveling, they allow many people to cultivate self-love, and consequently to become enterprising. Here again, the enormous sum of individual strengths, achievements and self-appreciation, newly made possible, allows us to foresee the magnitude of the changes to come.

More self-love is possible for everyone, even if you have the body, the thought or the heart bruised, you must realize that you are more than your body, more than your thoughts and more than the circumstances of your life.

The improvement in efficiency is cited as a result of the practice of several exercises in this manual. Being more efficient helps to improve self-love; while errors, omissions and failures (which cannot always be avoided) affect self-love.

If you compete with others, you will achieve better results by using the positive energy of the search for greater efficiency, and by avoiding the desire to dominate others that is loaded with negative energy.

The only fight that has value and you need to achieve is the fight to improve yourself.

## 027 - GUIDE to think positive

We are therefore beings who think, and not beings, only identified to our thoughts.

After realizing that we were thinking beings, we will now work at observing what we think. We will also work at observing what we say.

Our mind is very productive. Thousands of thoughts arise every day. However, our mind has a characteristic, which will allow the positive thinking technique, described below, to function. This characteristic is that we can think of only one thing at a time.

By observing what we think, we will then make choices. We will choose not to maintain negative thoughts, and to favor positive thoughts. The observation and the analysis of our thoughts will enable us to understand and to correct our thinking from negative to positive.

The following exercise will describe this technique step-by-step. And once again, here, the process is very exciting and playful, because from the first steps of this trip we discover beautiful landscapes that make us want to pursue.

♦

*'We model and we build ourselves with what we love.'*

Goethe

Before doing the exercises, here is a list of the examples of negative thoughts discussed in this manual:

- Suffering from a lack.
- Self-judging. Judging others
- To self-underestimate.
- To refuse the reality and the impermanence.
- Drowning in the past or in the future.
- Maintaining regrets and to betray oneself with hopes.
- Be impatient, resentful, neglectful, jealous.
- Be overwhelmed by bad news.
- Suffering from loneliness.
- To complain. To get angry. To be pessimistic.

Some of these points seem moralistic. Let us not be put off by this morality. It is not a morality derived from a doctrine, but a morality which authorizes our only possible way of life, the community life. And this morality at the same time authorizes our individual happiness.

♦

*'I often think that the night is more alive and more richly colored than the day'*                    Vincent Van Gogh

## Positive thinking technique

- Select a thought that gives you joy, such as remembering a happy moment, a scene, an element of your current situation, or a project you are working on.

- Observe when your mind is producing a negative thought.

- Replace instantly, this negative thought, with the joyous thought that you have selected.

- If you observe that you have just said a negative word, first feel the joy of having the ability to make this observation (and not the pain of having said it), then resolve to correct this trend. And finally feels satisfied to find that your correction is easy, fast and happy.

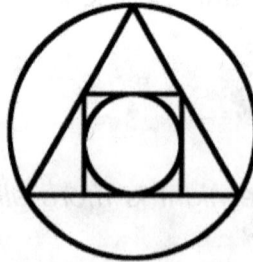

The negative thoughts are managed by algorithms comparable to those used by Internet servers.

If you get interested in it,
they harass you.

When you give up on them,
they become blurred then disappear.

Then,
to be happy,
let us avoid polluting our heads and our Web.

## 👀 Exercise 50 : The 24 hours experience

The day I discovered this practice of positive thinking, my life changed overnight. I started, as indicated in this exercise, a 24-hour practice. This practice has allowed me to realize its benefits. So, I continued the practice and I never stopped it. Thus, my happiness and my well-being have multiplied.

This exercise therefore consists in applying the positive thinking technique for 24 hours.

During these 24 hours, you will have moments of well-being and satisfaction, when you replace your negative thought by the joyful thought selected. These moments of well-being will be precious to you.

You will realize the ease to obtain the well-being, with the simple modification of your thought.

You will also realize the futility of the negative thoughts; And you will find that they present themselves more and more rarely.

You will be able more and more quickly to interrupt your negative thoughts to keep your positive thoughts.

Your negative thoughts will take up less space and generate less pain in your life. You will arrive at a constancy of positive thoughts.

You will be happier.

## 028 - GUIDE to be optimistic

To be optimistic is, to some extent, synonymous with being happy. This, is also demonstrated very well by its opposite, oppressive pessimism.

How does a pessimist use his time? It is obvious that the time spent being pessimistic, is not a time during which one is happy.

What does this pessimism correspond to? Pessimism is always a projection in the future, with reminiscences of negative events of the past assimilated to future projections, imagining an unfortunate outcome of a present situation. Yet, an optimist imagines him a happy ending of the same situation. Or, better still, an optimist may feel neither enthusiasm nor bitterness, in connection with the unknown outcome of a situation that may turn out to be either happy or unhappy. He knows that projections in the future are, for the most part, false.

So, in the same context the optimist uses his time to be happy and the pessimist uses this same time to be unhappy.

Let's be clear about this reasoning. The projection in the future is not reprehensible, when it corresponds to the feasibility study of a project. On the contrary, it is necessary. Then, we measure the resources available, we analyze the potential risks and we plan the activities. When one decides to embark on the realization of the project, one does it, considering having a good chance of succeeding. In this process, it is possible and desirable to remain continually optimistic, when planning, when deciding to embark on the realization of the project, imagining the sequence of events, and when the sequences are put in place. If our feasibility study leads us to abandon the project, it is a pity but a rational one, it must not permanently, but only shortly, undermine our optimism that we can be fed with the satisfaction of having learned useful things, and we will shortly, better equipped, study a new project.

If we embark on the realization of the project, unexpected events may also arise, we will face it, and we will demonstrate the constancy in our serenity and our joie de vivre.

Our optimism will give us more energy and better chances to succeed. In the event of failure, the optimist has a better chance of learning the lessons of failure and rebounding with greater chances of success, while, the pessimist, is likely to close even more on himself.

All great and small discoveries, all large and small projects start from an idea, a thought that is supported by an optimistic and enthusiastic vision. Without optimism, there is little chance of discoveries or achievements. It is easy to understand that an optimist has a better chance of succeeding in relational, loving and professional life.

An optimist also has better health than a pessimist.

Nowadays, every subject is the subject of numerous studies and statistics. These confirm the advantages of being optimistic.

An optimist knows these many advantages. He knows how to cope with the numerous imperfections in the human being. He knows that imperfections can be leveled. One can thus conclude that the optimist is more conscious, more present and has a better sense of reality, whereas some would sometimes try to make us believe the opposite.

That is as simple as that … in fact no,
it's not that simple.
It's simple for an optimist and it's complicated for a pessimist. And it's also complicated to know the roots of pessimism. There are certainly roots of education and other roots of experience. But there is also a natural individual character and propensity.

◆

'Optimism is the faith that leads to achievement. Nothing can be done without hope and confidence'

Helen Keller

◆

'Confidence isn't optimism or pessimism, and it's not a character attribute. It's the expectation of a positive outcome'

Rosabeth M. Kanter

## 029 - GUIDE to live here and now

Twenty years ago, when I was talking with my dear friend Gillou, with whom I still laugh a lot, I told him about the "magic" formula 'HIC AND NUNC'[19] that I had just discovered. The formula was magical to me by its depth and intensity, and by its refocusing power. Then, we continued our evening by tackling many other subjects. At one point, I had a memory gap, and could not find a word. Gilou then said to me, 'Are you going to find that word, Hic and Nunc?' Then a flash of lightning, like the light which, in a comic strip, lights up above the head of a mad scientist, I instantly told him that forgotten word. We laughed a lot. And we still laugh.

Here and now is a principle, a concept, which facilitates acceptance and anchoring in the present reality. The past with its joys and sorrows, and the future with its fears and hopes, do not exist, only the present exists[20].

This concept is a key to happiness. It was used by the Humanists, and by the Writer, of which Eckhart Tolle in his very good book best-selling 'The power of the present moment'. And, it is fortunately more and more used nowadays. Concentration on this concept brings depth and well-being, it also reduces anxiety and depression.

---

[19] ' Here and Now ' in Latin.
[20] Not to be mentioned that from a quantum point of view, the time does not exists.

And, we have a lot of scope to increase our presence in the present moment; effectively study in psychology is measuring that we are spending 98% of our time thinking about the same things, events from the past or projections in the future. Amazing! Let's first realize how much we are ourselves spending our time in such sterile way; then, let's us spend more of this wasted time focusing on the reality and fulness of the present moment. Breath.

*The excessive suffering of the past,*
*the lack of awareness of the present,*
*and forgetting potential of the future*
*are nonsense and outrages.*

♦

'*From time to time it is good to take a break in our quest for happiness and of just to be happy*'

Apollinaire

♦

'*There is no "next" in "I am".*
*It is a timeless state.* '

Sri Nisargadatta Maharaj

'A lifetime is not what is between the moments of birth and death.

A lifetime is one moment Between my two little breaths. The present, the here, the now.

That's all the life I get.

I live each moment in full, In kindness, in peace, without regret'

Chade Meng, poet Taoist

♦

'The human being thinks about the future forgetting the present. So that he neither live in the present, nor in the future. Finally, he lives his life as if he is never going to die, and he dies as if he had never lived'

Dalaî Lama

♦

'There is a fine balance between honoring the past and losing yourself in it. For example, you can acknowledge and learn from mistakes you made, and then move on and refocus on the now. It is called forgiving yourself'

"Being at ease with not knowing is crucial for answers to come to you".

Eckhart Tolle

Now is the only moment which exists.

The only moment when you are alive.

The only moment which has a value and a certainty.

Now is the only reality.

Where you can enjoy the silence.

Where you can feel and act.

Where you can breathe profoundly.

Where you exist.

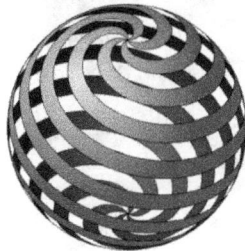

Repeatedly recalling to the present the memories of the past; to project the past inconsiderately into the future; and, constantly ignoring the present for the benefit of the future, are three common attitudes that are equivalent to denying presence, reality, truth, well-being, happiness and peace.

Once observed, these attitudes can be corrected, by the simple and powerful breathing. This famous breathing, which is restricted when chained to these same attitudes. This breathing can free us, by practicing one to three deep conscious inspirations followed by regular breathing.

By continuing to observe these three common attitudes, and responding in this way, these attitudes are transformed. They become less frequent, less painful and easier to correct. At the same time, we discover new attitudes.

When we live moments with these attitudes, the same phenomenon described above for the moments of stress occurs: we put ourselves in apnea (we stop breathing). Although we are suffocating, it is not easy to realize that, for a few seconds, we suffer from lack of air. Fortunately, the knowledge of this phenomenon of apnea allows us to increase its perception, and consequently to shorten these periods of asphyxia. At the same time, we increase our ability to perceive easily the moments in which we experience these three attitudes, and consequently make other improvements to our lives.

These two times, changes in our breathing, and the experience of our new attitudes, form a couple of forces that stimulates new existential dynamics.

Living in the present moment, is certainly very effective to be happy. That sounds easy. It is, in the sense that it is easy to live instantly in the present moment, even if you have done it only few times until now, with your hyperactive mind in the past and in the future. But the prolongation and the multiplication of those moments when you are alive and happy in the fullness of present happiness, will require you to follow a process:

o First, with deep inspiration, feel the good feeling of living without your life being conditioned by past events or projections of future events. Then, gradually prolong this happy sensation for a few seconds, for example during the 30 seconds of three deep inspirations-followed by slow expirations.

o Then, include these practices of few seconds in your everyday habits. You'll find that it is easier and quicker for you to automatically observe your thoughts and return to the present moment, especially after a frustration or after an incident.

o Then gradually increase these periods to several minutes.

You will realize that it is rather easy to focus on the Here and Now; especially when you use catalyst techniques (such as conscient breathing or focus on one action). Then you will realize that focusing on the Here and Now is bringing you comfort. The obsessional fears for the future and regrets from the past are dissipating. The eventual sorrow you are feeling for a missing person is also dissipating. While you could be spending days, years or your entire life in the discomfort of these thoughts you have the possibility to interrupt your distress and to live moments feeling to be alive Here and Now. The next moment will also be Here and Now; and the moment after. Instead of being oppressed, you are healing, you are feeling your ability to replace discomfort by comfort, in you are strengthening your ability to optimize your reaction to future events.

The focus on Here and Now is getting easier and easier. You are enjoying the feeling. However, all your life you will have, time to time, the tendency to return to the discomfort from fears and from regrets, therefore all your life you will have to remember to come back to the focus on the Here and Now.

♦

*'Learning is experience.*

*Everything else is just information.'*

Albert Einstein

## ◉◉ Exercise 51 : The walk Here and Now

Even after we tasted the wellbeing brought by the most valuable practice integration of the concept "here and now", the difficulty is to remember, or to not forget, to practice it. We shall take every opportunity and we shall follow each impulse to remember to practice.

Walking, alternately thinking and feeling presence Here on a step and presence Now on the next step.

During this walk, be fully aware of where you are, what you see, what you feel and even what you taste, if you happen to find a cherry on a tree.

During this walk it will also be advantageous to add optionally, and successively, other practices seen in this manual:

- Carefully unroll the foot from heels to toes.
- Think of the role of blood pump walking with blood circulation that goes in the direction of the heels to the toes. And think of your blood that continues to flow throughout your body. This helps to improve your blood circulation.
- Think about the points of walking 3 points.
- Think about the flow of energy through your chakras.

## 👀 Exercise 52 : 5 minutes here and now

Breathe consciously, concentrating on your spatio-temporal position here and now.

There are projections neither in the past nor in the future. When you come to the fullness of the present moment, you lack nothing, there is neither hope nor regret. For five minutes, your only consciousness is your breathing. If a thought arrives, you concentrate again on your throat, and you let it pass.

Renew often and regularly the exercise. In addition to a formal exercise of 5 minutes per day, seize the opportunities (e.g. waiting at a red light). You will be happy in these moments, to refocus on here and now.

Gradually, during the course of the day, you will experience the desire to enjoy this moment of peace and fullness, and you will be able to come back to it more and more quickly, and to stay into it, more and more at length. You will be able to change the scenario of your life, moving from a character inclined to spend a lot of time, anxious about the memory of past events and the fear of future events, to a personage happy to live, livelier and more capable to seize opportunities.

These positive results may seem difficult to achieve, but you can be confident, this simple practice, 5 minute every day, it's all what it takes to enjoy positive changes in your life. You will also find that you will manage to practice this technique automatically and repeatedly.

## 030 - GUIDE to unmask the complaint

When we observe our behavior, we see our great ability to complain. Whatever our situations, we find always reasons to complain. Then, these reasons become obsessions. We find it much easier to complain, than to rejoice in the many good circumstances of our lives. We more easily choose unpleasant circumstances than pleasant ones to define our identity.

To illustrate this behavior, let's take the example of our housing: we all tend to focus on its defaults (not enough light, or too much light, a more or less recurrent noise, it can also be a noise that rarely disturbs our quietness, or a heavy silence, a too small dwelling, a housing too hard to air-condition because too big, etc.).

Some of us complain even the whole time. It is a very unhealthy practice, which both harms the person who complains and the person who hears her complaining. People who complain, hurt themselves, and act like blood-sucking vampires, for those who listen, affecting their joys, motivations, creativity, trust, friendship or love. A person complaining also risks missing to see or spoiling a possible opportunity passing within her reach.

It is quite possible to eliminate all forms of complaint from your life. Just look at yourself and correct yourself. To observe how ungrateful you are to complain, rather than to rejoice in the good things that furnish your life (such as the comforts of your lodgings). Choose, then, the agreeable circumstances, to define your identity.

Of course, if you have the possibility of eliminating or reducing the origin of your complaint, it is not here, negligently, to resign yourself to living with, without making the effort to change it. But until you can eventually change it, it's better that you stop complaining.

In case the origin of your complaint is a side effect, indissociably accompanying an advantage that you desire to preserve, you will then have better to replace the opportunities to complain by the gratitude of benefiting from these advantages. Let the plaint then cross your mind at the speed of a flash, and your time be used rather with the pleasure of enjoying the advantages.

Takes the decision, now, to totally stop complaining. You will feel the immediate benefit. It is possible that for some time complaints come back. But, quickly, you will arrive at that the complaints become rare, to finally disappear. Quickly, you will also understand that your participation in the very popular and very common discussions that multiply the complaints, are useless and harm your comfort. In the course of this process you will realize, first of all, that you are complaining, the subjects of your complaints and the circumstances in which you complain.

This achievement will be rich teaching, because you may complain often without even realizing it. This achievement will allow you to correct this default, to perceive its uselessness, your ability to stop complaining and the well-being that this change gives you.

In the same way, you will realize that the subjects of the conversations in which you are participating are now different and much more interesting. The sterile tendency to complain has given way to constructive analyzes of problems, to the discovery of solutions, or to the discovery of ignored information. As a result, your life is now different, you are a different person, the events are different, opportunities arise, you are happier.

For example, it will be very easy for you to realize that at the moment when, in a conversation, you are expressing a complaint about a subject, there is an avalanche of complaints from all those present, and that avalanche drags. Similarly, you can do the second experiment, to express an idea on a positive, interesting, and perhaps even on which you want to have more information. You will then see the same avalanche of ideas expressed. And finally, you can do a third experiment: that of expressing an idea arousing interest on a completely different subject, in the middle of a conversation expressing an avalanche of complaint. You will then notice that it is very easy and beneficial to change a topic of conversation.

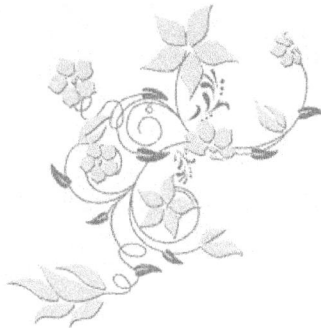

**Stop complaining - step by step :**

o Be attentive and realize the moment you complain.

o So, rather than feeding the path of your complaint, decides to stop it. And replaces this journey, by another path of ideas that awakens your enthusiasm, your creativity and your joie de vivre.

o Be satisfied, with the ease with which you have succeeded in modifying your attention and telling you that in your next complaint it will be as easy for you to change the path of your ideas and reap the fruits of your new reflection.

♦

*'I've had a lot of worries in my life, most of which never happened'*

Mark Twain

♦

*'Happiness is an attitude. We either make ourselves miserable, or happy and strong. The amount of work is the same'*

Francesca Reigler

## 031 - GUIDE to ignore the impossible

Never think that happiness is impossible
If we think that happiness is impossible, it is; and it is very likely to remain so.
Be conscious of, the wheel of fortune turning incessantly. The common misfortunes of life always disappear to leave room for happiness.
It is also common to observe, once past misfortune, that this one has positively transformed us[21]. This perhaps until, one day, when our wisdom allows us, not to condition our happiness to circumstances.

Similarly, it is never too late to be happy. And as our life expectancy and the longevity of our fitness increase steadily, we can be happy at the most advanced ages of life, provided we do not despair, remain active and not stop cultivating happiness. For example, it is interesting to realize, when we are fifty years old, that probably we are only half of our lives.

As for young people, seeing them pessimistic is a misfortune! They have all the time, every chance and every opportunity to be happy. Adults who live with young pessimists, must cultivate their own optimism, which will naturally be transmitted to these young people. The experience being much more powerful than the statement of the theory.

---

[21] Dynamic of the duality positive-negative (seen later in the manual).

## 032 - GUIDE to moderate your attitude

No matter what our trends and tastes, happiness is not the exclusive of intro or extrovert.

However, both can either indulge in a comfort zone, which barriers are desirable to break down, or have crises of their opposites that are desirable to moderate. Having a regular life, and having a life full of unexpected things, both have advantages.

It is thus important, to know how to alternate the pleasures of a regular life and the excitement of an eventful life. The first thing to do is, by observing ourselves, to realize the nature of your dominant tendency. If you are excessively extrovert, it will be beneficial to cultivate your introversion by making quiet and silent pauses. And if you tend strongly to be introverted, you will have an interest in making efforts to be more sociable, going out, seeing the world, going to shows, participating in clubs and associations, and making new experiences. You will then, realize the value and the teaching of the experience, which open horizons and that perfectly answers to our outstanding questions. Let us keep in mind, that we are free to act and react as we desire, and that the circumstances that prevent us from doing so, are rare.

♦

'Quiet people have the loudest minds'   Stephen Hawking

## 033 - GUIDE to remember impermanence

We build citadels, empires so solid, thinking they will last forever, to finally see them collapsing. We were rich, we are now poor. We were poor, we are now rich, but it is very likely that, one day, we will be poor again. Health is lost and is found again. Love and friendship are interrupted, new ones are born. Beliefs and truths change. We were young then years passed. We refuse premature death, making illusions about what life should be or should have been.

Impermanence is taught in all cultures. It is deeply rooted in popular cultures imbued with Buddhism. As for example in Japan, where impermanence is a very present concept, recalled in the symbolism of the paper house. But it is no longer a notion deeply rooted in western popular culture, where one is bathed in innocence and the playful aspect of childhood, with very little recall of impermanence, where the normality of death is ignored, and where, one is heavily influenced by the consumer society. Then, one is defeated, helpless and surprised, by one among many subsequent occasions to encounter impermanence.

Change is in the nature of things; it is good to remain aware of its reality. Not to be overwhelmed by the loss of a love or a friendship. To reduce the arrogance of our beliefs, our truths, our wealth and our successes.

*'Everything changes, except the change'*          Buddha

♦

*'As wave is driven by wave. And each, pursued, pursues the wave ahead. So, time flies on and follows, flies, and follows. Always, forever and new. What was before is left behind; what never was is now; And every passing moment is renewed'*          Ovid

♦

*'Try to not resist the changes that come your way. Instead let life live through you. And do not worry that your life is turning upside down. How do you know that the side you are used to is better than the one to come?'*

Rumi

♦

*'Old age is the most unexpected of all things that can happen to a man'*          J. Thurber

♦

*'The art of the life consists of a constant adaptation to the environment'*          O. Kakuzo

♦

*'Impermanence is a principle of harmony. When we don't struggle against it, we are in harmony with reality'* **Chodron**

♦

*'Remember that you are going to die is the best way to avoid the risk of thinking you have something to lose. You are already naked. There is no reason not to follow your heart"*          Steve Jobs

*'Your eldest son died? Love him even more. And above all, love others, those who remain, and tell them. Quickly. This is the only thing we learn from death: that it is urgent to love'*

E. E. Schmitt

♦

*'Death makes everything of enormous interest, gives value to everything, adds a dimension to everything'* J. Green

♦

*'A dead lion is not worth a midge which breathes'* Voltaire

♦

'The fear of death follows from the fear of life. A man who lives fully is prepared to die at any time' Mark Twain

♦

*'It is not death that a man should fear, but he should fear never beginning to live'.* Marcus Aurelius

♦

*'Cowards die many times before their deaths; the valiant never taste of death but once'.* William Shakespeare

♦

*'As a well-spent day brings happy sleep, so a life well spent brings happy death'.* Leonardo da Vinci

♦

'Some people die at 25 and aren't buried until 75.

Benjamin Franklin

## 034 - GUIDE to relieve mourning grief

It happens to all of us to lose loved ones, either because they have died, or because their reality has moved elsewhere. This creates a great void in our lives, just as it changes our identity, in which these loved ones held a large place, and gave us landmarks that have now flown away. We are more missing these landmarks than the person.

In some countries, death is sung as the end of a well-conducted period, and a passage to another experience. Some of us think death, that's final, while others of us believe in eternity. In some cultures, it is believed that the pain felt, causes the deceased to suffer. Others think that the acute suffering of mourning is necessary and even correspond to a right. Many only define death as clinical (breathing stoppage, heart failure, no muscle activity or reflex).
These beliefs are all conventional.

Death is a vast subject, extending from the finite to the infinite. But whatever our beliefs, physical life is undeniably impermanent, and physical death a reality.

And here again, prolonged suffering, following the death of a loved one, corresponds to a refusal of reality. Yet it is better that this pain lasts as little as possible and does not drag on for a great number of years. Once again, here is the technique of managing thought.

An excellent technique to reduce and heal the suffering of mourning is, to remember the love that we shared with the person now deceased. Suffering is then appeased. It will return, and the balm of love, the memory of shared happiness, may again relieve the pain.

The same technique works very well, to relieve and transform pain, when a romantic relationship, or a precious friendship, we believed to be eternal, has evaporated.

So what ?

Are we going to spend years of abundant regret? Or are we going now, carried by love, to turn the page and write the following, to have greater respect for ourselves, for the people now around us and for those who were around us.

There is also a tendency to forget the reality of our own death, sometimes suddenly, sometimes at night in our sleep, without being noticed and often surprisingly and unexpectedly.

For my part, I have been near death a very great number of times, following multiple accidents of bicycle, motorcycle, car and even, once, truck; As a result of diseases (not only tropical); Once, I fainted after a carbon monoxide infection produced by a generator. But also a very large number of other times, which I did not really remember, as a driver who loses control of his car and was at two fingers to touch me; During a walk in the mountains, the balance found when the bottom of the ravine was close; Several lost bullets, while working in war zones, electrical short circuits, falling objects, violent storms; Car accidents narrowly avoided as a result of a puncture or a snow slide; when many times I slipped into my bathtub. Many other times, I avoided suffocating as a result of food swallowed, etc.

Look also at your life and remember the number of times when directly and indirectly you have brushed against death. You will be surprised to find that this number is high. This reflection should neither frighten us, nor prevent us from taking the necessary precautions to reduce the risks. But, on the one hand, it must remind us of the fragility of life, and the normality of our death and that of our relatives and our friends, and on the other hand, it must encourage us to add up and give priority to choices, to live happy moments, alone or with our loved ones.

♦

- I have the feeling that all my life depends on this precise moment. If I miss it …

- I think of the opposite. If we miss this moment, we try the next, and if we fail, we begin again the next moment. We have all the life to succeed

Boris Vian

## 035 - GUIDE to be Zen

Let's stay Zen,

"Everything that happens to us happens for our own good"[22].

We realize, with hindsight, that moments of suffering, are the ones that have allowed us the most to evolve. One realizes, after having suffered, to be happier, being the new person that one has become. We realize the great opportunities that have unfolded, and that could not have been born if suffering or failure had not existed before. One learns to appreciate the reality of each moment, the pain as well as the joy. Suffering teaches us the difference, the impermanence, the flow of opportunity, the reality and the detachment.

In this capacity, paradoxically, one is, but without masochism, able to love pain as much as joy. One is able, to love life. And we are able, to accept, relativize and relieve our suffering.

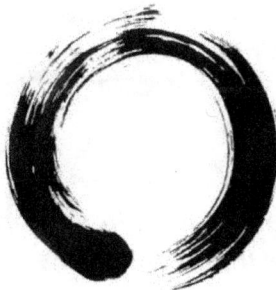

---

[22] Pillar of the Zen tradition

## 👀 Exercise 53 : Licking your wounds

Life involves emotional wounds for each of us, always in relation to impermanence, the difficulties of transitions from one situation to another, the difficulties of adapting to the new reality. Some heal quickly, others remain long gaping and infected. These wounds are, by human nature, inevitable.

A common process is that it is only after suffering too much that we can decide that we will no longer suffer, no matter what the circumstances.
However, thanks to our evolution, we now know, that it is only our thoughts that make us suffer. And so, we can avoid, reduce and eliminate our suffering. We can now achieve happiness, make the decision to be happy without having to reach those points of accumulation of excessive suffering.

The exercise consists in observing and touching deeply, one by one, your wounds still open and then realizing that it is better to accept reality and replace suffering with love and opportunities of happiness.

◆

*'I began to understand that suffering and disappointments and melancholy are there not to vex us or cheapen us or deprive us of our dignity but to mature and transfigure us'*

Hermann Hesse

## ☻☻ Exercise 54 : Relieve your pains

Physical pain is arduous. There is a technique to relieve it, described here step by step:

o Begin by making three deep inspirations, followed by long expirations. Then throughout this practice of pain relief, maintain regular and natural inspirations-expirations.

o Focus on the painful area.

o Now, concentrate precisely, on the most painful point of this area, the exact point of origin of your pain.

o Explore this point in depth.

o Now visualize the pain as not being felt only at this precise point, but as being felt by your whole body. Then hold this visualization for one minute.

o Repeat three deep breaths, then repeat this process several times (about 5), until you experience the feeling of relief of your pain, which you can then cultivate.

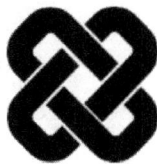

## 036 - GUIDE to avoid judgment

Every human being seeks the satisfaction of his ego, and progress in the fog, either walking on a trivial or on a courtly way. The realities of our lives teach us how to walk and make us visit in turn ungrateful or generous places.

No one knows the path of the other, his fears, the events that have forged his character, his scars, his passions, his joys and sorrows, his friends, his loves, his family, his readings, and all rest that shaped the person he is today, its facade, its intimacy, and its behavior. Everyone advances in the fog, tormented by the need to eat, the fear of missing and the ignorance of the meaning of life.

We spend a good part of our time, judging ourselves and judging others in relation to ourselves. That's our story. However, it is quite possible and beneficial to simply accept the reality as it is, and in so doing, to completely stop condemning ourselves and condemning others.

One can legitimately judge and condemn acts of criminality. Judge whether to support a cause. Or, measure whether we are going to stop or continue a relationship or an activity, so that we can use our time more effectively. We can also self-evaluate and judge our positioning with respect to an attribute. But in this case, if we evaluate the reality of a lower attribute than we would like to be, it is beneficial to quickly change our thinking, from the negative sensation in relation to this lack, to the serenity of accepting the reality, and to continue to breathe.

We must also, remain calm, when we plan to improve this attribute, if we can improve it. Then, we remain calm in our activation of this planning. And finally, one remains serene, continuing to remember to breathe, if one has no possibility of improving this attribute.

The same holds true when judging others; on their physical appearance (too small or too tall, too thin or too large, a too white or a too black skin, a too small or a too large a nose, tired clothing, too red trousers, a ridiculous hat or ridiculous shoes, a car too old, etc.); their attitudes (neglected, aggressive, lazy, out of the norm, reserved, eccentric); or their actual impermanent believes (atheist, fundamentalist, innocent, materialistic, satanic, sectarian, egoistic, or conscious that the properties of the matrix of our universe are homogeneous in all directions, as Albert Einstein said).

It is when judgments are erroneous or encumbered with aggressiveness, fears, dissatisfactions, jealousies, disgust, rancor, prejudice, assumptions or assumptions, that they harm our happiness and that they are good to avoid. Our judgments towards others, are like our judgments toward ourselves, fixing us, in an identification to an attribute, forgetting on the one hand, that our judgments are superficial, often false and impermanent, and that on the other hand, that we and the others are beings rich in multiple attributes and multiple limitations.

The least serious consequence is, that we make a mistake making us to suffer and to become isolated, but we can correct our error. What is more serious, but equally possible to correct at any moment, is that, being fixed in an attribute, we close the doors to the knowledge of many other attributes and opportunities.

By now reading and re-reading this paragraph you have the opportunity to improve your existence, because these reflections on judgment affect us all (unless we are among the few who have achieved great wisdom). These are very important reflections to enable you to become happier. They deserve that you linger and that you produce a sustained effort. Because they are complicated reflections. Indeed, we can first not perceive our ability to differentiate ourselves from our thoughts or our emotions. We may also have the false impression of feeling a certain pleasure in experiencing feelings such as anger, sadness, disgust, revolt, or others. We can consider as having the right to feel these feelings, that it is our duty, that it is our advantage or that it is a trait of our character that we cannot change. And, we can feel a blockage or even a repulsion to satisfy us with serenity and the absence of other feelings. In fact, we live a cocktail of all the features that have just been listed.

We must learn to self-observe, to know ourselves and to understand ourselves. For example: yes, I am currently angry (or any other feeling) but I am something other than this person who is angry; Yes, I am the first victim of my anger and the object of my anger is in no way improved; yes, that anger harms my health; Yes, I can reduce my anger to eliminate it; Yes, I benefit from thinking about why I am angry, this reflection will have as immediate benefit to reduce my anger, I will understand the deep reasons of my anger and understand why it is actually to myself that I I am angry and not the apparent object of my anger; and, yes, I recognize that it is nice to be serene and at peace, and it is a state that I will regularly seek.

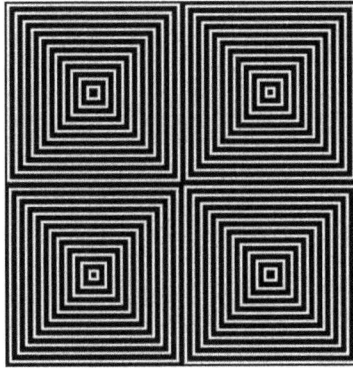

Thus, a very amusing thing to observe, in relation to judgment, is that what is accused of others is a judgment which one has towards oneself, and a punishment that one afflicts to himself.

The next time someone insults you, or judges you, and the next time you see someone insulting or judging another person, tell yourself that this person is, in fact, insulting or judging herself. This can be sometimes very fun, and informative!

And of course, observe eventual moments, when, it is you who insults, denigrates or mocks someone, then reflected, to what judgment to yourself it corresponds.

'The way you treat others is a direct reflection of how you feel about yourself'

Paulo Coelho

♦

*'A decrease in hypocrisy and an increase in self-knowledge can only have good results in terms of tolerance towards others; Because one is only too willing to relate to the other the wrong and violence that one does to one's own nature'*

C. G. Jung

♦

*'Don't judge a book by its cover'*          G. Eliot's

♦

*'Judgment, an impoliteness of self-love'*          R. Bielli

♦

*'Those we love, we do not judge them'*          J-P.Sartre

♦

*'The narrower our mind, the more severe our judgments'*

Bertrand Vac

## ◉◉ Exercise 55 : 24 hours without judgment

By remembering your freedom of thought, for 24 hours, does not judge any person, situation, appearance, behavior or speech. After these 24 hours, ask yourself, what effects the exercise gives you, if you want to renew it, and if you want to master this practice, in order to gradually continue to limit the judgments of your thoughts, until you succeed to completely eliminating them.

This exercise will provide you with immediate well-being. By adopting this new attitude, you will progress quickly in mastering it. And, your judgment toward others, being by definition a judgment toward yourself, you will denigrate yourself less, you will learn to know you better, and you will love yourself more.

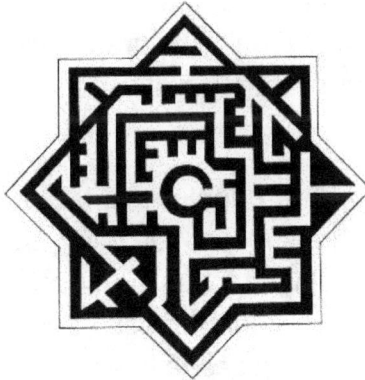

## 037 - GUIDE to not be jealous

Comparing oneself with others is natural, especially when one is young, beginning to know oneself, and in need to define oneself. However, it is a practice that must be measured, then eliminated.

Each person is different, with own qualities. Our modern societies forge a spirit of competition. It is desirable that we emerge from this competition, and that we practice the respect and cooperation of our complementary capacities. It is quite probable that our societies will succeed in adopting this practice, for the happiness and advantage of all. By adopting this principle of operation, we will find easily the ideas which will enable us, day after day, to improve it.

Do not be jealous of others but be happy seeing their success. There are illusions about the luck of one or the other; We see people who seem to have everything to be happy, but who are, in reality, in great distress; And people, who have to face great difficulties, that are nevertheless very happy.

Moreover, when you are jealous of the success of others, you take away the success of your future possibilities; While, now feeling joy, seeing the success of others, it is an immediate gain of happiness, and you give better chances to the opportunities to live your own successes.

In other words, in one way, you like the success, and on the other way you dislike the success. Moreover, the pleasure of seeing a happy person makes us beautiful and favors our success, while jealousy makes us ugly and promotes our failures.

♦

*'The only thing you should look in your neighbour's bowl is to make sure they have enough. You don't look in your neighbour's bowl to see if you have as much as them'*

Louis C.K.

♦

*'He that is jealous is not in love'*          St. Augustin

♦

*'Jealousy contains more of self-love than of love'*

*'Jealousy lives upon doubts. It becomes madness or ceases entirely as soon as we pass from doubt to certainty.'*

F. de La Rochefoucauld

## 038 - GUIDE to live beyond appearance

Pressed by changing, artificial and unreal beauty standards (Photoshop), it is common for many people to suffer from their physical appearances, to perceive themselves too small, too tall, too big, too thin, too beautiful, too ugly, too old, too white, too black, with such and such a defect, etc. Yet happiness is a state of mind that demands harmony between the three vehicles of existence: body, mind and action.

If we can work for the well-being and harmony of the body, then let's do it, and cultivate the satisfaction of the change obtained, which encourages us to continue.

To cultivate the love of our body, let us also stop focusing on details that we find too much this or too much that, and let us begin to focus our attention on those parts of the body that we can love[23], ideas that one is happy to have, and on the actions that one is happy to perform. Thanks to these new attentions, we become another person, happier. A person who laughs at the futility of having once been complexed.

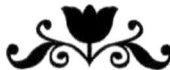

---

[23]Without arms, one cannot admire the beauty of the agility of a hand. Without arms and legs, it is even more complicated (I knew such man in Bangladesh. He is a beggar, a bright, permanent smile illuminated his face and rewarded him with a family. A good example of an extremely vulnerable and happy person, who has a place in society and who is generous in sharing his happiness).

## 039 - GUIDE to watch in the mirror

The others do not know who you are. Even your relatives do not know the complexity of your person. You do not know yourself who you are. The others judge you only on appearances, after a short time spent with you. Then they believe knowing you. Their imaginations gallop, to judge you, and to judge themselves, by comparing themselves with you, projecting their judgments of themselves.

Clearly, it is more comfortable that others have a good opinion of you. But, if they have, arbitrarily, prejudices and a bad opinion of you, do not be affected. Live your life. The priority, and the only thing that matters, is that you have a good opinion of yourself, and that you know how to justify it. Eventually, you can place yourself as an observer of the judgment of others and place yourself as an observer of the emotion you feel at these times. To be in equilibrium, in the analysis of the presumed cause of judgment, without the extreme oscillation of emotion, in the depth of the breath, and in the present moment, and returning to your thought of the realization of your ambitions, and of your progress in achieving it.

◆

'Anything that disturbs you in others is only a projection of what you have not solved in yourself'

Buddha

## 040 - GUIDE to protect your intimacy

To build one's happiness, is also to know how to preserve one's intimacy.

It is desirable to maintain and to often visit our intimacy, our inner garden, also called secret garden. It is a private place where we are safe, where we are sure to not be disturbed, where we can rest peacefully and where we can listen to our intuitions.
In these privileged moments, we realize that each of us, even when surrounded, is alone, alone in the face of his thoughts, problems, solutions and responsibilities. It is in the acceptance of this authentic solitude, freed from the illusions of our needs for validation, that we have access to our peace, our happiness and the good quality of our relations with others.

In architecture, gardens are built in the heart of houses. These gardens symbolize this secret garden, the inner garden of the individuals, compared to the precious intimacy in the heart of the houses. It is as important to maintain a strong inner intimacy, as it is to maintain intimacy in our family and in our home. Because here, at the heart of our private life, we evolve in a mixture of stories, confidences, love and a multitude of complex interactions. It is good to respect, and to defend our privacy and that of others.

One is grossly mistaken, thinking to give importance to himself, by revealing one's intimacy to others. It has the direct opposite effect, one gives oneself lamentably in spectacle and one wounds profoundly the persons unveiled.

These respects of our intimacy and the intimacy of the others are important behaviors in our quest for happiness. Because they bring us many advantages, and because, these are often behaviors that fail us, as evidenced by the popularity of exposure of private lives of more or less famous people. We, then, entertain ourselves, by seeing the mistakes and misfortunes of others, which give us an excuse to reduce our own.

These behaviors being so widespread, it is likely that you too, more or less, are behaving as such. Observe your behaviors, change them if necessary, and after feeling the well-being that these changes give you, continue your efforts to eliminate the behaviors that harm you and to favor the behaviors that make you happier.

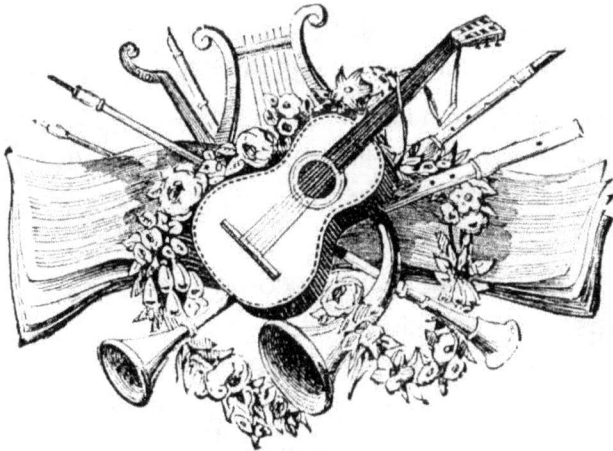

## 041 - GUIDE to enjoy being alone

Whatever the aspects and conditions of our lives, our ability to understand and enjoy the happiness of being alone with ourselves, while being happy with others, is of the utmost importance.

We have just seen that we are fundamentally alone. The fear of being alone is also natural. It is observed in the young baby, who weeps as soon as it is left alone.

The happiness of being alone, if not understood and cultivated, leaves a great place to this fear. This fear, which is with the failure to love oneself, at the origin of all abuses. It is also this fear of being alone, which generates our difficulty to be contradicted or ordered. And it is also this fear that disorientates us, when one passes, often abruptly, from a situation accompanied to a situation alone, when one has not built any benchmark of life alone, and that the only benchmarks one has are those in company with others; This disorientation, which is quite normal, can last for many years; Or one can quickly discover, and, enjoy the joys of living alone, and if one already knows these feeling, one can quickly find them.

Whether we are alone or accompanied, discovering the happiness of being alone with ourselves, enable us to be happier, and to be more effective and better actors, during our romantic, professional and social interactions. During these interactions, by being stronger, more self-confident and having removed this dependence on others, we then come to increase our presence and our contribution. We also manage to maintain our well-being, at the moment of leaving these relationships. In particular, we develop, the very precious mastery of the art of knowing to leave an assembly, or a person, in good conditions and at the right moments, a mastery that serves us daily. When leaving, we do not feel any discomfort or any fear, but we remain strong, stable and happy passing from one situation to another

In our professional life, we also increase our efficiency and success, whether in interactions with our team, with our employees, with the authorities or with our customers.

We are all very concerned with our happiness in our private lives. Our love and family relationships bring us intense joys. They also bring us, time to time, severe pains. We also feel intense joys and sorrows, in the comfort of solitude. On the other hand, we can live an unconditional and lasting happiness, independent of our romantic and family conditions, alone or accompanied, and in all circumstances, developing the feeling of being happy to exist.

The moments when one is alone, without looking at others and away from the gaze of others, are privileged moments that one must live fully, taking advantage of them to rest and take a step back from the tumults of life, enjoying our qualities, taking better care of oneself and loving oneself more, and to better loving the others.

It is as advantageous, to look for opportunities to enjoy solitude for short moments (by car, bus, metro or foot, when going to the bathroom), as during longer moments of introspection.

◆

'A little while alone in your room will prove more valuable than anything else that could ever be given you'

Rumi

◆

'The right to be let alone is indeed the beginning of all freedom'

William O. Douglas

◆

Universal Declaration of human rights, Article 12 :

'No one shall be subjected to arbitrary interference with his privacy, family, home or correspondence, nor to attacks upon his honor and reputation. Everyone has the right to the protection of the law against such interference or attacks.

◆

'Loneliness expresses the pain of being alone and solitude expresses the glory of being alone'.

Paul Tillich

◆

'Blessed are those who do not fear solitude, who are not afraid of their own company, who are not always desperately looking for something to do, something to amuse themselves with, something to judge'

P. Coelho

## 042 - GUIDE to accept

Acceptance of reality is a pillar of happiness ☺

Learning to accept reality, and choosing to be happy in this reality, is the most powerful progress, on which we must work, to be happy.

By definition, reality is our only truth, our only circumstance that exists, the present moment.

We should all be able to understand, and to accept, that our reality is changing, that after having been easy and gentle, it becomes difficult and acid, and then again becomes favorable. We should all, come to understand this, because it is a simple definition of life. Yet, it is our misunderstanding and our refusal of this simplicity that makes us unhappy.

When we accept the reality of life, we can decide to live happily, loving life, at every moment, in the morning when we wake up, when we are stuck in traffic jams, when we spend time with our colleagues and with our friends, when we meet a new friend, when this friend leaves us, when we bring our trash to the collector, when we sweep our flor, and in the evening when we fall asleep.

Let us take life with simplicity and lightness, love life and be happy.

♦

*'Happiness can exist only in acceptance'.*   George Orwell

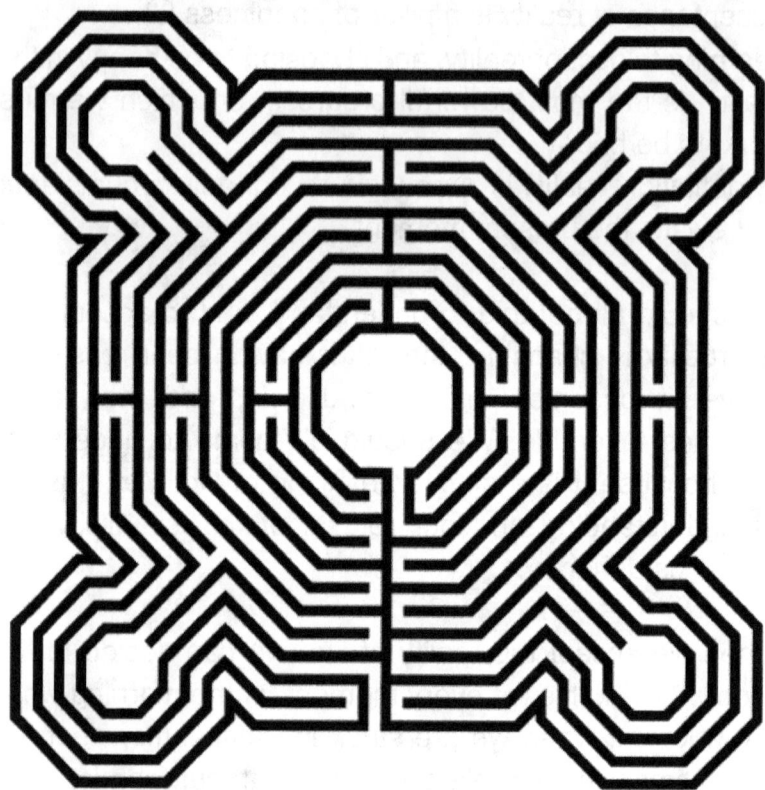

## 👀 Exercise 56 : The labyrinth of life

The motif of the labyrinth appears in many, if not all, civilizations and on all continents. It is already found in prehistory, and in ancient Egypt. It is found in cathedrals, where it is considered as a pilgrimage, especially for people who cannot physically travel. Today, we encounter new ones, in our parks, and in our architectures.

It symbolizes the initiatory journey of life. It contains obstacles, dead ends and complexities. It is not easy, but unavoidable, to arrive at the center, guided and never lost.

To practice this exercise, you shall use on the opposite side to the mine of your pencil, and follow, in the drawing of the opposite page, the course of the labyrinth, from the entrance to the central point, and then returning in opposite direction to the exit.

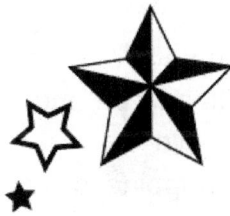

*'The initiatory journey of the labyrinth leads to the heart of oneself'*

Carl Gustave Jung

## 043 - GUIDE to be satisfied

Appreciate and be thankful of the good things furnishing your life, and of the good things happening to you. In other words, this corresponds to practicing gratitude. Gratitude, is, along with the emotions it generates, one of the feelings, the most powerful to be happy.

Even in the worst of situations, where one can be found, there is always something that one can appreciate and be grateful for. Life is Beautiful[24].

The joy of breathing, seeing, hearing, walking, contemplating the sun shining, I know where to sleep tonight and even that it will be in a bed. I have a roof over my head. I have a love. I have a passion. The nurse is very pretty and very kind. The doctor is very smiling, and he makes good jokes. 'There are people who have cancer, I have four'[25]. How beautiful it is, to drink this water, the beauty of this rainbow is transcendent, the happiness of the neighbour, etc.

By becoming accustomed to being grateful, one realizes to have many opportunities to be and to feel happy about it. These chances, that we used to live in indifference, become moments of happiness, which add up to all the others, which we learn to discover in our quest for happiness.

---

[24] Wink at Roberto Benigni's film

[25] Words spoken in private and with the enormous enthusiasm he always displayed, by the extraordinary Author-Composer-Interpreter and Philosopher Ricet Barrier whom I had the chance and privilege to know.

Happiness illuminates our face, and we are increasingly seizing opportunities to be lucky, in the same way that we have seen that enjoying success fosters success in our lives.

◆

*'Gratitude is not only the best of all virtues, it is the mother of all the others'*

Cicero

◆

*'The satisfaction brings the happiness, even in the poverty. The dissatisfaction brings poverty, even in the wealth.'*

Confucius

◆

*'To be happy, it is not having everything, it is to need nothing else'*

Zen

◆

*'We can only be said to be alive in those moments when our hearts are conscious of our treasures'*     T. Wilder

◆

*'As we express our gratitude, we must never forget that the highest appreciation is not to utter words, but to live by them'.*

John F. Kennedy

## ☻☻ Exercise 57 : Gratitude and lacks

First Part, managing gaps:

Let us also observe, the moments, when we feel, the pain of a lack. Let us then analyze this feeling of lack; We will often find that, in fact, we are wandering our imagination erroneously, for we do not really need what we lack (see also the Guide to desire), we live well with what we have, and we can be happy about it.

The same mechanisms of thought, which have already been described, come into play with the feelings of gratitude and with the feelings of lack (our ability to choose what we think, the addictive nature of what we think, and the disappearance of thoughts we do not cultivate). So instead of thinking about a lack, we can think positively, think about things for which we are grateful, and think about the natural abundance, until we eliminate this painful sensation of lack (such as, when paying for invoice, cultivating recognition of the chance and happiness of benefiting from what is paid, rather than being unhappy at the idea of subtraction in our budget, or fear of not having enough).

As for abundance, it is indeed natural. This characteristic can be observed, for example, in nature, with the ever-growing vegetables, the magnificence of the flowers, the trees giving a multitude of fruits year after year, or the sun, producing an enormous quantity of light and heat each day.

This abundance is also observed in the profusion of results obtained after our concentration and our action.

In the pursuit of happiness, which depends on a better knowledge of oneself, and a better consciousness of being alive, you will benefit from being attentive to your feelings of lack, for it is a complicated feeling. First of all, you have to understand that you are feeling it, then you have to understand the reason and the legitimacy or the illegitimacy of its presence, its effect, and finally your reaction in relation to its effect.

You can meditate on the fact that, if you are not happy of what you have, you will not be happy of what you will get, meaning that you may eliminate happiness from your life. While happiness is abundantly available to you at any time.


The suffering of material lack can also be very complicated, on two counts:

o   In some cases, it is real, as a lack of food can make us starve.

But this feeling of lack can be vicious. For, at the moment of eating, the fear of missing may come to spoil the pleasure of eating. We think, then, with anguish, that the plate will soon be eaten. Where we think that the pot of this very good jam, will soon be empty. Or, we think, that with what we have left, we will not last till the end of the week, or the month, or the year. One is even able, to suffer a lifetime from shortcomings, to later realize, never to have lacked.

o   We may also perceive, that we have often suffered from a lack of possessing something, and that shortly after having finally succeeded in possessing this thing, its possession gives us no joy, we neglect it, and we move on to another suffering of a lack of possessing another.

This analysis makes us better understand our interest, to observe and to know better ourselves, to better understand our needs, our lacks, our desires, our sensations, our emotions and our feelings. So, we reach a better health and well-being by optimally meeting our physiological needs, our security needs, our needs for belonging, our needs for esteem and our needs to fulfill ourselves. We understand better, how important and priority it is to be happy in meeting our needs, and to know the nature of our shortcomings in order to better manage them.

♦

If, on occasion, we possess something that is a luxury, beyond our needs. We will strive, to enjoy the use of this thing to the limit of our needs, to avoid the fear of losing it, and to avoid the pain when we lose it by remembering with gratitude the luck and the joy we had, as well as the possible opportunity to find it back.

<u>Second Part, listing gratitude</u>:


Remembering the good things, will give you happiness, will reduce the pain accompanying difficult things, and will facilitate your perception and the realization of new opportunities.

Regularly, seized the opportunity of a free moment, to think of being thankful and say, 'thank you' to life, for the good things happening.


**Practice:**


o For 30 days, with a playful attitude, write each day, on your computer or on a notebook, at least 3 things that happened during your day and which you are grateful for.

(You can continue this exercise for periods longer than 30 days. You can even do this exercise, a daily habit, for a very long time, as it will always be beneficial.)

o Play the explorer, searching for new reasons to be grateful in your daily life. This game will be very fun, and you will be surprised by your discoveries.

o From time to time, for instance in difficult times, you can re-read this list; This will bring you inspiration, well-being, physical and mental health.

## 044 - GUIDE to recover innocence

In the early periods of our life (Infant, child, adolescent), physical growth and the learning of life, like in all periods of life, involve their specific suffering. It is also in these periods that we feel, without hindrance, the greatest freedom and the greatest joys.

Faced with our efforts to become adults, and walking in the fog, just as our parents had done before us, we encounter sorrows, fears, regrets, shame, deception, aggression and failure. We then forget, our pure joy of living, our innocence and our unconditional childhood happiness, which are our true nature engraved in our subconscious. As adults, we suffer from dissonance with our subconscious ideals.

We encounter several difficulties here. When we are young children, everything is fine, and then we are influenced not only by the difficulties of life, but also, on the one hand, by our desire to assert ourselves as an adult, and on the other hand, by our entourage requesting us to be mature. Our innocence is thus suppressed.

Once we have grown up we will have great advantages in regaining the joys, the laughter, the lightness, the gratuitousness and the innocence which were very much part of our childhood.

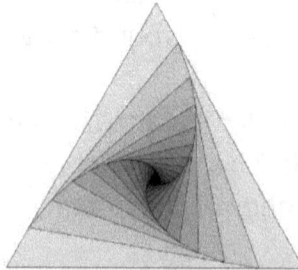

Let's take note here, of the too many cases, which are also evoked in another part of the book, where the child's innocence is unfortunately violated or abused, sometimes from an early age.

These victims will benefit even more from seeking, even if initially this seems impossible to them because persistent pain stifles happiness, the moments of innocent happiness from their childhoods and the innocence in their adult lives.

These practices will be for them, like a ray of sunshine that gives birth to the seed of the memory of innocence deeply buried in the ground; And they can enjoy the contemplation of the plant that grows and flowered.

Because the pain is acute, these victims shall not be offended, by the lightness of the image of the plant that flourishes, and that calmly, they can do this exercise of remembering innocence, trusting in the power of using positive thinking.

These victims shall get convinced of the priority they are giving to their happiness. And based on that priority, they shall be proactive in making theses prescribed practices. And they shall accept the shift from victimhood identity to happiness identity.

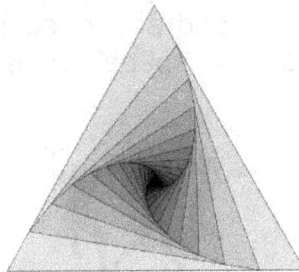

## ☻☻ Exercise 58 : Have a fit of the giggles

o   Take a moment and remember a moment when you felt an immense joy, when you burst out laughing.

o   Remember, in detail, this moment full of innocence.

o   This memory certainly brings you a lot of joy. Maybe you're even starting to laugh again. Savor the joy of this memory, this will allow the joy, to be more present in your life, beyond the only time of this memory.

For, here again, are at play the mechanisms often found in this book: an initial effort to live a moment of happiness, allows us to build a habit of living such moments of happiness, to be more attentive to the opportunities of living such moments, and to start of cascade of joyful events. Happiness, then appears, a question of multiplied effort and choice of activity, with the acceptance of changing our schedules and habits. Only the impulse is constraining, for as soon as the action begins, one feels one's pleasure, which persuades us to continue, and then to renew the effort of the impulse, until the new behavior becomes a habit and the impulse becomes natural. On the other hand, paradoxically, we have more difficulty, changing our personality, and accepting to be happy, when misfortune has become a definition of our personality.

The impulse to laugh and savor reunion with our child innocence, helps us to accept being free and happy again.

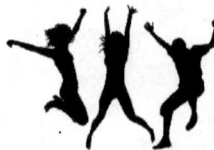

*'Unless artists can remember what it was to be a little boy, they are half complete as artist and as man'.*

J. Thurber

♦

*'Children are great sages: they know how to marvel, to have fun, to laugh, to concentrate on the present moment, to sleep when they are tired. They are simple and unprejudiced. We have a lot to learn from them '*

Catherine Rambert

♦

*'I left my childhood, as one escapes from a country in which one has suffered too much, vowing never again to backfooted, but it is this country that I miss all the most'*

Emilie Frèche

♦

*'A child can always teach three things to an adult: to be content without reason, to always take care of something and to know how to demand with all his strength what he wants'*

Paulo Coelho

♦

*'As soon as a child understands something, there is an admirable movement in him. If he is delivered from fear and respect, you see him stand up, draw the idea with great gestures, and suddenly laugh with all his heart, as in the most beautiful of games'*

Alain

## 045 - GUIDE to observe desires (34 questions)

Desire is paradoxical. The desire of the one is a disgust for the other. It is a vital energy. It can be ephemeral, and it can be excessive, to the point of becoming mortal. Happiness is sometimes defined as the satisfaction of desires, sometimes as the absence of desire. Some of us see no alternative to the lack of desire to live; While others conceive, to find happiness in the absence of desire.

We will benefit from asking us many questions about our desires. Fortunately, the guides in this manual help us to find answers. Here are some questions:

o  What do I desire to become and do?

o  If I do not know yet what I desire, am I able to desire to be confident that I will know soon?

o  If I am desperate, can I find a spark of vital energy, in desire and then in the joy of breathing, and watching the wheel turn?

o  Why do I desire this?

o  If I imagine living for some time with the object of my desire, do I like the picture?

o  Is it a caprice, or a fantasy without a future?

o  Is it an inaccessible desire?

o  Am I deceiving myself, by dwelling on thinking, that this desire gives me joy, when it makes me suffer?

Would it not be better to avoid it, and if I perceive it, to let it fly away, experiencing no emotion, except the pleasure of seeing it fly?

o What is this strange desire for this thing that does not please me, does not correspond to me, and even that would embarrass me, if I would possess it?

o Is my desire ambitious, as it should be?

o Does this desire give me the suffering of a lack?

And if it does,

- What could be the reason for this sensation?

- Once the feeling of lack has been assessed, whether it is reasonable to stop it. Can I, at this moment, live a happy moment, rather than suffering?

- Can I both cherish this desire and let it go?

- Can I be, together with this desired object, free to realize?

o Do I do what it takes to satisfy my desire?

o Isn't the right time, rather than being obsessed with my desire, to now breathe, and become stronger, take care of the priority, perhaps the one that makes me happy to walk towards the desired object?

- Have I done today, one thing contributing to the satisfaction of my desire?

- What am I doing now, contributing to the satisfaction of my desire?

  If I am distracted, could I do this other thing, which would make me happier, and give me the satisfaction of progressing in the direction of the desired object?

- When I have obtained the object of my desire, do I, now cultivate the pleasure?

  Does it last?

- How do I react when my desire is not satisfied?

  If, once again, carried away in whimsicality, I refuse reality and I feel pain:

  - Will it last long?

  - What is this pain?

  - Can I bounce back faster and faster?

  - Do I find satisfaction in what the failure has taught me? And if I got there, am I able to totally erase the penalty, to be only satisfied with the gain, with no further trace of the loss?

  - Do I enjoy this well-being at this moment?
    And in the next moment?

- Do I remember my previous dissatisfied desire?

  What do I conclude?

o   When I fail in obtaining a desire, am I, for a long time, like a snail, in a shell of sadness, shame or regret, prostrated, inert, with difficulty breathing?

Or, understanding my priority, remaining lucid, and looking at the true face of this sadness. So, to watch it evaporating. Allowing myself not to be, prostrated and asphyxiated before the spoiled desire?

o   Have I already tasted, satisfaction with what I presently have, free, without any imagination of a desire to change it?

Do I cultivate this satisfaction?

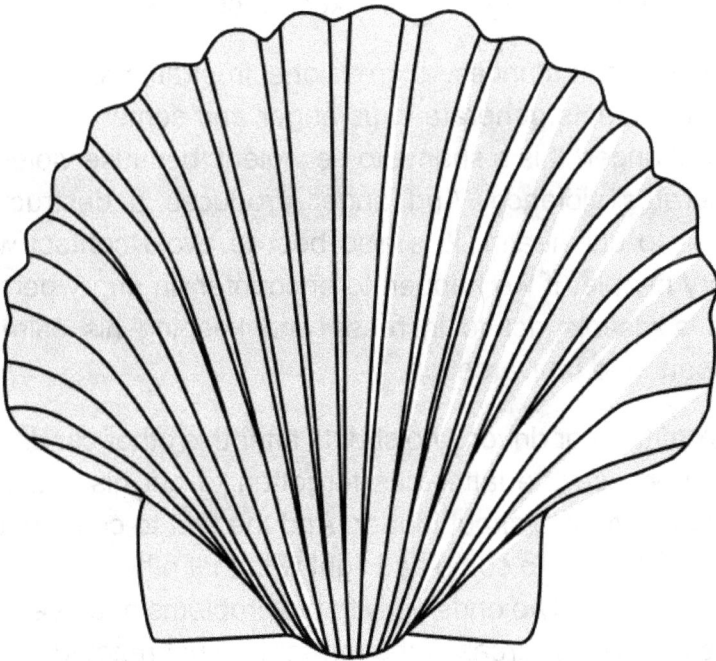

## 046 - GUIDE to never get angry

My shared experience here, is not an experience of anger, for I do not remember the last time I got angry. It is a lived experience of its observation.

What is most striking in anger, are the signs of unconscious inconsistency, which we can demonstrate: we can break our affairs, even our favorite objects; Hurt the people we love, and leave them; Give a degrading spectacle, even to frighten an assembly; Use violence without measuring consequences; Stop doing something or leave a place we love, and even compromise it, and so on. These inconsistencies, which affect us, even in the smallest and the shortest angers, are powerful incentives to convince us to suppress the anger of our experience.

Certain circumstances, aggressions, frustrations, insults or disagreements generate in us anger and sometimes even violent anger. It is a shame to be violent, because violence generates violence. And anger produces a destructive stress to our health. It is also best to avoid contact with angry people. If we happen to encounter an angry person it is advisable not to increase and keeping his calm to suspend the conversation.

Look at this car driver who shouts after this other car driver, only because the latter has forgotten to put his flashing. And this other to shout louder. And the first to come out of his car abruptly to come and fight with that other. Then one is hurt and the two ends up with big problems and see their lives tumble. Whereas, if the former had not reacted to this minor inconvenience, or if the latter had not increased, life would have continued quietly, towards possible and most probable better circumstances.

It is also good to avoid approaching people who are perceived being in a state of crisis or possibly under alcohol. If the person in crisis is a friend or relative, we should ask her if she needs something and then wait for the person to calm down, but without ourselves lose our composure. The person who assaults us, uses us as a mirror to express his discomfort, his loneliness or any other of his problems. As we are his image, the person is very sensitive to our reaction. If, for example, we react with contempt, the angry person feels contempt and his anger is likely to increase. If, on the contrary, we react with calm and respect (without any disdain), his anger diminishes.

When traveling or working in Asia we are advised not to get angry. Anger is much rarer than in the rest of the world. Being rarer, they are also more serious, in the sense that it is difficult to regain the confidence of a person against whom one became angry. A person who gives in to anger feels deep shame and loses respect for others.
This geographical and cultural difference is proof that anger is not inevitable and can be eliminated.

♦

*'Anybody can become angry - that is easy, but to be angry with the right person and to the right degree and at the right time and for the right purpose, and in the right way - that is not within everybody's power and is not easy'.*

Aristote

## 047 - GUIDE to know how to say 'no'

As if to justify the many days spent, suffering the insipid speech, the cruel gossip and the incessant repetitions of Marcel, Corinne replied 'I cannot say no'.

When one accepts, reluctantly, to do this or that, or to meet this or that person, sometimes in a repetitive way, it is not only a lack of sincerity and honesty that will stir up the flaws reproached to this person, but it is, for us, a great source of stress and a waste of time, which go against a happy life.

'I cannot say No', this is not an immutable characteristic like 'having green eyes' or 'five fingers to one hand'. One can very well, and very easily change this trend.

However, it is not so simple, because Corinne, in her uncomfortable comfort zone, continues to have this type of relationship with Marcel.

Our generosity in helping a person in difficulty is certainly a very positive thing, and even a source of happiness. But, only if this is done, with good-heartedness, and with a solid and stable intention.

On the other hand, it is a mistake to think that acting or interacting reluctantly is beneficial. It is very likely that this will have a detrimental effect on oneself and others.

Here again, in our quest for happiness, we will consider the good management of our time and how we furnish our time.

So, rather than spending time doing a thing that stresses us and makes us uncomfortable, it is best to use that time to take care of another person than Marcel or of ourselves; or to do a exciting, enjoyable, relaxing and rewarding thing.

And if you have trouble finding this thing to do, you must look. The saying 'When one seeks one finds' is correct. And, if one does not find directly, at least one is satisfied to progress.

Corinne, like all of us, desires freedom and happiness. To obtain them, it is necessary for her to make an effort to learn how to say 'no', and to correct this tendency, which until now gave her a sensation to exist, to replace it with another tendency which will make her happier to exist.

◆

*'When you say "yes" to others, make sure you do not say "no" to yourself'*

Paulo Coelho

## 048 - GUIDE to tell the truth

The recommendation to try to speak the truth may seem moralistic. It is, however, strongly justified to have a happy life, in our heart and in our community. For lies and dishonesty, generate guilt, discomfort, suspicions and conflict.
Just as water always finds a way to flow, lies and dishonesty are always discovered and are thus the cause of loss of confidence, loss of esteem and even breakdown of relationships.

When we lie, we lie to ourselves first, so we suffer a loss of confidence and self-esteem.
Truth, is more powerful than falsehood. And, if the lie has the illusion to wins one or even several battles, it always ends up being loser. Truth is reality, with its purity, its ease and its limpidity. Lying, denies reality, with chaos, qualm and consequences.
Lying is useless and easy to avoid, we have other opportunities to explore our weaknesses. To get there, just make the decision to stop lying, and then maintain that decision.

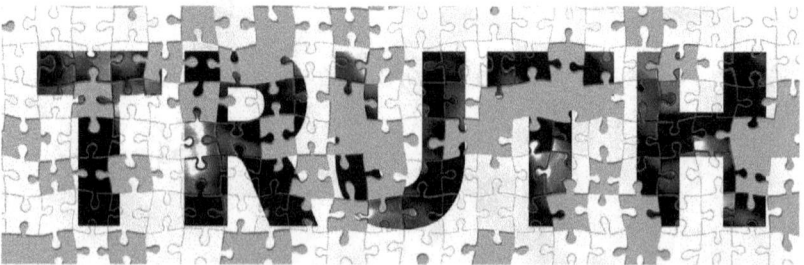

You may be used to lying, or that you lie about a specific point, without really realizing it, being resigned or without giving importance to your actions?

Truth is a powerful fuel, which naturally activates your other positive behaviors and happy circumstances of your existence. The lie is just as powerful, it leads you, without you noticing it, into the drunkenness of other negative behaviors, and in finding yourself, to live unhappy circumstances.

Be attentive to the observation of these dynamics (the ease with which you add up the actions and the happy circumstances, and, the blinding drunkenness that leads you to add up the destructive actions harming your happiness and making you live a series of unhappy circumstances), for they are more powerful than your will (A hormonal influence, then directs the triangular dynamics of body-thought-action).

On the other hand, these observations will enable you, naturally and easily, to strengthen your will to change, to live happily with better actions and better circumstances.

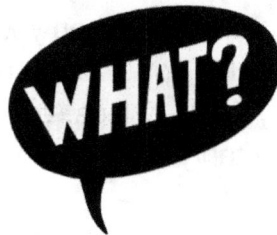

WHAT?

## 👀 Exercise 59 : Do you lie?

Here is a new opportunity to have fun:

### First exercise :

Observe the possible moments when you lie to others. Then, explore in depth the reasons why you lied.
Once touched, the reasons can be corrected and come out of the game, and you will again be able to observe and savor the delicious fluidity of the truth.
Observe also the reality of the profits and losses engendered by your dishonesty and draw conclusions.

### Second exercise :

Observe and question your beliefs, to understand when you lie to yourself.

Thus, it is useful to continually observe the opposites or contradictions of your beliefs. As a result, your beliefs will either be consolidated or modified.

This can be a bit difficult, because your beliefs are the arms and legs of your mental body. When you discover the need to change your beliefs, you will feel the happiness of walking better with your new legs, but it is likely that you feel fear, and momentarily pain, when amputating the old ones.

It is not right to justify the lie on some occasions.

Imagine, to demonstrate it, our lives in a world without lies. Where relationships are clear and confident. Where everyone has understood that the biggest victim of a scam is the crook. Where we appreciate transparency fluidity and reality. Where we don't lie to ourselves.

Such a world, may seem a utopia, however, it is the one, in the direction of which, leads us our evolution.

You can, now, choose to act in this direction and to contribute to the dynamics of our evolution.
The first result will be, instantly, that you will be happier.

Note that this also involves other personal development work to avoid behaviors that will require you to lie.

◆

*'Three things cannot be long hidden: the sun, the moon and the truth'*

Buddha

◆

*'Truth belongs to the past and lies belong to the future'*

Anonymous

## 049 - GUIDE to rub with positive shoulders

You will benefit from meeting happy, vibrant, dynamic, enterprising, smiling or fun people.

Happiness is contagious, so let yourself be contaminated, and contaminate others.

Like all research, it requires you to be curious, open and enterprising.

It is also desirable and important that, before and during these meetings, you feel love for yourself, rather than relying solely on your happy interlocutor to increase your well-being. This will help to improve the encounter and your contribution to happiness. This will allow it to grow and renew itself.

We are like sponges, The feelings and behaviors of others influence us and without realizing it, without even wanting to, we adopt these feelings and behaviors. This is a powerful truth that is good to remember.

◆

'The love, the friendship, it's above all, to laugh with the other, it is to share laughter that to love one another'

Arletty

## Plan a visit

o   Now, think of one of your friends or a member of your family who exudes happiness, then arrange an upcoming encounter.

o   Consider this visit as a privileged moment of happiness, during which, you will be as generous as attentive.

o   During this visit, do not talk about negative things, and quickly change the subject if your interlocutor touches on a negative subject, so that this visit can be purely positive and you both carry happiness.

o   Renew often the exercise.

◆

*'Wholesome friendships are the ones which stimulate, which liven up, which increase our vitality, which awaken in us spark, eloquence, courage, which make us stronger and better'*

Henri-Frédéric  Amiel

## 050 - GUIDE to be steadfast

Some of us are unhappy chronic. These people are weak to love themselves. They are in a constant search for attention and validation. They commonly see life in black. And they can repeat the same problems over and over again. This behavior has become the precious definition of their identities and their lives.
Their attitudes should not affect you.

It is natural, that with your natural empathy, and with your naturally generous personality, you feel the desire to help them to get out of this situation. Do it then, remaining solid and stable in your balance, your inner serenity, your love for yourself, your well-being, and your life goals.

In addition to being the way to keep your happiness and the pursuit of your goals, it turns out that this will also be the best way to help unhappy people.

Let us make an analogy with a vibratory state. At the quantum level, where everything is vibration, we have a quantum body, with specific vibrations differentiated from the vibrations of our surroundings. Quantum physics has shown us that we influence the vibrations of our surroundings. Consider, as an analogy, that your well-being and your happiness correspond to a state of high vibrations. And that conversely, the discomforts correspond to low vibrations. Then consider the influences of these vibrations on yourself and on our surroundings, the relations with the unhappy chronic and each of your relations.

We shall therefore consider that the unhappy chronicles vibrate at low frequencies. At the moment when you are experiencing pain, alongside these people, your vibratory state has shifted from high vibrations to low vibrations (those of sorrow), placing you at the same vibratory level as the unhappy chronic.

You are mistaken, if you think your prolonged pain is the correct answer of your compassion. It is desirable, on the contrary, in these situations, that you quickly retreive, and maintain, your level of vibrations at high frequencies (your well-being). Then, you will observe, that the answer to your compassion, is more effective, for the pain of the unhappy chronic will thus be relieved. You will thus observe, that these unhappy chronic, cease to relate with you their problems and become themselves happier. And, you will observe that your eventual action, which is motivated by your compassion, will be more effective and will also make you happier. Rather than joining the unfortunate, at his uncomfortable level of low frequencies, naturally and without effort, you will have give him a lift, allowing him to reach you at your comfortable level of high frequencies.

When you meet a unhappy pathologic, victim of an accident of life, or after an accumulation of circumstances difficult to carry, you can adopt the same technique. This will be the best you can do. In most of the cases the technique will succeed, but it is sadly known that, in certain extreme cases, nothing sufficient can be done; The unfortunate is then the only one who can find the strength to get out of it, and sometimes he does not find it.

Probably, by reading the previous chapter, you thought of this unfortunate or unhappy chronic, in your circle of friends, your family circle or your socio-professional circle, which you regularly encounter, while experiencing pain. Well, the next time you meet this person, start by approaching this meeting, after having eliminated the a prioris on the negative attitude of your interlocutor and on yours. Decide to remain stable in your well-being, then observe what is changing in this relationship. Your interlocutor will stop abusing you, and will stop telling you his sad stories. You'll both be relieved.

In case your relationship is old, and also in the case where your stability is still fragile, it is possible that the behavior change of your interlocutor is minor and transient. It is important that you are attentive to the perception of this change in attitude and to the perception of the improvement of your well-being and that you continue to do the work of refocusing on your well-being During this meeting and during the following ones.

In this process, and after this meeting, evaluates the evolution, feels satisfaction for progress, remember that it is a mistake to accuse yourself of weakness or imperfection.

Interpersonal relationships are complicated because, bearing the heavy burdens of history, and having difficulties to adapt to new evolving paradigms, respects, dignities, freedoms, cooperation, justice and love. You, can work at this adaptation, to become a modern person.

When you practice this exercise, there is a risk that your interlocutor may interpret your stability for arrogance or contempt. In order to avoid this risk, you must be careful not to feel arrogance or contempt, and to include a sufficient dose of humility and consideration. But do not worry too much, because your good balance will serve the purpose.

(However, in some cases it will be beneficial for you to space your interactions with these people, and possibly to stop seeing them, if the expected progress, using the technique described here, is hardly perceptible, and if the encounter is draining you toomuch. As already mentioned above, in certain extrem cases you have to resign ourselves to our inability to satisfy our desire to help a person you love, or it can be very long, and requiring a great deal of patience, and the time for the persons to make progress on their own.)

❖

Remember, as you read previously in this book, the technique and best practice to approach each encounter, having previously focused on the love of yourself, and on the desire to have the best possible meeting. The same analogy, with your vibrational state, can be made, considering that this concentration on the love of yourself places you at a level of high vibrations.

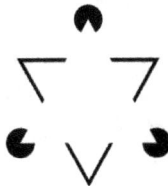

## 051 - GUIDE to be happy unconditionally

Human rights are being flouted. Thousands, or millions, of people are murdered. This ecological catastrophe is now spreading, over thousands of square kilometers. Billions are diverted. Corruption distorts the value chains. Officials are not tried. Thieves, rapists, abusers, crooks, bankruptcies, losses, conflicts, illnesses, premature deaths. This is a beautiful reality!

And my little self, in all this?

He would have many reasons to be nauseated, to be sad, wounded, disgusted, misled, disillusioned, desperate.

Fortunately, I am a conscious being who thinks. I know, that my nausea comes from my thinking. It is neither the crimes nor the other events that, with their little hands, which are turning my stomach.

I did everything I could. There are other things to do, I will do. I do not have nausea.

Besides, these thoughts, these negative thoughts, sterile and distressing, now that I realize it, I will avoid them. I can put them in a drawer and get them out if I need them. And most importantly, I can put them in this drawer, right after doing what I had to do, to quickly return to the happy thoughts that have become my priority.

It's not the situation that gives you sorrow, but your perception of the situation. Do not condition your happiness to circumstances that may, or probably may not occur. Or to the ones that did occur. Or, even to the ones that are currently occurring. While a positive attitude, which cannot be corrupted by sad memories, imagination or circumstances, brings happiness, makes it possible to progress, to remain attentive and effective, to find possible solutions, and to see the new opportunities.

Whatever the conditions of our lives, we live moments of fear and doubts. And it is still the capacities we gain, in our practices of the quest for happiness, which allow us to return, more and more easily and more and more rapidly, to happy feelings of love, trust and of well-being.

So, to our delight, we got to engage in action and we trust in the positive developments that we can or even cannot influence through our action. The latter, like the negatives, have chances of realization. Meanwhile, now it is better to be happy, and to fully live our lives.

◆

*'Life is 10% what happens to us and 90% how we react on it'*                                                      Irvin Berling
◆

*'I became a rose petal and you are as the wind which carries me. Take me to make a tour.'*
*'What comes, will leave. What is found, will be again lost. But what you are, is more than to come and to leave, it is indescribable. You are it'*                                                      Rumi

*'I am not what happened to me. I am who I choose to become'*

Carl Jung

♦

*'The best thing you could ever do for yourself is to become unconditionally happy'*

Edmond Mbiaka

♦

*'There is no path to happiness. Happiness is the path'*

Buddha

♦

*'It is necessary to manage to rise until understanding that real love is universal love put down everywhere in profusion, love which one can drink and breathe non-stop'*

O. M. Aïvanhov

♦

*'He who is not contented with what he has, would not be contented with what he would like to have.'*

Socrates

♦

*'Joy is not a thing; it is in us.'*     Charles Wagner

♦

*'Our greatest happiness does not depend on the condition of life in which chance has placed us, but is always the result of a good conscience, good health, occupation and freedom in all just pursuits.'*

Thomas Jefferson

*'The significance of a man is not in what he attains, but rather what he longs to attain.'*

Khalil Gibran

♦

*'(...) Look every day at the world as if it was the first time. Then I followed and applied this advice. The first time, I contemplated the light, the colors, the trees, the birds, the animals. I felt the air passing in my nostrils and making me breathe. I heard the voices rising in the corridor as in the vault of a cathedral. I was alive. I shivered with pure enjoyment. The happiness of existing. I was amazed.'*

Eric-E. Schmitt

♦

*'Every intense desire is perhaps a desire to be different from what we are.'*

Eric Hoffer

♦

*'For after all, the best thing one can do when it is raining, is to let it rain.'*

Henry W. Longfellow

♦

*'Accept - then act. Whatever the present moment contains, accept it as if you had chosen it. Always work with it, not against it.'*

Eckhart Tolle

♦

*The basic root of happiness lies in our minds; outer circumstances are nothing more than adverse or favorable*

Matthieu Ricard

## 052 - GUIDE to not be proselyte

Seeking to convince a third party to adopt our beliefs, is an attitude often encountered. It responds to a need for validation of beliefs. It shows that one is neither free, nor convinced, nor sincere. For if he was, he would not need this validation of others.

It also happens all the time, that we are wrong, or that our beliefs are transformed, or even that we come to believe the opposite of what we had previously believed. It is a normal process that allows us to evolve. It is good to know that this is a normal process, for then, one can, by acknowledging, his errors, and, the normal process of the evolution of his thought, not be proselyte and not feel regret, even shame, to be deceived.

The earth is flat, it is well known.

Your interlocutor is, as free to have his beliefs, as you are free to have yours. Humanity has suffered greatly, and many continue to suffer, to obtain this freedom. In no case, can it be violated.

♦

*'Only fools never change their minds'*                    Proverb

It is easy to understand that the need for validation is powerful. It is again, the frenzy desire to exist. And, there are many beautiful stories, giving us feelings of existence that we may feel the need to validate.

But proselytism remains mysterious.
For it is practiced, and trampled on, by believers, and even more by fundamentalists in doctrines and religions, all of which contain the prohibition to practice it.

On the other hand, this enigma illustrates the difficulty of abstaining from proselytism, and the interest of observing when it happens that we do so, to simply stop doing it, without feeling ashamed we did.

Do we need validation to be happy, or rather to respect others, and respect ourselves?

♦

*'For at least two thirds of our miseries spring from human stupidity, human malice and those great motivators and justifiers of malice and stupidity, idealism, dogmatism and proselytizing zeal on behalf of religious or political idols'*

A. Huxley

## 053 - GUIDE to not be afraid

To be afraid, is natural and instinctive. Fear is the expression of our survival instinct. It accompanies each of our gestures. What varies is our perception of fear, and our reactions to fear.

We can feel fear so fleetingly, that we would swear, not feel it. In this case, we see no risk, and, we analyzed having the physical and mental capacities, to perform the action. The elimination of risk is then naturally integrated into our action. We do not consider that we can fail.
In other cases, we feel fear. We assess our ability to take the risk. We are committed to get into action. And we have two possibilities. One, is to forget the risk, and to perform the action by making the best use of our abilities and feeling the maximum pleasure. The other, is to cultivate the shadow of fear, which then darkens our abilities and our pleasure to act.
At other times, we would have the ability to perform the action, but fear prevents us from doing it. A greater analysis of our abilities, daring, the elimination of the fear of failure and the love for the action, could allow us to perform the action and enjoy the pleasure of doing it.

These fears interfere, since the action is assimilated to a past accident or to a past failure, which continues to spoil our lives.

In all cases, risks and abilities are realities, and fear is only a reaction. We can modify our reaction and avoid the fear, so as not to suffer unnecessarily, and to retain our full lucidity to assess the risks and our capacities; By including in this analysis, the possibility that they can be overestimated or underestimated.

Let us take an example of frequent fears: a parent who is afraid that something will happen to his child. Accidents happen, but they are rare. The parent has spent, in vain, a tremendous amount of time being afraid, while perhaps no accident occurred to his child, who has now reached adulthood. Or maybe, too anxious, the parent forgot to make an important recommendation; that could have avoided the accident. Or else, this parent has passed on his anxiety to his child, the child has suffered, he became clumsy, he was blinded by his fear and his blindness was the cause of an accident. And finally, the child will transmit this fear to his own children, who will then transmit it to theirs.

One could go over many examples, where a fear prevents action and performance. It always does.

However, our experience of the fears, depends on our character, which is both forged by our experience and innate. So, we will feel the fears with more or less frequency and intensity; and we will manage them with more or less ease. It may not be the most comfortable, but we can live with our specific level of fear.

It remains important that we observe our fears, when they occur and to find out how we can live more comfortably with them (again breathing will be a suitable solution).

This beginning of the observation of our fears, will allow us to realize the most important thing: when the fears prevent us from being happy, because we limit our actions. Then, we shall focus our attention on removing these obstacles.

This will be done by pursuing the observation of the fears and analyzing:

- o Failure in our past, exiting our imagination of failure to the present action. If we discover such past failure, its observation will contribute to reducing the fear. We may even, become able to overcome the fear, and become free to engage into the actions.

- o The rationality of the fear regarding the risks and our capacities, and how we can cope with them.

- o Our experience of the fear when we make efforts to overcome it. And,

- o The value of the missed results from the inaction, compared to the value of our effort to exit our comfort zone and to engage into the action.

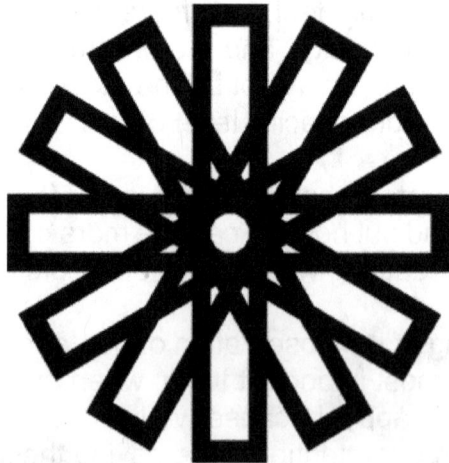

*'We stopped checking for monsters under our beds when we realized they were inside us'*

Darwin

♦

*'Inaction breeds doubt and fear. Action breeds confidence and courage. If you want to conquer fear, don't sit home and think about it. Go out and get busy'*

Dale Carnegie

♦

*'What would life be if we had no courage to attempt anything?'*

Vincent van Gogh

♦

'Our greatest glory is not in never falling, but in rising every time we fall.'

Confucius

♦

*'Fear is only as deep as the mind allows.'*

Japanese Proverb

♦

*'The only real failure in life is not to be true to the best one knows.'*

Buddha

♦

*'Most great people have attained their greatest success just one step beyond their greatest failure.'*

Napoleon Hill

## 054 - GUIDE to be fully available

Do not bring your personal problems to your workplace, nor your work problems at home. Then you gain in serenity, in efficiency and in joy of living. Because the relationships with your loved ones and with your co-workers are improving.

Your family, your colleagues, your friends and your other relationships, deserve, when they are with you, to enjoy your full availability (you will instantly observe, that all will be, as well, more available to you, and that the new quality of your relations brings you happiness).

We see again here, the importance, of the management of thought, and of the management of time, in our search for happiness. It is totally sterile to constantly twirl problems in your head. That will not bring you the solution. While, after you have stopped ruminating on these problems, thinking of something else, or doing something else (such as being happy), you realize, that the solution of the problem simply appears. You also realize, that in this diversification of activity, lived fully, these solutions appear unexpectedly. In the case where there is no possible solution, it is likewise unnecessary, to deceive yourself thinking about the problem, and useful, to move on living fully other activities and giving a chance to new opportunities, keeping in mind your intention to maintain happiness.

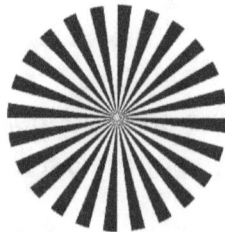

And we see again here, how the choice of a new behavior, quite simple enough to make, is capable of generating a cascade of positive events.

It is likely that you realize that you effectively have this attitude at home, at work, or in your circle of friends. Decide then to work to improve it, starting now, by the most obvious case in your relations, then extending your exercise to your other relations. Here again, observation of the outcome of the exercise will be important to give you the motivation to continue exercising it and to continue to correct this attitude until a new, happy attitude of full availability at every moment has become your new normality.

If for this exercise, as for all the exercises in this manual, you say 'I am incapable', 'It's stronger than me', or 'It's easier said than done', well, you are mistaken, for it is as easy to say as to do. Your personality and your usual behavior are in no way frozen. And you can change them at any time. The methodology to be happier, remains the same: it is enough to increase our awareness of being alive, to improve the experiences of our lives; starting by being attentive to the observation of our behaviors, realizing that such behavior is not optimal, and starting, while remaining conscious, the change process.

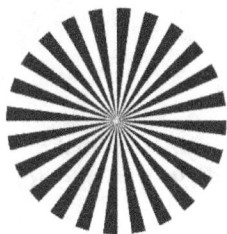

## 055 - GUIDE to be discreet

One can observe, that some of us have a compulsive desire to speak incessantly. Therefore, automatically, the monologues contain unnecessary and heavy errors and repetitions.

This excessive desire to speak is a sign of a desire to be recognized and approved. It is also the sign of an emotional lack. And, finally, the mark sign of a fear to not exist, if we stop to gesticulate.

However, the result obtained is contrary to expectation, by speaking too much, one loses the interest and the esteem of his audience. One also loses, the advantages that one could gain by listening, including that to embellish this furious desire to exist.

This is a defect that is difficult to correct, because people who talk too much have a hard time realizing that they are doing it.

Again, it will be important for you to become an observer of your actions and to correct a possible tendency to talk too much.

♦

*'Before opening the mouth, assure that what you want to say is more beautiful than the silence'*

Confucius

*Before you speak, let your words pass through three gates.*
*At the first gate, ask yourself, "Is it true?".*
*At the second, "Is it necessary?"*
*At the third gate ask, "is it kind?"*

Soufi proverb

By practicing the principles of this Sufi saying, you will be able to see that your happiness and the quality of your relations will be markedly improved.

If your current interactions do not usually pass through one of the three doors, you will find much happiness in passing through it, and the desire to persevere. Be patient, indulgent towards yourself, and persevering, when you observe an occasional failure in these new practices, for this exercise is harder than it seems.

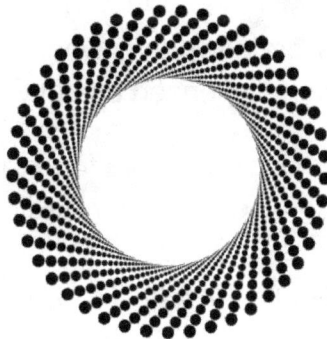

## 056 - GUIDE to be humble

Being humble is beneficial in our relationships with others. Each person is unique, and there is no justification for feeling superior or inferior to anyone.
We will seek to accept, without pretension or shyness, our reality and those of people, as they are, with their strengths, weaknesses and complementarities.

Being humble, allows us, to have better romantic, social and professional relationships. Being humble allows us to benefit from synergies reaching common goals.

If it is important to be loved, to be confident and to have ambition, it is also important to be balanced and to feel humility towards ourselves, our desires, our certainties and our ambitions (even the big ones). Then, we can seize opportunities to learn. Humility allows us to be freer.

Our modern society pushes us to compete. It is, however, possible and desirable, to be both realistic, confident and humble.

Material wealth is praiseworthy, when it is gained in an honest way and then dispensed usefully.

Poverty is sometimes glorified (as for example in Zen, Sufi and other cultures), when it is then assimilated to humility and to the measure of thought. With this poverty, one becomes rich in the essence of life.

In case you find a justification of your superiority, it will be very beneficial for you to observe it and to dissect it.

◆

*'There is nothing noble about being superior to some other man. The true nobility is in being superior to your previous self.'*

Hindu Proverb

◆

*'Humility is not thinking less of yourself; it's thinking of yourself less.'*

C. S. Lewis

◆

*'Pride makes us artificial and humility makes us real.'*

Thomas Merton

◆

*'Only humility knows how to appreciate and admire the good qualities of others.'*

Sri Chinmoy

◆

*'Be like the bamboo the higher you grow the deeper you bow.'*

Chinese Proverb

## 057 - GUIDE to be patient

Driven by, our ardor, our desire to succeed, and the masses of bad news from the media, which project us into a frightening future generating dissatisfaction of the present moment, we forget our history. Where we come from. The tremendous progress that has been made, so far, since only a few decades, which are ongoing, and which are promising in a near future, with an exponential rate of progression.

We also forget, that the only moment when our fervor and desires can be realized is, now.

We forget that the process of change, even when accelerated, remains a slow and rarely instant process.

Our impatience makes us unhappy.

And once again we realize that the obstacle to happiness is our refusal of reality, and even that our impatience is a fight against the reality.

These words will have you already anchored in the present. There are also in this manual many other techniques and exercises that anchor us in the now, and our feet on the ground.

For this chapter, I wanted to offer you, a new exercise of anchoring in the reality.

I then thought about the practice of sound OM. Then I was embarrassed, because my desire, in writing this manual, is that the techniques and exercises, besides being beneficial, are attractive, practical and enjoyable for everyone, whatever their beliefs (so that everyone can be happier and can improve his participation in the construction of the new world, and that this sum of abilities, allows us to live in a world as beautiful as we deserve). I was afraid to frighten away those who refracted the sacred. And the sound OM is very rich in sacred and symbolic concepts.

I finally decided to propose the exercise of sound OM, starting with the vibratory feeling, which is the most interesting of this practice, and that is accessible, playful and beneficial to everyone.

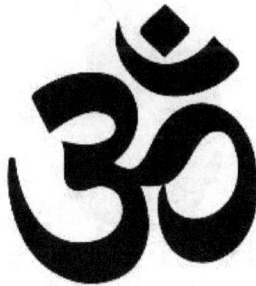

26

---

26 OM

## ◉◉ Exercise 60 : Vibrate with OM

OM is considered as the primordial sound of the universe, the first sound.

It is a combination of three syllables "Ah", "Oh", "Um", and the silent syllable. OM pronounced in continue during a long expiration emits a strong vibration which we feel easily in the entire body.

- As we say "Ah", the lower portions of the body, up to the stomach, are vibrating.

- As we say "Oh", the chest area is vibrating.

- With "Um", the face and the brain are vibrating.

- And the last syllable is the deep silence of the infinite.

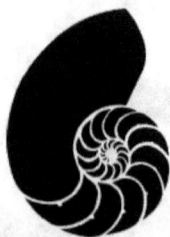

The exercise consists in playing with the sound and its vibration, to make the sound deeper playing with the bass, to feel it spreading in the body, to fill the whole-body vibrating. Below are several optional and chronological suggestions (make 5 sound exits for each). You can, depending on the quality of your feelings, do only the beginning of the exercise (the first two options) or else follow the next steps and stop when you desire it, or else chain to the last:

o Focus on pronouncing the sound OM.

o Think that the sound filled the whole body.

o Think that the sound filled each cell.

o Think that the sound is unified to planet Earth.

o Think that the sound is unified with the ambient energy field.

o To think that the sound is unified to the cosmos.

o To think that the sound unites to infinity.

o To think that the sound is unified with the unknown.

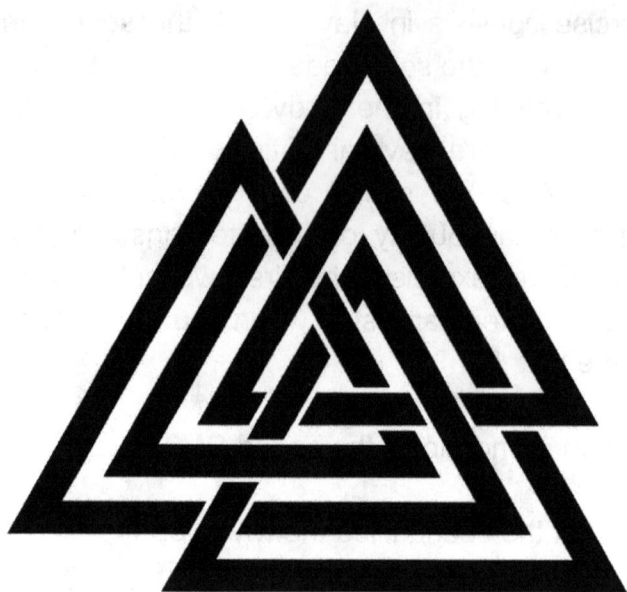

*'All human errors are impatience, a premature breaking off of methodical procedure, an apparent fencing-in of what is apparently at issue.'*

Franz Kafka

## 058 - GUIDE to forgive

Forgiving is one of the most useful things to get happiness.

What is paramount, and may be enough, is to think and to sincerely feel the forgiveness.

On the one hand, be indulgent and sympathetic to cultural and generational differences, and to the lived experiences that have led the offender to make the fault they are accused of. In some cases, we must also be indulgent with ourselves, for the possible responsibility that we may have in the conflict, for it was the best way we were able to act at that moment. We must also be realistic, and not, assign us responsibility, when we have none, as we are only victims.

On the other hand, love is once again the solution that will enable us to forgive, to feel the welfare of forgiveness, and to take out from our memory the painful memory. The technique is to seek and then feel the moments of love, which must have been there somewhere, before the fault to forgive.

After having forgiven, that one has the desire, or the possibility, to change something, depends on the circumstances. It is possible, that it is now impossible, to renew links. It does not matter, forgiveness has healed our wound, and we have evacuated resentment, remorse, regret and suffering, even if they have been intense.

But which are, as we shall remember, only thoughts. One can easily, or perhaps with the necessity of renewing several times the practice of the technique, make the decision not to keep thinking about them. And to do this to replace them, first by the welfare of forgiveness, and then, allowing new thoughts to live in the space made free by the disappearance of painful memories and bitterness. These new thoughts will fill us, and they will make their way. Roads, which we would never, otherwise have discovered. The space made free, will also have the opportunity, to remain empty, making us enjoy the well-being of the silence of thought.

♦

Let's take an example, which is unfortunately, both among the most difficult and among the most frequent. A child who has been mistreated or abused by a parent, or by a third person. It is a deep and painful wound. We meet elders, arriving at the end of their long life, having always kept this acute pain. Often even, a strange and false feeling of guilt, comes to graft and comes to contribute to the pain. Thus, these people see, in some way, their lives wasted. What a pity! The unfortunate event is past, only its memory is nourished by thought. Sometimes, for a lifetime, we keep biting ourselves with our thoughts, for we believe we cannot forgive. Yet it is enough to arrive at the decision. The sentence remains so acute that such a decision may seem impossible. Nevertheless, the stakes deserve to try, and to keep an open mind to the practice of this technique the memory of moments of shared love. There must be such moments, even with, for example, a father who has raped us and who has broken us twice, also deceiving our trust, love and references. And then, even if we really cannot find a single moment of love, rather than keep a pain for a lifetime, it will be better to think of self-love, innocence, to the new people around us, and to future years that it would be good to rid of the persistence of pain.

(This said, sexual abuse on children, even though they are diminishing, due to developments in the status of women and the condition of childhood, are still very present in all communities and may even be the case in all extended families. Then, it is very likely that you are or that you know a victim. It is necessary, for you to find the solutions to stop this criminal situation, as quickly as possible. If you are underage, or if you feel too weak, broken, helpless or scared to stop the crime, then find someone responsible to help you.)

There is another case, which everyone experiences, more or less intense, at the time of the death of a loved one. Then, strangely, one reproaches, and one cannot forgive the person for having left us or even to have abandoned us. This suffering also can last for years. Yet the same remedy, remember love, can be used. And as soon as possible will be the best. The technique is even more rapidly effective in this case than in a case of violence of the innocence of a child, for death, even if premature, is part of the normality of life.

*'Holding onto anger is like drinking poison and expecting the other person to die'*

Buddha

♦

*'When you forgive, you in no way change the past - but you sure do change the future.'*

Bernard Meltzer

♦

'I believe forgiveness is the best form of love in any relationship. It takes a strong person to say they're sorry and an even stronger person to forgive.'

Yolanda Hadid

♦

*'Forgiveness is the giving, and so the receiving, of life.'*

George MacDonald

♦

*'Forgiveness is not an occasional act; it is a permanent attitude.'*

Martin Luther King, Jr.

♦

*'Forgiveness is a reflection of loving yourself enough to move on.'*

Dr. Steve Maraboli

♦

'Forgive others, not because they deserve forgiveness, but because you deserve peace.'　　　　Jonathan Huie

## Your new stability

o Now, observe your feelings for the people you have trouble forgiving.

o Research, even if they are well hidden, moments of love with these people.

o Replaces rancor with love, while letting go of rancor with the wind.

You can repeat the exercise if there are still a few crumbs of bitterness or if there are hints of painful feelings of resentment. But it is not even certain that this is necessary.

You will succeed in erasing, one after the other, all the memories of the painful moments of your past, which are for obstacles to your happiness.

Perhaps, in reading these lines, you tell yourself that these painful moments are part of your personality, and that you would lose something if you forgot them? It is not so. Your personality is immensely greater than these bad memories, which in fact, prevent you from exploring and experiencing the dimensions and possibilities of your personality that are hitherto unknown to you. By thus managing the bad memories of your past, you will certainly see them, little by little, disappear. But in case you have a desire at some point to remember one of them, which gives you a kind of stability, you would only have to open the drawer where they are stored. For, shortly after, carefully fold and store them again. Little by little, you build your new stability, without having to resort to these painful landmarks.

## 059 - GUIDE to be compassionate

Compassion is rich and subtle, as it must simultaneously contain, the sensitivity to the pain of others, the desire to remedy it, and the commitment to the remedy that can be realized in the measure of constraints. But it is essential, that compassion contains neither pity nor suffering. Pity, whether it comes from self-pity on one's fate, or on the fate of another, is a feeling that is not only unnecessary but also harmful, for it is associated with an erroneous notion of inferiority of oneself or of the other. Pity and suffering prevent engagement in a possible corrective action. Explore this subtlety, measure the quality of your feelings and your possible remedies during the exercise of your compassion. And enjoy, without moderation, this new way to exercise your compassion.

◆

*'A human being is a part of the whole called by us universe, a part limited in time and space. He experiences himself, his thoughts and feeling as something separated from the rest, a kind of optical delusion of his consciousness. This delusion is a kind of prison for us, restricting us to our personal desires and to affection for a few persons nearest to us. Our task must be to free ourselves from this prison by widening our circle of compassion to embrace all living creatures and the whole of nature in its beauty'*

Albert Einstein

## 060 - GUIDE to ponder responsibility

Some of us feel responsible for everything and are very unhappy about it. Wars in the world, children dying of hunger, dolphins smothered by plastic, and so on.

These events are regrettable, especially as they should, and could, be avoided. On the other hand, the feeling of uneasiness, while not being among those who make the decisions, feeling responsible and disillusioned with the bad game, without even being a player, or without even having access to the chessboard, is a feeling that is not only erroneous and inconvenient but counterproductive, because, it limits our availability to seize the possible opportunities to contribute to the changes. Contributions, even the smallest, that make us happy.

The only responsibility that befalls you is that of your acts. It is a mistake and an illusion, to suffer, as a human being, from responsibility for the faults and sufferings of humanity. Especially since then, we contribute to this suffering.

♦

'The responsibilities of the bad leaders towards the Republic are disastrous. Not only do they take charge of their vices themselves, but they permeate the city '

Cicero

Perhaps you felt an emotion reading the text above, thinking of something for which you feel responsible for. If this emotion is passed at the first reading of the text, then everything goes very well in the best of all worlds. If it returns, despite your acknowledgment of the error, then say and repeat yourself, as many times as necessary:

*I have no responsibility in this thing.*

*And I have no reason to feel an emotion for a breach of my responsibility.*

*If, now, I think of an action that I can do to contribute to resolve this thing, then I go there*

*'Freedom is the will to be responsible for ourselves.'*

Friedrich Nietzsche

♦

*'Wherever you are, be there totally. If you find your here and now intolerable and it makes you unhappy, you have three options: remove yourself from the situation, change it, or accept it totally. If you want to take responsibility for your life, you must choose one of those three options, and you must choose now. Then accept the consequences'*

Eckhart Tolle

♦

*'You cannot hope to build a better world without improving the individuals. To that end, each of us must work for his own improvement and, being to aid those to whom we think we can be most useful'*

Marie Curie

♦

*'Government is like a baby. An alimentary canal with a big appetite at one end and no sense of responsibility at the other'*

R.Reagan

♦

*'If you own this story you get to write the ending.'*

Brene Brown

♦

*'I think 99 times and find nothing. I stop thinking, swim in silence, and the truth comes to me.'*

Albert Einstein

'Time and silence are the most luxurious things today.'

Tom Ford

♦

'The quieter you become the more you are able to hear.'

Rumi

♦

*'Have you not noticed that love is silence? It may be while holding the hand of another, or looking lovingly at a child, or taking in the beauty of an evening. Love has no past or future, and so it is with this extraordinary state of silence'*

Jiddu Krishnamurti

♦

*'The tree of silence bears the fruits of peace.'*

Arab proverb

♦

*'Silence is your best friend.'*          Libyan proverb

♦

*'Silence is the wisdom of all wisdoms; look, see, and shut up.'*          Moroccan proverb

♦

'If you understand, things are just as they are...
If you do not understand, things are just as they are...'

Anonymous

♦

*'I often regret that I have spoken; never that I have been silent.'*          Publilius Syrus

## 061 - GUIDE to practice the silence

According to our culture, our relationship with silence is very different. In my country of origin, sweet France, the place reserved for silence is important, as well interspersing a conversation, as in private life.

On the other hand, I have worked and lived in countries where the inhabitants are very afraid of silence, where they cannot stand a moment of silence, and where they should speak without interruption, even repeating many times the same things, during a brief conversation.

It is however, so profitable, to intersect a conversation with silences, as well as to bathe individually in the void of silence.

In the city, noise is considered the primary source of pollution. And all its inhabitants, more or less fortunate, are concerned, the noise of traffic, police sirens, ambulances and firemen, horns, aircraft or passing trains, noisy neighbors, other noise attacks. Solutions can be sought to reduce or eliminate these noises, but often there are none. And this is very frustrating. The first remedy is to be careful not to escalate frustration. A possible adaptation is to use the noise, as an indicator, in order to return to the consciousness of the peaceful inner silence, in the same way that the sound of the gong does during a meditation. But above all, this frustration must be remedied, by ensuring periods of complete silence. Suspend our exposure to noise. Go to the countryside, or in a quiet place of the city, like a park, a library or a soundproof place. And even more, one enjoys then, to savor also the silence of the word, to say nothing and to hear nothing. And at the same time, to practice the inner silence, which corresponds to suspend thoughts.

This practice of total silence is particularly useful when our exposure to noise is important, in our workplace or in the home. It is also useful, if we live in the middle of the desert. It is a pose in the tumult of life (Yes, the tumult of life is also at play, when living in the middle of the desert). It allows thoughts to settle. As a result, after the exercises, our thoughts are clearer, and our ability to learn, understand, find solutions and expand our horizons is enhanced. Our life is simpler, and we are more relaxed. We feel new sensations that make us happier.

These statements may seem strange to you if you are carried away in a whirlwind of a life full of responsibility and/or entertainment that seems to satisfy your existence, or even if you live without existential questions. But, here, we are dealing with new sensations, and we cannot imagine that they will make us happier before we have experienced them and felt them. Our curiosity, our interest to make new experiences and even our taste for entertainment, can then, with happiness, allow us to access unknown territories. Once we get the glimpse, we have a desire to continue to explore them.

In addition to the necessary and useful remedy for our excessive exposure to noises and thoughts, we have found an occupation of our time, which satisfies us more than those to which we were accustomed.

**Practice the inner silence :**

(For 5 minutes). Practicing inner silence means silencing thoughts about the past or the future, emotions, desires, plans, judgments about others and about oneself.

To help you practice this kind of inner silence you can at the same time practice Exercise 4, Conscious Breathing. Then a sustained attention on your breath and your throat, as in Exercise 6, will make your practice of inner silence easier. Indeed, when your attention is thus on your throat there is no room for what was listed above (past, future, emotions, desires, ...). You can return to all these thoughts, after this pause, if you wish. But, by practicing inner-silence, you will naturally experience less desire, in your daily life, to torture yourself with painful thoughts.

This present moment is yours, take advantage of it, enjoy and relax.

It will be quite normal, for thoughts to come to your mind during this practice; Just let them pass, as if you let them go with the flow of the river, or, as if a thought was a bird that you watch to fly and then disappear; And each time come back to the attention brought to your throat.

I can assure you, if you repeat this practice, 5 minutes, every day, for a week, you will feel new sensations of which you will be satisfied.

## ◉◉ Exercise 61 : 24 hours without speaking

If you live alone, it will be easy for you to choose a period of 24 hours, to practice this exercise.

If you live in a couple, with or without children, you can decide to do this exercise together, by having a clear understanding of the benefits you will explore. Then, if rare communications would be necessary, they can be made, writing messages on pieces of paper.

It is also possible, that you live with other people, who are not interested in this exercise. Then, you will inform them of your desire to practice it. They must not speak to you, and they cannot expect you to speak.

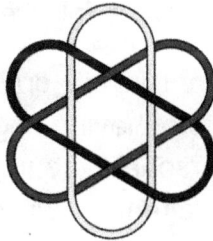

## Conclusion chapter HAPPY IN YOUR HEAD

Let's be clear. Having negative thoughts is very normal, contributing to the construction of our being. Would it be pain, disgust, grief, greed, jealousy, fear, impatience, envy, dependence, judgment, or the like.

However, we benefit, being attentive to these thoughts rather than being annihilated. Because their observation reduces their scope.

And, the time we spend having this kind of unpleasant thoughts is manageable. It can even be shortened, until it becomes imperceptible, like a lightning flash, by developing our ability to return to well-being in the present moment, while benefiting from the building materials of our being, and by learning to know the new building, even in its nooks and crannies.

Along the way, we experience feelings of happiness and wholeness that are entirely new, unknown, and that we cannot describe until we have followed the process.

We should be persistent in the practice of the process, because our bad habits of having negative thoughts, have so far defined our personality, our way of life, and our stability. And it is easy to remain, without realizing it, and to suffer, in our familiar comfort zone.

Better habits quickly turn us into a happier, more vivid and more effective person.

All that has just been said about negative thoughts applies equally to the stress.

Stress is quite normal. And being aware of this normality allows us to live our stress with serenity.

We see in this manual many possibilities for managing the duration and intensity of our stress; also, to eliminate it (until it comes back, and we can manage it again).

Stress can be useful, and knowing its normality, we can use it as a food for our vitality.

And finally, the regular practice of these management and use of stress allows us to master them.

By nature, we are very complacent about our negative thoughts and about our stress. Because it is easy and it gives us the impression of living, while it damages our lives. We must make a journey and maintain a state of consciousness to modify these complacencies and replace them with happiness, serenity, health, love and efficiency. At first, we must understand that our natural tendency is to take pleasure in being unhappy. Then we must observe our thoughts and emotions in order to identify our negative and stressed trend. With a little attention and practice we get to know ourselves and to recognize, then to correct, the times when we embark on an unhappy path. This is, in a way, the definition of our life, because it is an approach that we must be aware of every day and at every moment.

# Action

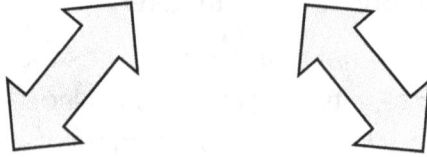

# Body 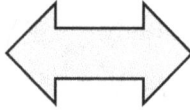 Mind

## 3.3.  HAPPY IN YOUR ACTIONS

In this chapter, we will learn to identify two mistakes that we are able to make:

o The mistake of believing that the action is not necessary.

o The mistake of believing that inaction is neither necessary nor productive.

We will identify, the comfortable inertia, that follows the start of the action. And consequently, you will become happier being more efficient and more active, using the impulse of starting-up actions

We will see, the importance of loving oneself, of loving what we do, and of loving ourselves when doing what we love to do.

And, we will see, several behaviors and several techniques that also make us happier and more efficient in our actions.

## 062 - GUIDE to be active

*'Nothing happens until something moves'*

*'Life is like a bicycle. When you stop pedaling you fall'*

Albert Einstein

Much is said in these two truths enunciated by Einstein.

Furthermore, the start of the action creates the event and produces ideas. The first event generates the next one, the next one, and so on, including conducive events, encounters, new ideas, and the machine is running. We then realize, that everything connects with great ease.

The main difficulty, which can easily be overcome, is to start.

Furthermore, studies in psychology[27], which measure the level of happiness, have found that the level of happiness is higher, when one is engaged in activities requiring concentration, and less when one is engaged in passive activities (such as watching television). We can verify it by experience, managing our time differently, giving priority to the motivating activities in which we are focused and that bring us the greatest happiness.

---

[27]Psychology studies use questionnaires completed by thousands of people.

## 👀 Exercise 62 : Immediate launch

Reading this text above, may have made you think of an activity, you've always wanted to do, but never started.

Now, begins to focus your attention on this activity, and then pursues this attention in the following days, ensuring regularity and initiative, taking notes and engaging in activities (even small ones) that contribute to the realization of your wish.

You will be surprised and satisfied, observing, the amount of progress made during a day, and, the amount of joy that you lived. Then fully enjoy these satisfactions and surprises; For it will nourish their continuities, their progress and your happiness in the following days.

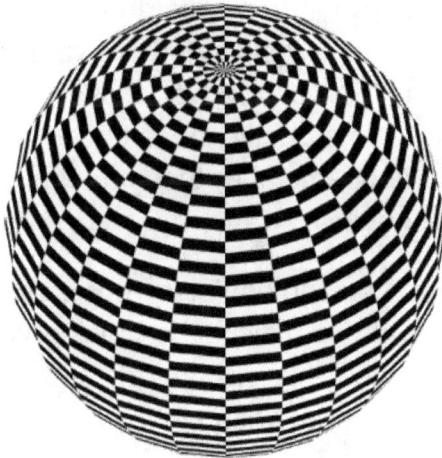

## 👀 Exercise 63 : What should I do ?

If you do not know, what is the best goal you could achieve now? You can start by, asking yourself precisely the question. You can be confident that, by taking the time to listen, your powerful subconscious mind, aware of, your best interests, and, your greatest desires, will give you the answer.

Similarly, if you do not know where to start, to progress towards achieving your goals in the medium or long term (even if you have no idea what these goals are), again, ask yourself precisely the question. In response, one or more ideas of action will come to your mind. Take the habit, without prevarication, of getting into action to realize the idea that you feel the easiest, most accessible or the most attractive of the moment (The results of these actions will correspond to short-term objectives). If you do not yet know what, in the medium or long term, to pursue, the activities that will come to you in this way, and which are the most favorable for your well-being and for your evolution, will contribute to make you discover these objectives soon. You can cultivate your trust in these upcoming discoveries, to facilitate them. (Remember that you can use the tool of lists, see next chapter).

An action, which you find useful to your project, may seem to be difficult, and this difficulty is making you uneasy. In this case, overcome this discomfort, and engage in this action, paying all your attention to it.

To help you overcome this discomfort, and now to avoid succumbing to the desire to escape into a distraction that seems easier and more comfortable, remember that the times when you are active and passionate, bring you more happiness than distractions.

You will soon notice, that your commitment in this action effectively gives you pleasure and satisfaction.

You will feel, that this action is finally not as difficult as you had (sometimes long) imagined, and that often it is even surprisingly easy.

You will take care, to linger to experience the pleasure regarding the progress made, and to cultivate the esteem of yourself, in the face of a success that seemed to you out of reach. Again, according to the mechanism identical to that seen in the previous chapter, the feeling of this satisfaction will enable you to consolidate your confidence and your mastery in your newly acquired capacity. To linger to experience this pleasure, will also arouse your enthusiasm, to enchain the following activity that leads you towards the realization of your objective.

(However, as we will later see the value of the inaction, you will also practice comfort, during necessary periods of rest and relaxation to the gestation of your ideas and plans. As well as, during seemingly barren periods)

On the other hand, you will also notice that when you are committed to achieving an objective, it is not only the process and the action that give you happiness, but also the fact that, with a clearly defined perspective, you enjoy a pleasant freedom of mind (without wandering thoughts), for the duration, until the completion of the goal (1 hour, 1 week, 1 month, 1 year or 1 life).

Be attentive to the next time you feel such determination, such freedom and happiness. And print those feelings in your memory. This will facilitate your commitment to action. You will abbreviate the empty passages; and you will avoid gloom.

This process is worth insisting upon. And it is worth for you to be attentive at multiplying these moments of full consciousness. It is possible to reach this state from the time you wake up in the morning till the time you start your night sleep.

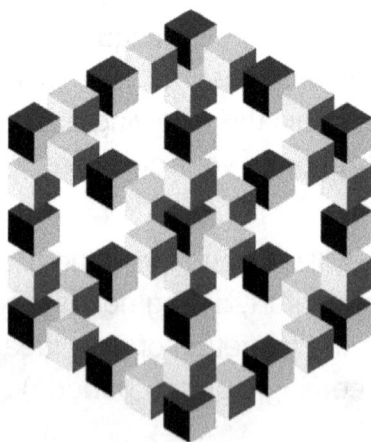

## ☻☻ Exercise 64 : Making lists

Lists are very useful tools, that allow us to find and develop ideas, to be better organized and to remember the steps to be taken.

There is an infinite amount of list that you can do, according to your tastes, and according to your experiences. When you think 'what list can I do?' Then an idea comes to you, and you can start writing this list.

Some lists are particularly useful:

o  10 quick and easy things to do to achieve one's goals;

o  10 more complex actions to achieve objectives;

o  The positive and negative aspects of a proposed action or choice;

o  Things to do during a period;

o  Topics I would like to know more about

o  Good resolutions; etc.

Regularly you will be able, to return to a list, and to enjoy, to check and savor the progress made, to draw inspiration seeing the actions still to be done, and to note the new ideas. In these regular reviews, you will also enjoy observing that your choices are evolving and improving; You become more creative; You have more inspiration; You get to do more things; You are better organized, and your life is more interesting and happier.

## 063 - GUIDE to set targets

An important goal in our quest for happiness is to know what we really want. This applies in all areas (eg work, relationship, property, health, time use, milestones, etc.).

Realizing what you really want is not easy and requires a lot of questioning. We must make detours through mistakes, failures, doubts, impatience and despair. All these difficulties, which are rich in teaching, allow us to correct, clarify and develop our ideas, and which make it possible to progress to succeed at knowing what we really want, to be satisfied, to love ourselves and to enjoy what we do.

The important thing is always to continue, to avoid, being unhappy at length, or stagnating in a sterile indifference, but rather, to be constantly aware that happiness is a state of mind that is possible to live or to reach at any moment.

Being active, and highly conscious, is the best thing you can do. Its opposite is not to be alive, a kind of state of death. You will have to keep a good frame of mind when you are not really satisfied with your life situation, by accepting reality, remaining active in thinking, planning, setting goals and acting to improve this reality. You will have to accept failures, to accept the pain of failures, to get up and walk again.

Your goals must be realistic but ambitious.

These may be short-term goals and objectives (the next hour, today, tonight, tomorrow ... I would have accomplished this or that), or medium-term goals, such as changing behavior, or Long-term goals, such as life goals or business goals.

When an action is over, or a goal is reached, you can rejoice, without moderation, and then move on to the next one. Learn how to shorten, and then eliminate, these moments of transition between two goals, during which you risk succumbing to a long period of relapse in entertainment or gloom.

If the achievement of the goal is delayed, compared to the time you have imagined, do not be upset, but measure and rejoice in the progress already made. Pull in this satisfaction the energy to continue.

It is very normal and frequent, that over time, objectives are changing, because circumstances or ambitions did change. You will observe, that for a time you are very excited, very happy and convinced that this or that is good for you. So, you invest in its construction. Then some time later, you're excited about a new thing, and you realize that this new thing, is finally much better than the first. You realize then, that it is very beneficial that this first thing did not come true. This first thing, however, having the great value, of having led you to this news. These changes may even occur several times.

Be indulgent towards yourself, learn to recognize, the normality of the successive phases of the process of evolution, and learn, to remain comfortable, and to maintain the love for yourself, your enthusiasm and your vitality.

Learn also, how to shorten, until they are eliminated, the depressive episodes that follow a frustration or a failure. You will achieve it by rapidly focusing on the next action, finding the pleasure of being active and regaining the pleasure of the success.

You will have advantage, in the organization of your timetable, to give priority to the activities of your list, which will lead you to the realization of your objectives. This attitude is paramount. Certainly, it will be necessary for you to change your habits, to make choices to eliminate certain activities, certain behaviors and certain distractions. These eliminations, will, at first, appear to you, difficult or painful. But it will be a mistake. Because, the other activities, will prove to be easier, they will bring you a greater well-being, and the satisfaction to progress towards your objective. Then you will not feel any attraction or envy for these past activities, behaviors and distractions. You will become passionate about the new ones. You will be so enthusiastic, that you will even have to force yourself to make poses, and to make sure that you do not become intolerant or proselytizing.

You will be happier.

*'Choose a job you love and you will never have to work a single day in your life.'*

Confucius

Note: this say from Confucius maybe disturbing for you, in case you feel stuck in your actual situation, without any perspective of alternative. You will improve your happiness, as well as the developments of the situation, by focusing on the things you like in your job, instead of focusing on the things you dislike.

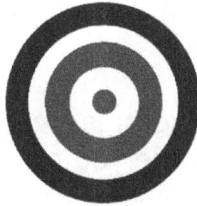

*'I have been impressed with the urgency of doing; knowing is not enough; we must apply. Being willing is not enough; we must do'*

Leonard de Vinci

♦

*'If you hear a voice within you say, "You cannot paint" then, by all means, paint, and that voice will be silenced'*

Vincent van Gogh

## ☺☺ Exercise 65 : Explore in great details

Choose an object of desire. It can be a romantic relationship, a friendly relationship, an ideal job, a leisure activity, a reasoned purchase (e.g. home, car), a place to go for holidays, a goal a form or a physical health, or anything else.

Make a descriptive list of the characters, appearances, colors, specificities, etc. In making this list, describe the object with many details.

By doing this search for details, you will discover many useful information, which will bring you closer to the object of your desire.

Also, very often during this research, you will learn information, that will make you change the object of your desire, for a better.

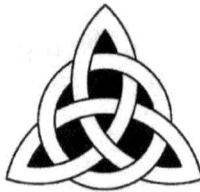

*'Work out the details in achieving your dreams'* S. Adelaja

◆

*'Peculiar I say, how so often the smallest, most seemingly insignificant details later unveil their faces as vital means for progression.'*

Criss Jami

330

## 064 - GUIDE to go from bitterness to action

It happens to most of us, to remember dozens of times, with bitterness, that we should do this or that task, which we are still dragging to do.

We have this attitude, both for activities that are enjoyable and contribute to the achievement of our objectives, and for activities that are a priori obtrusive, even if these activities are contributing to the achievement of our objectives (for example: housework or administrative tasks).

Such a waste!

A significant amount of time wasted repeating 'oh I have to do this or that', or 'I am not happy doing this or that'. It also represents a significant amount of bitterness.

This is very paradoxical.
Because the time spent doing this activity, is often much shorter, than the sum of the small moments, when we have suffered from our negligence.

Moreover, in completing it, and once it is completed, this action brings us the satisfaction, the pleasure, the happiness of the work done and well done. It is thus obvious, that it is preferable to neither lose our time, nor our chance to be happy.

On the other hand, by immediately taking an action born of an idea, the completed action allows us to progress. While we realize, that dragging things, unfortunately we forget and spoil ideas and inspiration, things are not done, we stagnate, and we remain unhappy.

We can easily agree with these realities. We must, however, make the effort to remember it, to put it into action and to change our habits.

♦

Let us return to these a priori daunting tasks, such as the many domestic and administrative tasks.

We have a still greater tendency to retard them, to suffer during these delays, and to continue to suffer when we are executing them.

We can change these destructive scenarios. Again, we can think of the priority we give to our happiness and live these moments lightly. It is possible, for example, to live a moment of pleasure, peace, even meditation, sweeping with minutiae the floor of our house.

♦

Our happiness lies, when one of our objectives is reached, and during the journey that leads us to achieve our objectives.

In addition to the fun that one finds in actions, we can, incidentally, still increase our pleasure and enthusiasm by the visualizing the positive energy of the achieved goal.

## ◉◉ Exercise 66 : To not forget

By not letting things be dragged on, we suppress the impropriety of important omissions.

However, not all tasks can be started immediately, if for example, you cannot interrupt what you are already busy with. So, the risk of forgetting important things, is not yet totally eliminated.

It is possible to build our confidence, that we will remember, at the right time, things that we risk forgetting:

○ Just start by stating this trust.

○ Then, to be happy and satisfied whenever we realize that we are remembering the right information at the right time.

○ By following this process, it becomes more and more reliable.

If, on the contrary, we cultivate the fear of forgetting an important thing, we increase the risk of forgetting it, and we build the identity of a person who forgets important things and who is unhappy about them.

Cultivating this process, can be assimilated to cooperating with our powerful intuition, and to cultivating the constancy of our consciousness.

## ☯☯ Exercise 67 : Cultivate autonomy

We have already seen three advantages of cultivating autonomy: in the appreciation of being alone, in the existential independence in relation to others (They do not belong to us), and in relation to events (unconditional happiness).

There are also many advantages and satisfactions in cultivating autonomy in our actions: to do, what we wish to do, what it is necessary for us to do, to be painstaking when doing, and to make efforts to learn how to do the things we do not know (within our reach, despite a primary doubt, without requiring the intervention of a specialist). By thus cultivating our autonomy of action, we are always surprised and satisfied, by the quality and quantity of the things we can do. By increasing theses quality and quantity and by learning new techniques, we increase our perception, our ability, our confidence, our satisfaction and our community contribution. We also get better contributions from others, who do not waste any more time or who do not feel frustration assisting us.

Some people in our communities have more difficulty becoming self-reliant. Evolutions of knowledge about happiness in many fields (sociology, economics, humanism, development, etc.) have unanimously concluded that it is in our greatest interest, individually and collectively, to help the weakest among us to become self-reliant.

You will be able to recognize, on what point cited above it is desirable that you pay your attention for improvement.

*'A journey of a thousand miles begins with a single step.'*
Credited to Confucius and to Lao Tzu

♦

*'When we start walking, is when the road appears'* Rumi

♦

*'Find the autonomy in your work. Autonomy is key to feeling good about the work you do, no matter what kind of work it is.'*
Jean Chatzky

♦

'Control leads to compliance;
autonomy leads to engagement.' Daniel H. Pink

♦

*'Autonomy is the whole thing; it's what unhappy people are missing. They have given the power to run their lives to other people.'*
Judith Guest

♦

*'Adults don't know how to respect and really love their young ones. Often love is confused with possession. You say "this is my" about your child, without taking into account that you're dealing with a real person with his/her own personality, rights, and autonomy, even when very young.'*

Dacia Maraini

## 065 - GUIDE to accept empty periods

Time to time, a feeling of lack of energy or enthusiasm, is something quite normal, natural and necessary, especially after a passage rich in events (roller-coaster effect, with its ups and downs), a bad digestion or strong emotions.

Depending on our personality, the circumstances, the level of our commitment and our habits, we live more or less well, and more or less quickly these passages.

Some of us have a hard time accepting them, and they shall be particularly attentive to correct this bad habit. For others they are very short, even imperceptible. And finally, for some of us, they last for months or years.

We will benefit, according to our needs, to improve our management of empty periods.

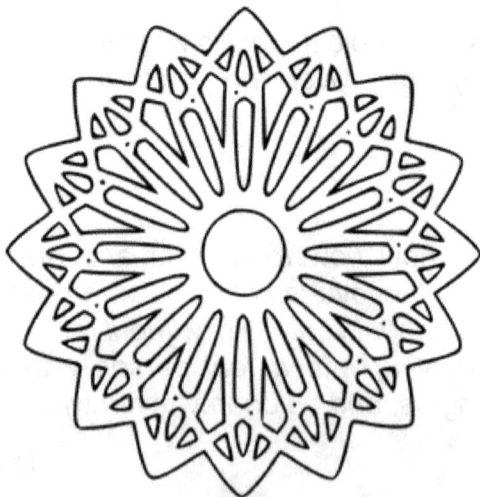

Managing empty periods: we must first accept the normality of sometimes lacking energy or enthusiasm, and also accept the normality of not being constantly to the best of our creativity or our productivity. And we must know that, like everything else, these moments will pass.

Rather than to suffer from these moments, it is good to love them, to live them fully (even if they correspond to a full of emptiness), without guilt, and to seize the opportunity to practice introspection, to rest, to do other attractive things and to let things evolve (as we will develop later in the chapter doing-not doing).

If we are bogged down in a long period of inactivity, the first thing to do is to regain confidence and self-love, the second will be to engage in any kind of activity (such as, for example, one of the exercises of this manual), which will generate experiences and opportunities, and one begins to perceive that they will certainly bring us more happiness and vital energy than does passivity.

We must observe ourselves. What are our actions? What are our thoughts?

We must also observe our behavior in order to know whether we accept and respect the normality of empty periods in others. Then, if such period occurs, it is better to accept and adapt.

◆

'Patience is not simply the ability to wait - it's how we behave while we're waiting.'

Joyce Meyer

## 066 - GUIDE to temperate the perfection

Here are two anecdotes: 'The day I lost my illusions' and 'The day my illusions turned into possibility'.

The day I lost my illusions :

was about thirty years ago. I was completing one of my first humanitarian operations, and I was at the headquarters of the international organization I was working for, doing my final debriefing.

My interlocutor said to me 'Thank you for sending your final mission report in advance, this allows for more clarification and this makes the final debriefing's meetings more substantial and livelier.'
I was very surprised hearing this comment, because, sending the report two weeks before the end of the mission, was an obligation stipulated in the regulation attached to the contract of employment that I had signed. And I considered this report as a not only normal but also an important component of the operation.
So, I answered with astonishment that I found it normal.

The organization was professional and serious. The operation had proceeded smoothly. We had, with my colleagues been conscientious in our work. I was very far from thinking that I could hear the answer of my interlocutor, who then said to me:

"Oh! But in reality, many people give their reports only on the debriefing day, or several months after their returns, or not at all."

That day, I lost my illusions about the quality of men's involvement in their professional activities.

In the following years, I observed behaviors in all types of job, and unfortunately, I got confirmation of the high frequency of the workers' very low commitments. Even, I could observe that most of workers were not happy to be at their workplaces. As if, they preferred to cultivate sadness rather than happiness. However, I also saw many people who were remarkably committed, creative and effective in their work.

However, things are changing, as for example, thanks to the progress of standardization and data processing, and if individual commitments too often fail and hurt individuals, these failures are decreasing.

I later recounted this anecdote, to several serious and committed young colleagues who were worried about their professional future. Telling them, that by continuing their serious commitments, they had every chance of succeeding because the competition was, unfortunately, rather erased. I also told them that, beyond the frustration of meeting people tortured by their professional disgust, they would also have the opportunity to collaborate with other workers sharing their enthusiasm.

<u>The day when my illusions were once again transformed into possibility</u> :

The following years were very exciting.

I participated to the beginning of the knowledge revolution; worked on the first desktop computers and then, around the age of twenty-five, with the first laptops; contributed to the progress of standardization of working methods; worked on the first databases, their analyzes and the standardization of the resulting methodologies; and worked at including, previously ignored parameters (such as environmental impact, carbon weight, water weight, measurement of user and stakeholder satisfactions, risk analyzes and solutions to reduce them, and sustainable development).

Then my illusions were again transformed into possibility. Eradication of poverty was no longer a utopia.

We now had the know-how and resources allowing us to include all the parameters in the equation, and to allow the machine to turn for the good of all.

New methodologies, technologies and techniques had reduced constraints and obstacles. They offered many opportunities. And while the task remains huge, we now have the ability to organize and to manage it.

Our evolution had also helped us, to understand, that only the eradication of poverty and its misdeeds, with particular attention to the poorest[28] among us, could give its strength to the base of the socio-economic pyramid, making shine this pyramid, and bringing comfort and prosperity to all of us. The good life, for all men, had finally become a possibility.

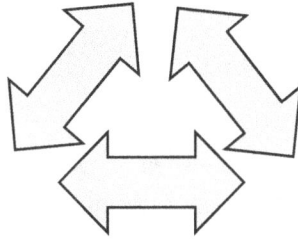

When committing to doing something, it is good to spend the time allotted to this activity, being as conscious and effective as possible.

---

[28]The most deprived persons are often the most generous, and hospitable people. They are also rich with other remarkable human values which are often forgotten by the people living in comfort. A poverty eradication program must preserve these values. However, poverty is also accompanied by a great deal of suffering, such as child marriages, human trafficking in the sex industry (third source of crime income after arms and drug trafficking), domestic violence, days with a single meal, lack of water, hygiene and housing, great ante and postnatal mortality, lack of school education, criminal oppression, and so on. Which can and must be eliminated to enable these people to live a dignified and integrated life in society.

People who do not do so, are obviously unhappy, because disliking their job and having the right feeling to waste their time. Recall that happiness has been measured greater in the moments of concentration than in moments of passivity (ref. Value scale, in the psychological study questionnaire). These people also suffer from their dishonesty, and consequently from their low self-esteem, producing a result below what is expected of them. And the colleagues who wait for them are also embarrassed by this failure. This is at the origin of conflicts end loss of respect.

To be happier these people have three solutions.
The first, is to cross the barrier of doubt and paralysis, and to engage properly in their activities, where they will find, thereafter, interests and happy interactions.
The second solution, in the case where the repulsion is too powerful, rendering these people incapable of engaging in the activity, is to change activity.
The third solution, for those of us who do not see a possible alternative to their daily suffering, is to approach every beginning of the day, when waking up, no longer with the suffering of the projection of a new sad day, but immersing, for 30 seconds, in the well-being of the present moment, and then working at extending, maintaining and renewing this feeling of well-being, during the day.

This 30 second technique is simple and immediately very effective in changing our reality, it becomes even more effective after working the sincerity of the feeling of well-being.

Some of us have difficulties, carried away by the impetus of their strong commitment, to accept a result other than perfect. There is even suffering in this non-acceptance. It is a shame because not only is it unnecessary and unrealistic, but it is also counterproductive. In order to be happier these people have to do a job on themselves, in order to accept the reality of the constraints.

These people can reassure themselves, knowing that a strong commitment always produces (except in rare accidental cases) good results. And even when short passages or moments of less enthusiasm intervene, the predominance of strong engagement always produces the same good results.

For yet another category of us, the quest for perfection lies in the planning phase. And this unresolved search becomes an obstacle to the start of the activity, sometimes even becomes an excuse before a fear of starting. For these people, the situation is uncomfortable and painful. The solution for these people is still to start, taking into account the time constraint, satisfying a minimum of vision and planning, and knowing that the start-up has the ability, which it generously honors, to generate experience, movement and speed.

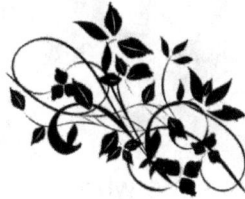

## ☯☯ Exercise 68 : State of consciousness

The state of consciousness is a state in which we feel the happiness of being alive. While in a state of unconsciousness, during which we perform our tasks in a robotic, under duress, or reluctantly, is a moribund state, in which we asphyxiate.

By learning to recognize the state in which we find ourselves, we know whether we are dead or alive. If we are dead, it is in our interest to resurrect, returning to a state of consciousness and careful attention to detail, to scenes, to our well-being, to our thoughts, to our gestures, to our words, to our body posture and to our breathing.

The exercise consists in taking the daily habit of observing the moments when you are in a robotic and unconscious state, as well as the moments when you are bruised by refusing reality, then take a deep breath, and return to a state of consciousness of being alive, in a life where you have resolved to live at best and happily every second.

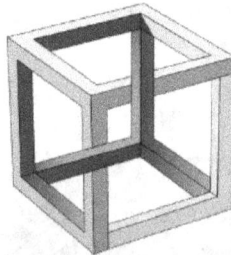

They tell the story of a sage who, passing beside a corpse of decaying dogs, exclaimed "that his teeth are white and beautiful! "

## ☻☻ Exercise 69 : The perfection of others

To think that everyone should be perfect, in relation to a projection and judgment of oneself, in relation to our variable conception of perfection, through empathy or impatience, is also a painful tendency which is often observed a lot of us. We must work our acceptance of each one's reality of constraints, characteristics and capacities, and in doing so accept and compose between our expectations and the reality. When we have an interest in accepting our imperfections, it is natural that we accept the imperfections of others.

We also shall ensure at doing our part, leading by example.

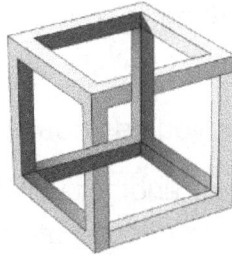

Observe to what extent you are subject to such suffering, and work to reduce them. Rather than focusing on the defects and thus giving them importance, you can focus on the qualities (including human qualities), which will also become more important. Rather than suffer, you will rejoice, and your relationships with others will become better, because of your joy and as others will feel the respect and esteem you bear, not your discomfort, your disdain, your disgust or your pity.

## 👀 Exercise 70 : Five Senses Exercise

This exercise is to practice and to strengthen your mindfulness.

It consists in noticing experiences with the 5 senses, consecutively and in the following order, spending 20 seconds minimum with each sensation:

o   Notice five things that you can see.

Choose preferably things or details you usually do not notice.

o   Notice four things that you can feel.

For instance: your clothing, a spoon, a glass, your skin, the table, an object, etc.

o   Notice three things you can hear.

For instance: a plane or another vehicle passing, a bird, a neighbor, the fan from your computer, etc;

o   Notice two things you can smell.

For instance: from nature, from food or from pollution; etc;

o   Notice one thing you can taste.

Therefore, you should be choosing a timing for this exercise when you can have access to something to put in your mouth.

## ☯☯ Exercise 71 : Leverage moments of "waiting."

Often, we must wait. Would it be in a waiting room before an appointment, in a queue at the cashier, at a traffic light, waiting the train, the metro, the bus or the elevator, waiting because of a slow internet load, waiting an advertisement to end, etc.

In these moments, we can tend to get nervous, impatient or disgusted.

With this exercise, you are going to transform these unpleasant and disturbing moments into pleasant and beneficial moments. The complete achievement will be attained step by steps, practicing using those moments as timely triggers to take a bowl of mindfulness and positive vital energy.

o  Close your eyes and take a deep breath.

o  Continue, for the time you must wait, practicing conscient breathing, and with a positive thinking observing thoroughly your surroundings.

o  Eventually, if relevant, while maintaining breathing, you can review your readiness to the next event (for instance: what you are going to say and what will be your attitude during the coming meeting).

## Imperfection and feelings

Each person is different and automatically each person does not fully match our current ideals.

But there is a difference between judging a person as racist, cruel, or this or that, even if this person is violating our freedoms, and feeling a long painful emotion by seeing the actions of that person.

Emotion, in the face of imperfection, is not only painful, but it is also useless because it does not change anything and handicaps us by limiting our eventual ability to react to contribute to an improvement.

Become accustomed to observing the moments when you feel such painful emotions and remember that this external reality is different from your inner reality that you desire serene and happy. Then continue your activity serenely. With practice, you will come to much shorten these times of perception of the painful emotion, to quickly regain a serene state and to rapidly recover efficiency in your activities.

We can also often hear, in the daily discussions of many of us, reactions of disgust or revolt in the face of cruel, racist, sexist, perverse, xenophobic, homophobic or corrupt, criminal or simply clumsy. (Recall that, because of the commercial interest of the mass media, we are often the spectators of such actions by a public figure or a stranger.

Most of this information, in addition to be rehashed, is false, deformed or amplified. And our sensation of existence is more direct, rapid and easy, by means of negative stimuli than positive excitations).

This disgust and revolt are often addressed to society, to the whole of humanity or even to existence. And so, we use, rebellious, our time in a sterile, uncomfortable and degrading way.

However, our true nature is innocent, loving and positively evolving. And the pseudo-guilty of these actions, condemned justly or unjustly, constitute, despite the great space they occupy in the media, in our conversations, in our emotions, in our thoughts and in our lives, a very small one minority of us.

Observe your behavior. Eliminate this kind of gossip, mockery or revolt from your subjects of conversation. Use your potential activist energy, to verify and possibly expose false information or information that should not be ignored, and especially, if you have the opportunity, to help the victims of these evil acts.

Use this same time, to share and act according to your true positive nature which deserves to dominate the space of your life. Also, use this time, to observe and address your own deficiencies tempering your happiness.

## 👀 Exercise 72 : Admit your errors

The human society to which we are entitled, and which we have the capacity to obtain, is a society in which individual actions and transactions bring satisfaction and interest to all the parties concerned. And that in no case may a party be abused.

We are not supermen; we can be wrong.
And since the satisfaction and legitimacy of each other's interests is now the way of life we have adopted, we must be loyal and admit our mistakes, and thus, increase the chances that our errors can be corrected, rather than being at the origin of a cascade of problems.
Our interests and our satisfactions, individual and common, are thus preserved and our time is well used.
In addition, errors and failures are very natural.
Practice getting into the habit of admitting your mistakes.

◆

*'Recognizing one's mistakes is a mark of courage and intelligence'.*                    Pierre-Marc-Gaston de Levis

◆

*'Happy is he who, after having lost his way, can find himself and acknowledge his error'.*                    M.de Puisieux

◆

*'A fool who looks at himself in a mirror does not recognize himself'.*                    Sophie Arnould

## 067 - GUIDE to not suffer from impossible

*Do not try hard
to change things
that your action
does not have the possibility of changing.*

*And do not suffer
from things
which you cannot influence.*

## 068 - GUIDE to do one thing at a time

The evolution of communication technologies (including mobile phone, internet connection 24/7, email, SMS and social media), our interlocutors expecting for an immediate response to their multiple communications, the increasing demands of productivity at work places, our enthusiasm our curiosity, and our desire to escape in these new electronic virtual worlds, lead to do faster more and more, and many things at a time.

Yet, our brain can only perform one task at a time. And, we are more efficient, and globally faster, and more productive, when we focus on one task at a time, without being interrupted by another.

We must adapt the management of our time and our reactivity to do only one thing at a time, eliminating the distractions by making it. For example, it is preferable to reserve periods of exclusive responses to emails; We will also benefit from being conscious when we eat, without being distracted by television; We will not use our mobile phone when driving a vehicle to avoid the likely risk of accidents. We can also design to cut our phone the time of an action.

Multitasking has been fashionable for a while, until we realized monotasking was more efficient.

What is happiness?

Perhaps, we have forgotten what it is to be happy?

Perhaps, happiness seems impossible to us?

To define happiness, we name equivalent sensations, such as: well-being, satisfaction, safety, lightness, freedom, joy, comfort, balance, carefree, strength, love, ease and naturalness. Sensations, that we first learn to know, then, that we recognize, with increasing certainty.

These short moments, during which we are occupied with only one precise task, are particularly favorable moments for exercising a maximum feeling of happiness, discovering new intensities of these named equivalent sensations.
In these moments we can, with a light heart, concentrate exclusively on this task, with the desire to perform it at best, without thinking of the next task, and without thinking of anything other than action, freedom, and to the happiness of living and breathing.

We will do the same during the next task, between tasks, and so on.
As we perform our tasks to the best of our ability, they are successful. The few errors and the rare failures no longer affect our happiness, for it becomes more and more strongly, at any time, our priority. We are discovering new dimensions of the named equivalences, it is enjoyable, and we are getting used to it.

## 069 - GUIDE to remember achievements

Naturally, we all have the desire to evolve. Culturally we are impatient. Our obsession with the goal or the ideal to achieve is oppressing us. We forget where we came from. We lack the legitimate value of progress made and progress being made. Again here, we are insufficiently aware of the reality. This results in dissatisfaction, contempt, stress, and insecurity. Paradoxically, it is our impatience to be happy and our enthusiasm to do well, which make us unhappy and which handicap our action.

First, we must realize that we are impatient. We must then, remember the initial statuses of the things we are working at. We will recognize that change is a time-consuming process. We will cultivate our conscious presence in the present moment, rather than in the projection into the future. We will feel satisfaction, by observing the progress already made. And we will leave the necessary time for the progress in progress, to be realized. Thus, we will realize better and greater progress, and we shall be happier in doing so.

◆

*'The important thing is not the destination, it's the journey'*

Stevenson (The treasure Island)

Some of our accomplishments bring us dissatisfaction:

o This may be after a failure, where disappointment can even be devastating. It is then recommended, to quickly remember that failures are a valuable learning, and open the doors to better opportunities. Immediately after the failure, here are step by step the remedies we can use:

- Immediate relief is obtained by accepting the normality of the discomfort and dissatisfaction. Here again, it is useful and effective, to observe and to avoid apnea.

- The infallible remedy is love: Love, love and laugh with your parents and friends. Contemplate, easily during a walk in exuberant nature. Recreational activities conducted with care and without apnea. Create, watch, listen, feel, taste and touch art (music, photography, exhibitions, films, cooking, etc.).

o Sometimes our satisfaction of having completed a task, is mixed with the dissatisfaction of thinking that we could have done better.

There are then two scenarios: it is no longer possible to modify our action, then the best thing to do is to focus on satisfaction, or else, it is still possible to correct our action. In this second case, we can again feel embarrassment, not knowing how to correct it, in this case, the priority again is to stop feeling dissatisfaction, then relax and allow our rich and powerful subconscious to bring us this best solution.

## ◉◉ Exercise 73 : To enhance your progress

In application of qualities developed in this book,

- The Balance;

- The driving force, and the multiplying effects of, motivation, positiveness, initiative, and self-gratification;

- Benefits of loving oneself, with comfort and lightness and without pretentiousness, shame or hindrance;

- Enjoyment and fruition, from the preferred choice of action contributing to the achievement of an objective;

- Self-observation, and, self-knowledge;

- The benefits of clarifying and nurturing the intention,

here are two examples, of the tools I used, in my project of writing and publishing this manual, to follow and to improve the results of my work.

These examples will help you to develop your own tools for monitoring progress in your projects, and for building dynamic of happiness and success.

## First tool :

I started to write on a daily journal the accomplishments of the days.

I cultivated the satisfaction for the quality and the quantity of the accomplishments.
And time to time I could return to the journal and further cultivate satisfaction when reading it (as we already saw, the satisfaction energizes further progress).

I paid attention to have stable days, equilibrated with components of happiness in body, in mind and in action. And to monitor this optimal use of my time, I used the five icons listed on the following page. There is a big number of different combinations of icons (exactly 3125) depending on the physiognomy of the day, much more than we need.

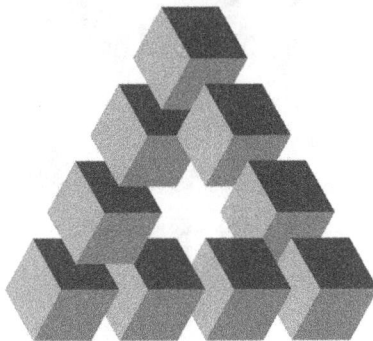

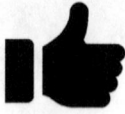

This icon to represent achievements in my project.

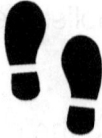

This icon to monitor relaxing physical activities (usually walking in nature, collecting mushrooms in the forest, or swimming in a lake).

This icon to signify activities or event enriching my intellectual knowledge. (meditation being one activity represented by this icon).

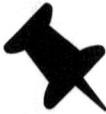

This icon to represent the necessary administrative or domestic tasks that I strive to make happy moments.

This icon to represent family, friends, entertainment and relaxation.

In my daily journal of the accomplishments of the days, I added five columns, in which I inserted a combination of icon representative of day.

Usual combination was: 👍 👍👍 ‼ 💡
to signify a fruitful day for my project (with qualitative or quantitative achievements, often both), with a time for physical exercise, a time for intellectual enrichment (including social media, arts, entertainment and meditation) and a time for administrative (not project related) or domestic task.

To make the game even more fun, I added a parameter. Some days, the progresses of the book project were better than other days. And sometimes progress was particularly great. To cultivate my satisfaction and enthusiasm, I began counting and collecting this particularly advantageous progress.

For each, I added a green background to the icon 👍.

I made sure to use these green funds for legitimate reasons. And I noted these reasons on my journal.


Then, I got very good surprises!

Days started to happen, when I put three green backgrounds. And the day after these days, I had the happy surprise of being able to put again three green backgrounds (amazing and unexpected! Another fantastic day!). Such great surprises multiplied.

In addition to being very amusing and surprising, it was very exciting, satisfying, effective, productive, dynamic and motivating.

The performance had given rise to a taste for performance. The use of this new parameter created an additional inertia of progress, success and joie de vivre.

I started to live less and less days, when I was not fully satisfied; Then, I even managed to eliminate such days. I became, a different person, happier, more active and healthier.

Sometimes, I was surprised, I met a slight difficulty in recognizing myself, in this new panoply. But the discomfort was brief, and I got used to it, because instantly I remembered my goals, to live, fully and happily, and to maintain my curiosity and my openness.

Happiness firmly settled into my life.

Playing with this tool and with the second one, and focusing on my goal, I could progress while transforming, durably, doubts, fears, sterility and dissatisfaction, into, confidence, love, fertility and happiness.

## The second tool :

On another sheet, I listed and updated the tasks remaining.

And after finishing one, I could choose from this list, more or less respecting priorities, the new tasks that attracted me the most at time.

Systematically writing new ideas of task, allowed to not forget any of these new ideas carried away by the win. This also allowed, to keep this tool much alive, and to perform a big number of tasks toward achievement of my goal.

It could happen that some days I was not very enthusiastic at focusing on any task. Then, I took the habit to give my attention to start a task picked up from the list, and I realized, with great pleasure, at the end of the days, that these days have been among the most enjoyable, productive and fruitful ones. When the initial feeling was, these days are going to be sterile, or even sad, they end up becoming 12 hours of happy focus and love to be alive.

This allowed me to build the intention, to live exclusively satisfying days, shaped with occupations carried by the dynamic Body-Mind-Action. I verified that I was far happier when focusing on doing things that were bringing me the greatest satisfaction, and de facto doing less of these things that were bringing me lesser satisfaction. So, I looked at the ways to find the greatest satisfaction in all I was doing (Including in domestic or administrative tasks that before could easily arouse lassitude or disgust in me), allowing me to find the happiness of having my days and my life well filled.

## 070 - GUIDE to see best always being done

We do the best we can, at any time.

When we intend to do well, then we do the best we can at that time.

If we are making progress; it may be not the perfect one, but we are learning how to sharpen our intention, and we are learning to shift our focus to maintain satisfaction of progress and to eliminate frustration from imperfections.

If we make mistakes, they surprise us, because we thought we were truthful, we were certain to succeeded, but we were not able to think and to do otherwise, because we did not know yet how to function properly.
It is entirely normal, that with the experience we acquire every day, we increase our ability to succeed. We are more capable today than yesterday.

When we are not able to intend to do the best, it is also, now, the best we can do. The next moment will be different, and maybe it will be the moment when we will have gain sufficient experience and capacity to be able to have that good intention. Maybe today we are finding the trigger allowing us to improve our happiness, our efficiency and our liveliness.

This teaching is very powerful. It is also very comforting because it avoids the painful and disabling sensation of regrets, loss of self-esteem, stress and depression. We perceive then that it is totally useless to feel bitterness for past mistakes.

When we integrate this concept, our thinking is more capable of progressing. We develop our ability more easily, to learn from our mistakes, and to avoid repeating them. We can also, more easily, come out of difficult times, during which we lack the desire to act. This truth also allows us to be more indulgent towards the mistakes of others.

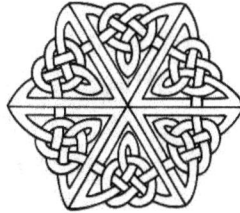

This powerful truth takes its full power, when it is associated with our anchoring efforts in the present moment, which is the only one that exists, the only moment we act, and therefore, the moment when we do the best that it Is possible to do.

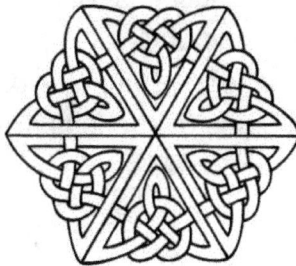

## 071 - GUIDE to develop self-esteem

To lower self-esteem, is a tendency often observed in the behavior of everyone.

The value of not lowering self-esteem, is a value that is taught in very varied fields, such as for Communication, Marketing and Personal Development.

For example, in conversations, we often hear phrases like "I feel incapable of doing that.", "I'm awkward.", "I'm not good at ...", I I'll never remember that. ',' That's really not my specialty. ',' I've always been nil at that. ',' That's a guy's job. ',' That's a girl job. ',' I'm too small to do that. 'Or' I'm too old to do that. ',' It's too complicated ',' I do not have time' and so on. These expressions freeze our personality thus artificially devalued.

Other examples of common expressions are showing underestimation of one-self, lack confidence and disbelieve in success: when we are using the verb 'to try'. As for example, in 'I will try to set up a company of ...'. Here, the person wants to express that she has made the decision to set up this company. But the use of the verb 'try' expresses fears and doubts about her commitment to achievement and the success of the company. These underlying fears and doubts are paradoxical, as they intervene even, in cases, where the commitment is very strong, and the first signs of success are encouraging.

Similarly, in the expressions: 'I will try to stop smoking '. 'I'll try to stop drinking sodas or alcohol' 'I'll try to be less shy'. It is preferable in these examples to think and say, 'I'm building a business ...', 'I quit smoking on January 1', 'I do not drink alcohol,' or 'I decided to be less shy'.

In general, the thoughts and ideas that are expressed in a grammatical negative sentence, have a negative character. As another example: it is better to say 'I can meet you in 15 days' rather than 'I could not meet you before 15 days'. It is also preferable to use conjugation in the present time, which is more real and dynamic, rather than the conditional time which expresses the condition, for example it is preferable to say, 'I wish to meet you' rather than ' I would like to meet you.

These beliefs, expressions, identifications, erroneous conceptions of politeness and habits, often come from our childhood.
They can also be cultural traits.
They imprison or limit our potentials.

Similarly, Marketing studies, advise against using negation in slogans and advertising campaigns. And personal development teachings place an important place on the development of self-esteem and the struggle of underestimating oneself.

You will benefit from exploring in your thoughts, your conversations and your writings the possible uses of such phrases, and all the qualifications you attribute to yourself with severity and belittlement.

This exploration will first enable you to realize this defect, which you can then systematically replace by cultivating your confidence and love of yourself.

This exploration will have to be durable, so that you manage to correct your bad habit to underestimate yourself.

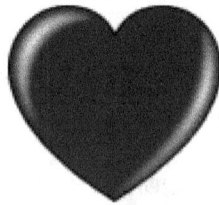

Have no fear, in this process, about the risk of overestimating yourself. On the one hand, this fear is also a way of belittling you. On the other hand, a dose of overestimation will not hurt you, as underestimation does. You can even play with the overestimation and with the feeling of pride; It will be beneficial for you to cultivate a certain pride, while being safe with realism and humility; Like the pride of what you do, the pride of a task accomplished, the pride of a skill you have, and the pride of life you lead.

Just as when, you cultivate love for yourself, be patient in this very important process of cultivating your esteem; You will have to seek confidence, lightness and comfort, and to avoid pretension and shame;

You will become a different person that you will have to learn to know, to accept and to esteem.
You will have confirmation that you are progressing well in this evolution, at the time when you will feel the happiness and a natural comfort to have a good esteem of yourself, and you will then be able to continue evolving in this direction.

◆

'Until you value yourself, you won't value your time. Until you value your time, you will not do anything with it.'

M. Scott Peck

◆

'To love oneself is the beginning of a life-long romance'

Oscar Wilde

◆

*'You are very powerful, provided you know how powerful you are.'*

Yogi Bhajan

◆

*'The real difficulty is to overcome how you think about yourself.'*

Maya Angelou

L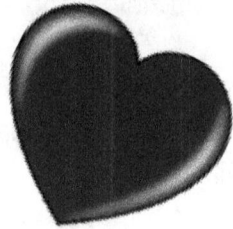

V E

## 👀 Exercise 74 : Hello beauty!

Every time you meet your eyes in a mirror, a showcase or in any other reflection, say to yourself:

' Hello beauty '

At the same time make a big smile, and feel a sincere esteem for yourself, joy, and the satisfaction of existing.

If you have some difficulties, to sincerely have these feelings, be even more diligent with the practice.

Practicing and renewing this technique will bring you immediate and lasting happiness. Together with increasing your self-esteem, you will also increase (with the help of an increased production of neurotransmitters) your confidence, your efficiency, your joie de vivre, the quality of your relationships with others, and your success.

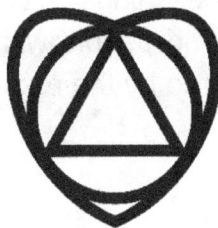

## 072 - GUIDE to be on time

I remember a popular saying, addressed to me, when I was a teenager: 'Only people who have nothing to do are late'.

I had at the time, found this reflection relevant, because I was late, and indeed it had been by negligence, because I had nothing else to do. In the years that followed.

I continued to observe my behavior on this subject, and I realized that, if it happened to me (seldom, because I do not like it) to be late, it was most often by the same negligence, when I had nothing to do.

Apart from the rare people who already master the art of not judging hastily, the ones you meet, make a first opinion of you, based on the only items immediately available, such as your appearance, your look, or the character of your hand shake.

Another basic element of judgment is your punctuality.

Each person, whether she is busy or not, gives much value to her time. Or rather, everyone has a hard time accepting someone wasting their time. Your punctuality gives the image of a person you can count on, a person who is organized, and who does things on time. Be punctual brand and inspire respect. And people with whom you have an appointment are flattered by the respect you are showing.

Arriving to an appointment at the right time, is also a success, which gives you a personal satisfaction.

Your delay gives the opposite image. When you are late, and consequently in a hurry, it creates stress in you. This also creates stress in the person who is waiting for you once the scheduled time has passed. This is not in favor of the quality of your appointment (and may even make you miss an opportunity). If at your job, you are regularly late, you will be blamed for your lack of reliability, productivity and legitimacy. A delay is also felt as the failure to be punctual. It can be a punishment you are giving to yourself. Well, it can happen to be late, for a good and exceptional reason. Then, the best practice is to warn the person you must meet, and that you are fully available, as soon as the meeting finally begins.

If you are regularly late, it is highly desirable that you correct this trend, which is a handicap for the smooth running of your life and for your happiness.

♦

*'Better three hours too soon than a minute too late'.*

William Shakespeare

♦

*'Method is the very hinge of business, and there is no method without punctuality.'*

Richard Cecil

Here are some tips to make your punctuality easier:

- Plan and coordinate your activities. Where necessary, priority is given to important activities.

- Uses the alarms functions of your mobile phone.

- Go with sufficient lead (even take a margin of safety). Once you arrive at the place of your appointment use your possible time in advance to make some deep breaths, to relax, to concentrate and to think of your appointment.

- For an important appointment (if possible) mark in advance the place of your appointment.

♦

*Punctuality is the first step towards success.*

Nishtunishaa

♦

*'I never could have done what I have done without the habits of punctuality, order, and diligence, without the determination to concentrate myself on one subject at a time'*

Charles Dickens

## 073 - GUIDE to schedule the next day

Knowing the day before, your program for the next day, you will sleep better, and as soon as you wake up, your day will begin in a more fluid, dynamic and efficient way. You will be able to plan activities that satisfy equilibria between your work, and your physical and mental health.

A few pages ago, we saw the technique of the 30 seconds, during which you will immerse yourself in the well-being and in the power of the present moment. Upon awakening, you will be able to use this technique to immerse yourself in the prospects of comfort, efficiency and pleasure that your scheduled activities are going to bring to you.

If your program of the day includes an activity that will require a great deal of concentration, during these 30 seconds you will be able to cultivate your trust in your optimal availability, clarity of mind and efficiency.

If your program of the day includes an activity, a priori daunting, you will, during these 30 seconds, cultivate your priority choice to live happiness, serenity and vivacity. Visualize yourself doing this activity while living these states. Also visualizes the benefits and satisfaction of the outcome of the surly activity carried out.

You will seek to maintain your positive thoughts, beyond 30 seconds, until you live an entire positive day.
This 30-second technique, of positive thinking and conditioning, when waking up, is very effective to optimize the profile of your day.

Conscious breathing is still an ingredient you can add, and that will allow you, during these 30 seconds, to optimize and to vivify your confidence, your availability, your clarity of mind and your efficiency.

◆

Again, and always, you will be convinced of the effectiveness of the technique, only after practicing and feeling the dynamics of its components, body-thought-action, balanced.

◆

If you needed extra motivation to start practicing the attitudes described in this technique, let's see the effects of practicing the contrary attitudes: when awakening, you begin to cultivate perspectives and sensations, doubts, confusion, reduced breathing, painful constraints or failures, they will persist, and they will continue to influence, your mood and the events of your day.

It is equally advantageous, to prepare the day before, the clothes you are going to wear the next day, and the things you will need.

This advice seems simplistic and innocuous, yet, when I applied it, after having received it myself, I could taste its great advantages. By adopting this simple mode of operation, you also ensure greater efficiency, by avoiding stress at the beginning of the day. You also reduce the inherent risks and disadvantages of being late, forgetting something, or deceiving yourself.

Again here, is an example of being happier by avoiding what makes us unhappy. It is also, an example on how simplifying life is bringing happiness.

And we continue to cultivate our happiness, adding up the happy moments and subtracting the unfavorable moments.

◆

Programming for longer durations, than only one day, is also beneficial. Similarly, we are more comfortable and more efficient in our body in action, in complete freedom, fully engaged, without the concern of knowing whether we are right to do this activity, since we have already decided, and since we will verify it. We are more efficient, in the defined succession of activities framed. And we are then, also freer, more efficient and happier in the other programmed activities (private and professional).

◆

*'A goal without a plan is just a good wish'*      St Exupery

◆

'If nature is called abundance, the society must be called providence'.

Victor Hugo

◆

*'The foresight of evils is the great art of weakening them before they arrive.'.*

Voltaire

◆

*'Plan your work and work your plan'*      Napoleon Hill

## 074 - GUIDE to stop the excuses

The normal process of the mind, when one has the idea of undertaking an activity that is deemed to be good and realistic for us, is, at first, to feel excited, joyful and dynamic. Then, immediately, in a second stage, the mind sets in motion, and, finds a whole list of bad reasons and excuses, for not undertaking this activity. Then, possibly through ease or fear, one rejects or abandons the idea.

It is important that you observe this normal process of mind activity, and to realize that it is working that way.

Then, you can undertake another mental process, which consists, after this second period of fear and doubt, to explore again the parameters of the idea, to re-evaluate your good reasons for undertaking this activity, the way in which you will operate, in an objective manner the obstacles that could possibly be encountered and whether these obstacles can be crossed.

Then, you must be bold, and engage in the activity, with total confidence, or being comfortable accepting a dose of unknown.

Your experience will be enriching, it will enable you to achieve our objective, or it will give you new information for new objectives.
You will observe that events, opportunities and actions are linked, are flowing together and bring you satisfaction.

If, on the contrary, you stop, at the excuses or fears, nothing happens, only dissatisfaction persists. And, as excuses and fears are part of the normal process of thinking, and intervene for each of your ideas, you may find yourself stagnant, frightened and paralyzed, constantly, and for a long time.

## Measure your excuses

You are now invited to observe, realize, reflect and react on the normal process of thought for each new idea: excitation - contradiction - excuse.

Begin with the concrete example that currently holds your heart. So rather than yielding to the ease of the excuse that immediately makes you abandon your project or your resolution, you can continue to analyze ideas, measure their feasibility, and watch them developing. You will correct the illusion, that the excuse brings you comfort, well-being and security, while it brings you the opposite. And you will enjoy the happiness that action gives you.

Seek to analyze your motivations every time you give yourself an excuse.

As if, from now on, an excuse is triggering an alarm signal to start your reflection.

## 👀 Exercise 75 : Love or Fear

There are only two basic feelings, love and fear. And all the other feelings are flowing from one of the two. This is perhaps a new fact for you, that may require your meticulous reflection.

It is a very strong reality.

Think about it, analyze your feelings in defining your choices of behavior, relationship and action.

You will be able to dispel many fears, to engage in avoided activities, and to carry out your activities with love.

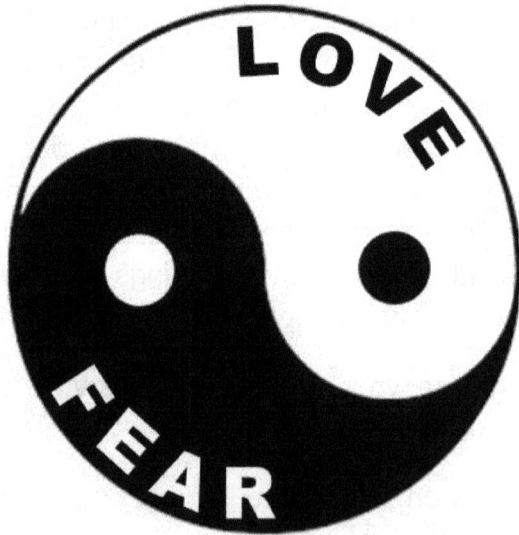

## 075 - GUIDE to give and receive

Knowledge of the principle of giving before receiving is present in many traditions. This truth is very vivid in Asia, but in the West, although it remains present, it is a truth that seems forgotten or even illogical and improbable.

Yet this truth is easily demonstrable, with examples like friendship, love, a smile, help, respect, attention, compassion or esteem; It is also verified that the best way to learn is to teach. It is also a truth that is verified, by its opposite (something that one does not give, one is unlikely to receive it in return). This truth also applies for our negative behaviors, such as, for example, violence, disrespect, hatred, which one sees escalating, following the same principle: I give you - you give me back, then I give you back, and I give also to someone else - and so on (again, the butterfly effect, the cascade effect and the snowball effect are on, and they are going to travel a long way).

There are of course the emotional, social, moral and spiritual benefits gained when one gives, but the benefit is also material. And it is love and emotions (our emotional body balanced with our action) that allow the boomerang effect of the gift.

You can have fun experiencing it, with the following Exercise (86), and see that it works.

By being attentive to this mechanism, which gives an order to the events, you will be able to influence a positive unfolding of the events, and to improve your existence.

Naturally, the events are predominantly positive. It is this majority that allows the functioning of the universe. Without this majority, chaos and self-destruction would have been dominant. Through your actions and thoughts, you have the power to energize the positive process of your existence. This power also works, in most of cases, however, it is dangerous and erroneous to consider this power as infallible. The reality is very different.

Similarly, matter, with its constant proportions, is ordered. Science has also allowed us to understand that matter can be chaotic, but with a statistical order (Chaos Theory).

Synchronicities also indicate that events can be ordered. (Remember, reality of synchronicity is not debatable, after the case documentation begun by Carl Gustave Jung.)

(The phenomenon of synchronicities is difficult to understand and to believe, when one has never experienced it. And in this case, it is even more interesting to be attentive and to experience the phenomenon.)

It is also not debatable that our actions and our positive thoughts favor the success of our actions.

However, we must beware, of believing that the success resulting from our actions and our positive thoughts are infallible, or that one can succeed while excluding the action, or else that one can receive without giving. The believe of infallibility, is false, inconsistent, and irresponsible. For reality is not conceivable, without both failures and successes, which can only exist with one another. Without the inevitable difficulties of life, we could not recognize the favors and the simple and ecstatic happiness of life, and we could not make the progress that leads to success. However, it can be disconcerting to observe, in some circumstances, the possibility of modifying our reality in an extraordinary way, by the quality of our thoughts and emotions (as, for example, in Exercise 87, "The world is beautiful").

Cultivating the components of your triangular body-thought-action dynamics will be much more useful for achieving the successes you desire. While becoming comfortable, with the surprising mechanisms of, the synchronicities, and the dynamics of positive impulses, and with acceptance of, the delays due to failures, and of the impossibility to apprehend the absolute.

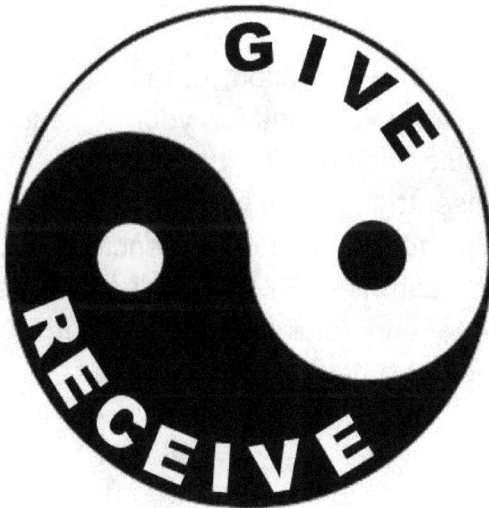

## ☻☻ Exercise 76 : 5 Experiences

**Experience 1:**      The dynamic 'giving - receiving' is logical in some cases. But it remains difficult to believe, if one has not experienced it, that this dynamic may have an extraordinary dimension (comparable to the extraordinary synchronicity).

With this exercise, you will be able to experience this extraordinary dimension. You will give your attention, and you will receive a favorable event.

o For a few days, during your free time, give your attention, and take notes, to a project that is close to your heart (details, atmosphere, actors, calendar ...). If you do not have a project in mind, start by writing a list of outstanding activities, and pick one.

o Without tense expectation, be attentive to a favorable and encouraging event for your project, or for your picked outstanding activities. When, the favorable event presents itself, you will recognize its extraordinary character, more than a coincidence or a chance, and you will be surprised. For example, it will be a perfectly appropriate and totally fortuitous meeting, or useful information or other timely events.

o When this event occurs, be not afraid or refractory, for lack of habit, observing this extraordinary character (as, for example, in my childhood, I was scared watching synchronicities). But on the contrary, be happy to admire, once again, the beauty of existence. This will allow it to expand, and to this kind of experiments to renew itself, with power and lightness, and to your advantage.

o   If you feel uncomfortable awaiting this favorable event, it will not happen, because your emotion is the sign that your project requires more reflection and maturation, or that your skepticism prevents this opportunity.

You'll have to think again, to cultivate your patience and your trust. And, to repeat the experiment.
Be confident, curious, open and patient, and give a chance to the experience.


**Experience 2:**     Adopting the same attitudes as in the previous exercise:     attention, observation and absence of expectation, doubts or impatience, you will note extraordinary events in return from a help that you give to someone, and in return from any other expression of your generosity.


**Experience 3:**     You will be attentive, to the return of a simple positive thought. This one is fun and subtle.


**Experience 4:**     You will be attentive, when teaching or when transferring knowledge, not only to the benefit of improving your knowledge, but also to this kind of extraordinary and favorable events.

## Experience 5: The world is beautiful

You will reserve the practice of this exercise, to the next time you are in a state of ecstatic happiness. It can be, at moments of immense happiness because of success.
In these moments, the world seems, more than usual, beautiful to you.

Then, observe the unusual events, in relation to your usual daily reality, the contemplations, the encounters and the occurring events. It can be: the joie de vivre expressed on the faces of many people you meet, laughter of children or adults, a rare opportunity to hear children talking to each other, synchronic events, a panorama, etc.

And become comfortable with these surprising mechanisms.

◆

*'Generosity is a mark of bravery, so all Sioux boys were taught to be generous*

Luther Standing Bear

◆

*'Honesty, sincerity, simplicity, humility, generosity, lack of vanity, ability to serve others - qualities within the reach of all souls - are the true foundations of our spiritual life'*

Nelson Mandela

*'Hatred must be overcome by love and generosity'*
De B. Spinoza

◆

*'Generosity means giving without expecting anything in return'*
E. Banovac

◆

*'To be born is to receive an entire universe as a gift'*
Jostein Gaarder

◆

*'The true generosity toward the future*
*Is to give everything in the present'*　　　Albert Camus

◆

*'We make a living by what we get, but we make a life by what we give.'*
Winston Churchill

◆

*'For it is in giving that we receive'*　　　St. Francis of Assisi

◆

*'Of the various kinds of intelligence, generosity is the first'*
John Surowiecki

◆

'Abundance comes from generosity'　　　　　D. Mridha

## 076 - GUIDE to consume intelligent

It was quite normal and legitimate to be excited when our first vacuum cleaner, washing machine, electric iron or our first car, made it possible to simplify a long and tedious task, leaving us more time for better activities. Similarly, when our first television or our first trip, opened a wonderful window, in our boring daily lives.

It was also quite logical that, faced with this craze for consumption, traders were eager to sell, as much of their products, as possible. What is no longer logical, but irresponsible, is when short-term profit is planned, knowing that it is going to jeopardize long-term profit.

The consumer society offers many temptations for all ages. Thus, one observes, capricious children and adults who think they can only be happy, after having bought this or that thing. We, also, often see, dusty things on the shelves, which had been so much desired and so quickly forgotten, almost immediately after they had been possessed.

These things acquired capriciously and irrationally, have been to the detriment of something else more useful. The money, that allowed to buy this useless thing, and the effort to earn that money, was spent in vain, wasted. Our disproportionate consumption affects our wallet, our environment (with the environmental footprint of production and waste) and our happiness. While adopting intelligent consumption, it is possible to correct this unfortunate development of our society. We now have the knowledge and the means to consume and to produce without polluting. This will be achieved through information, behavior changes, innovations and opportunities, by producers and consumers.

We can rely on the powerful evolution process of the consciousnesses we are currently experiencing, the power of ideas, and the instantaneous propagation of mass information on a planetary scale, to soon reach this ideal. We can also consider, becoming strong enough, to force our legal Human Rights to be endorsed.

**Improve your consumption**

Review your consumptions (food, water, gas, electricity, transportation, accommodation, culture and recreation), list the improvements you can make, considering your better health, your budget and the preservation of the environment. Implement these improvements.

It should be remembered, that it was only after the first oil shock in 1973, that a great deal of thought was put into place to avoid waste of energy (insulation of homes, reduction in electricity consumption, reduction of the fuel consumption of the cars, etc.). Before that, because these consumptions did not represent a large part of our spending, we used to waste a lot.

Having lived in the 1990s in several countries of the former USSR, where gas and electricity were billed very cheaply, it was similarly striking to observe, in the middle of winter, the enormously heated houses, with the windows remaining opened all day.

## 077 - GUIDE to travel

I lived for some time, in the country, in a charming little village, populated by only 160 inhabitants.
One day, in 1986, I was discussing things and others, with my kind neighbor.
She said, 'No, I never saw the sea. And I do not want to.' When you see what is happening ! '.
As, I had already traveled a lot, this comment was quite surprising and amusing.
My neighbor, had lived, in another time. An era, where it was normal, to spend a life without leaving the borders of the village or the region.

Today, transport is easy and fast. The world is now compared to a village.

Whether traveling to another village, another region, another country or another continent, travel is rich in experiences. We meet some very interesting people.
These encounters can have a magical side, in the sense that we are amazed to know things that we did not know before; And often we encounter people in unexpected circumstances, and it turns out that these people allow us to answer, with exactness, a question which trotted in our heads on the preceding days; Or, we meet exactly the person who will solve our current logistical problem.
Lifestyles and cultures are very different, from one place to another, and being exposed to it makes it possible to realize that life is much more than what we are accustomed to.

We also realize that people with customs and resources very different from ours have the same needs, the same questions, and the same feelings than we have, whereas in our sort of isolation, we thought having exclusivities. Together, it is much easier to find answers, lessons from the present experience, and sharing past experiences.

We realize, how unusual experience produce unusual results. We come out of our shell and we realize that it is good we did.

## To plan for a travel

Finance is not an obstacle to travel, because there are many ways to travel cheap, and even, spending, as much as, in everyday usual life.

Do not be scared at the idea of traveling alone, as traveling alone, is recognized, as being the most interesting and most conducive to interesting encounters.

If an opportunity to work, in a place far from your present residence, presents itself, seize it, without fear. You will be very happy to enrich your life. And, you will benefit from, the famous benefit of getting out of its comfort zone.

Now, plan a trip, short or long distance, for a short or a long time. Go to discover new shores. Go to make new discoveries.

## 078 - GUIDE to gift

What a joy to give and to receive gifts!

A carefully chosen gift; Or even, simply a drawing made quickly by a child; Or the help that one gives to a friend and the one received from him.
A gift carefully chosen, and long appreciated, or an improvised gift that lasts for a short moment, produces a great happiness.

In fact, a large amount of happiness surrounds a single gift! The donor's pleasure, when he imagines the special gift, then when he offers it, then when, he thinks about these two pleasures, and revisiting and sharing again the happiness with the beneficiary. The happiness of the beneficiary, when it receives it, and whenever seeing the gift, he rethinks to the love shared with the donor.

In these moments of happiness surrounding the gift, donors and beneficiaries, will feel a pure love, a wish for the best things for the other, feeling the ecstasy of the best moments spent with the other, without any thought of regret or hope does interfering and tainting the love.

The stimulant of the ceremonial (which will be seen in the Guide of the Still Position), marries very well gift giving. It can be a nice packing, or a staging.

As seen in the next exercise, making gift can be helpful.

## ☻☻ Exercise 77 : Free and valuable

This exercise will not only allow you to practice giving gifts, but also to empty your head, your cupboards, your shelves and your attics of things that are no longer useful to you, things that you never finally used, and even things that are hurting you (reminding you of bad memories). It will also allow you, to make room, for more freedom and for new ideas. It will allow you, to enjoy the lightness of the refined decoration of your lodging, or else, the space freed will be filled with objects carrying new joys and new memories.

In this exercise, gifts, will not require financial expense, but only a happy use of your time.

o   Look in your storage, for those things that are not useful to you, and for things that needlessly remind you of painful events.

o   With each new thing found, ask yourself the question to know to whom this object could please.

o   Then, act on it, and surf the wave of the gift happiness.

o   Back home, surf the waves of happiness, seeing your clean environment, enjoying your simplified life, and discovering news events replacing painful and useless memories, including the joy of the gift beneficiary.

o   Surf with the exercise at regular intervals, doing spring cleanups.

## 079 - GUIDE to rub children & seniors

While children learn from adults, adults also have a lot to learn from children. This second truth is often ignored. Indeed, it is beneficial to seize the opportunities to listen to the individual, brilliant, natural and singular arguments of each child, as well as the prospects of their still unconditioned innocence. It is also good, to be able to benefit from the qualities, the specific life experiences, of the older people. In fact, it is beneficial to seek opportunities to exchange points of view, with all generations other than ours.

Sure, to spend more time with your own children or parents. And, for example, to communicate with people of all ages during community activities.

You will also seek, to promote the opportunities, for various age groups, to express themselves.

As we have seen in the technique of brainstorming, the people of each generation will share ideas and perspectives unknown to other generations.

As, in our present-day, generations are experiencing far more changes than previous generations, the sharing of experiences, cooperation and updates is becoming more and more substantial, precious and beneficial.

Moreover, in their planning efforts, adults must ensure the participation of young people, who will be the ones who will live according to the plans.

Currently, from one generation to the next, children are more and more awake, capable and educated.

With the new longevity of our lives, with our dynamism and our physical form, which we are able to preserve for longer and longer, and with the face of the world of work that will significantly change in the years to come, seniors are increasingly available to participate, and to play important and changing roles.

This require, opened mind and capacity of adaptation, for all ages, to reach best practices and ease, in the changing roles and interactions.

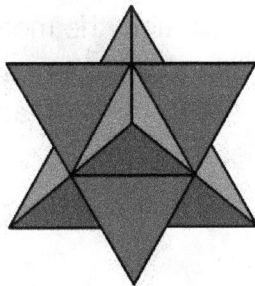

## 080 - GUIDE to smile and laugh

As happiness makes smile and laugh, smile and laughter bring happiness.

Indeed, when you smile or laugh, several muscles of your face contract. Try now, you will feel the muscles of your face contracting even to the ears. This combination of muscular contractions sends information to the brain. The response of the brain is to initiate the secretion of endorphin, the neurotransmitter of happiness, which acts on the opiate receptors. Thus, effects are produced, comparable to those produced by an opiate (including opium and morphine), happiness, which can go as far as euphoria, and the relief of pain.

Smile and laughter also increase the production of white blood cells and resistance to disease. These effects, which therefore have only a mechanical origin, and which are obtained, as well with artificial smiles and laughter, as with naturals. [29]

The more you smile and laugh, the more you will smile and laugh, as an addiction to happiness. Your face also changes, the smile is drawn and replaces the expressions caused by your worries.

---

[29] All the chemical reactions described during a smile on our face also happen when we happily see a smile on someone's face.

Smiles and laughter are contagious and enhance social and professional relationships.

When you laugh, contractions of the belly muscles facilitate digestion and relaxation.

We must look for opportunities to laugh and smile more often.

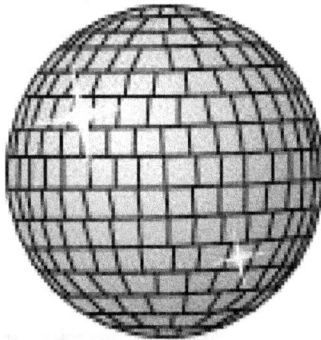

Optionally, we can add an extra dimension to the practice of the smile, as to that of laughter. It is to be considered that they are not only on our lips, but that we smile and laugh with the whole body.

## 👀 Exercise 78 : The trick of the car

Choose an event that occurs several times in your day. Like for example, every time you see a car from a specific well-known brand.

Then, make a beautiful smile, every time this event occurs.

Laughter is rarer than a smile. It is more difficult (and yet just as beneficial) to laugh artificially. Then, to practice artificial laughter, you will select an event that occurs less frequently. For example, you can choose a brand of car less widespread, and decide that every time you see a car of this other brand you will laugh artificially for a few seconds.

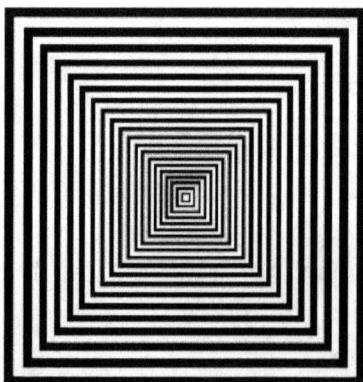

**Watch comedies**

I have great respect for people with a sense of humor, the right word at the right time, the ability to make people laugh. Whether these people are professional actors playing in movies, of course writers scenarios of comedies, or friends and encounters.

Seize the opportunities to see a comedy of good taste whether in cinema, theater, television, internet or social media.

(Avoid jokes of bad taste, because they are accompanied by a suffering that affects you).

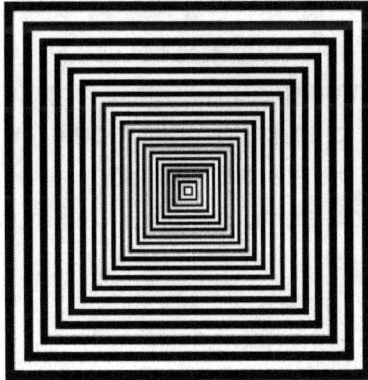

## 081 - GUIDE to rub shoulders

It is beneficial to seek to spend more time with family and friends.

Of course, it will not be here the chronically bitter relations that it is better to space. So, by definition the relationships that we will choose here as a priority, will bring us a singular happiness. These intimate, open and trusting relationships then allow for rich relationships that are catalysts of happiness.

## Some suggestions

- o Take interest in your children's homework.
- o Head to head with child and with your partner.
- o Family breakfast.
- o Reading and listening sessions
- o Activities during leisure time. (Going to a concert together, playing games, doing a picnic, regular or occasional practice of a sport or other exciting activity such as swimming, camping, biking, cooking together, climbing, going to pick mushrooms in the forest, take pictures and create an album or evoke memories by flipping through a photo album, visiting an exhibition).
- o Celebrations. Surprises.
- o Messages on pieces of paper.
- o Gifts (not just commercial).
- o Listening. Support. Debates.

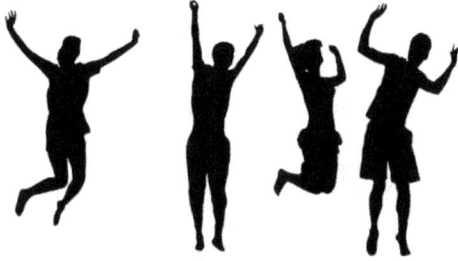

- A walk after dinner.
- Together, a commitment to a voluntary charitable activity.
- A phone call to a friend or relative (e.g. grandparents).
- Watch a sports competition.
- Go to the movies, or to the ice rink, do-it-yourself or gardening.
- Make a day picking blackberries and then make jams.
- Make a modeling project (such as building a glider aircraft and then flying it).
- Making a nap together.
- Hold together a notebook of memorabilia, such as admission tickets to the cinema or other leisure activities, train or plane tickets, a restaurant business card, sand grains photos, newspaper headlines, a postcard, a recipe for a new dish, wedding and baptism announcements, drawings, quotes, and anecdotes.
- Teaching your child how to drive a car.
- Together, listening to their favorite songs.

## 082 - GUIDE to celebrate

When we celebrate, we laugh, we see friends, we exchange ideas, we share good times and we meet new people. We make, unexpected experiences.

When you are a child, then a teenager, you have great ease and a great desire to party. As an adult, the occasions and the desires to celebrate are dispersed and sometimes even disappear.

It is important, for the sake of happiness, to preserve, throughout life, a light and festive heart. Parties are opportunities to experience lightness, innocence, joy and love. It is good to look for opportunities to celebrate, with family or friends, for various celebrations, renewing contacts with people lost from sight, celebrating the positive events of the day ...

We saw, that it was good for our happiness, to develop our community life, our family, friendly and professional ties. To do so, the celebrations are quite appropriate. These can be spontaneous parties or celebrations of promotions, birthdays, spring festival, music festival, themed parties, innovative festivals.

In the same way that we have seen before, and as with all relationships, put yourself in condition, before beginning the encounter, to be at the best of your energy, your positivism and your love. And, takes the resolution to maintain this optimal state throughout the party.

We also saw previously, the mastery of the art of knowing how to leave, in good conditions, and at the right time. You will benefit from practicing this art, when leaving a party, without any greed frustration for the ending good time that would spoil it, but as a culminating level of happiness. Also, making sure to thank your host or your guests for the good moment.

## Plan for a beautiful party

This exercise is for you to have a party soon. Now think about what party you could do and organize so that it will soon become a reality.

During your next parties, get used, little by little, adopting the new behaviors above

♦

*'The more you praise and celebrate your life, the more there is in life to celebrate.'*

Oprah Winfrey

♦

*'Celebrations infuse life with passion and purpose. They summon the human spirit.'*

Terrence E. Deal

## 083 - GUIDE to live with aestheticism

We can neglect to look after a corner of our home or workplace, which could be arranged, put in order or cleaned (because we have never given any importance to this discomfort, or we resigned to it, or we get used to it, or we are lazy to react). Whenever we look at this corner, consciously or unconsciously, we feel an embarrassment or a devaluation of our person.
Another corner is acceptable, but with a little effort and creativity, we could embellish it, and feel a pleasure, whenever our gaze arises on it.

The aesthetics of our places of life influence our ideas. Great or beautiful spaces are favorable to great and beautiful ideas; they promote our pride, the pleasure of our eyes, our valorization and our love of ourselves. On the contrary, a dirty or disorderly place favors lack of ideas or black ideas.

Thus, improvements in the appearance and cleanliness of your private and professional environments will bring you happiness.

In places where you usually spend time, makes storage, cleans (including, for example, inside your car), improves, embellished with decorative objects.

As you think about these possible changes, ideas will come to mind. Activate yourself to implement them.

These can be small things, that you will benefit quickly. Or tasks that will require more efforts. Anyway, just start the implementation of these embellishments. You will feel pleasure, working on the embellishment, at the sight of the finished work, and then every time your gaze will cross the improved place.

The effort is worth it, because your gazes are posed on these places several times a day.

Note also that your happiness capital will be increased when you take the habit of doing these 'domestic' jobs in joy rather than being depressed.

Note, finally, that, for the elements making the place beautiful, and for the elements making it ugly, as for all things, apply the addiction, the habit and the zone of comfort. So, you can suffer, and become complacent to suffering by living in a degrading place. Or on the contrary, become more and more happy, seeing the aestheticism of the place improve. You shall be attentive to this point, because you may, not consciously, be living in a not conducive environment for your happiness, while, a little action could significantly improve the situation, making you happier and more efficient in your life.

If you are living in a place totally lacking aestheticism, and there is no much you can do about it, still search regularly exposure with aestheticism, visiting parks and monuments.

## 084 - GUIDE to interact with community

Over the last fifty years our lifestyles have changed enormously. Urbanization has been galloping and has become a great transportation's time spender. Jobs have become more and more short-term, and we are increasingly changing jobs, sectors of activity, places of residence, even cities, regions or countries. Time spent on individual leisure activities (television, social media, electronic games, access to information) has increased significantly. Local commerce and relations with the local shopkeeper have greatly diminished after the appearance of supermarkets (in the 1970s).

While all these changes have their positive and negative side, they all correspond to a damaging scarcity of our community interactions. We spend less time with our friends or with our neighbors. There is also less mutual help. The lack of experience and the lack of diversity of experience, already seen previously, are still the cause.
By increasing our individualism and reducing live sharing, we are cowering, and we diminish the happiness opportunities.

It should be noted, however, that periods filled with satisfactory individual activities and experiences may, for the time being, justify isolation.

**Be proactive.** According to your possibilities and to your place of residence, now, begin to establish relations with your neighbors, the small proximity tradesmen, the clubs of your quarter, or the associations.
Then, naturally, let yourself being carried away by the dynamic multiplying this kind of activities.

See also if you can do training courses or become the initiator of a new community activity.

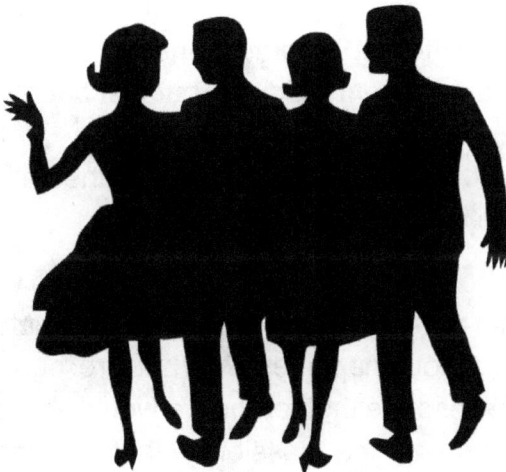

## 085 - GUIDE to make happiness a priority

Let us make sure, during our choices, to not forget the paramount parameter of our happiness.

Some of our choices may be motivated by what we feel as a necessity, desire, fear, ambition, someone else's opinion, habit, conformity, appearance, ease. Sometimes we are mistaken, thinking that our choices are motivated by love or responsibility; We are either blinded by desire and our actions are excessive, or on the contrary we feel constrained to limit our action. Sometimes even, none of this motivates us, our days pass, neither happy nor unhappy, without leaving room for a possible different choice. Or, on the contrary, ceaselessly, we cannot prevent ourselves from seeking a different choice, a different opinion or a different comment, never stepping back or really living the present moment, but just babbling.

Happiness is a good indicator during the reflection that precedes the choices.

Are we able to assess whether or not a choice will make us happy? What are our favorable choices and factors that are unfavorable to our happiness? What are our intentions? How can we describe the person we would like to become? Are we observing the possibility that we may lie and deceive ourselves? Is this other choice an unfortunate escape? Is this the moment to be happy? Simply because we may seek other ends, but we will find none better.

## 👀 Exercise 79 : Intuition

Our intuition is powerful. And, it is beneficial to develop it.

*Our thinking comes from*

*the surface of our knowledge.*

*It is often misleading.*

*Our intuition comes from*

*its totality.*

*It is wise.*

To develop intuition, you must start by using it and trusting it.

You can use your intuition starting by asking a question calmly, for example, when you have a decision to take. Then learn to listen to the answer. If the decision is legitimately urgent, listen to the instant intuitive answer. If it is not urgent, be confident that an answer will soon come to your mind at the right time.

Here, for example, is my experience of using intuition when writing this manual: during the first few months of writing, when I felt dissatisfied with the expression of an idea or another, it created a discomfort that could last several weeks. Little by little, I realized that each dissatisfaction was finally resolved, thanks to the discovery of the satisfying words. These words could appear at any moment, such as during a walk, at bedtime, or even in the middle of the night. Every time I was surprised, amused and happy to see this idea emerging.

Gradually, the confidence, that I will finally find the suiting words, grew, and I stopped feeling uneasy at such dissatisfactions. I had thus, the confirmation of the correctness of the functioning of my intuition.

This lived example of the use of intuition, can make it more comprehensible. It can also give you ideas to practice yourself, experience and develop your intuition.

Our intuition is naturally present and active.
But we cannot hear it without believing it, before perceiving when and how to listen, and becoming at ease newly using this capacity untapped till now.

After looking for this perception, we realize that it had very often accompanied us in the past. It is easier to listen to it in the present. And one is inclined to take the habit of listening to it.

It is quite good practice and good learning, leading to a mastery, in order to add the use of intuition to our ability.

For example, you can begin learning your intuition, with the simple, direct and practical technique, described in Exercise 20, intuitive diet, ask yourself the question 'What will I enjoy eating in what is available? '. Then exercise yourself freely, with pleasure and lightness, and without procrastination, to follow the first idea that comes to your mind. You will then be able to identify the nature of the intuition, this idea that comes to mind, without a priori or limitation.

♦

During the writing of this book, as an artist-author I could feel the immense pleasure of being the spectator of my work.

This feeling is often described by artists, because their activities are greatly, deeply and intimately creative and expressive.

However, the strong perception of this feeling, of being a spectator of my action, also allowed me to realize that I had already felt it during previous professional, social, leisure and domestic activities.

It is possible, for you, to make the same observation, to enjoy the same conclusions, gaining confidence, ease, inspiration, support and serenity. This observation will also allow you to better know yourself.

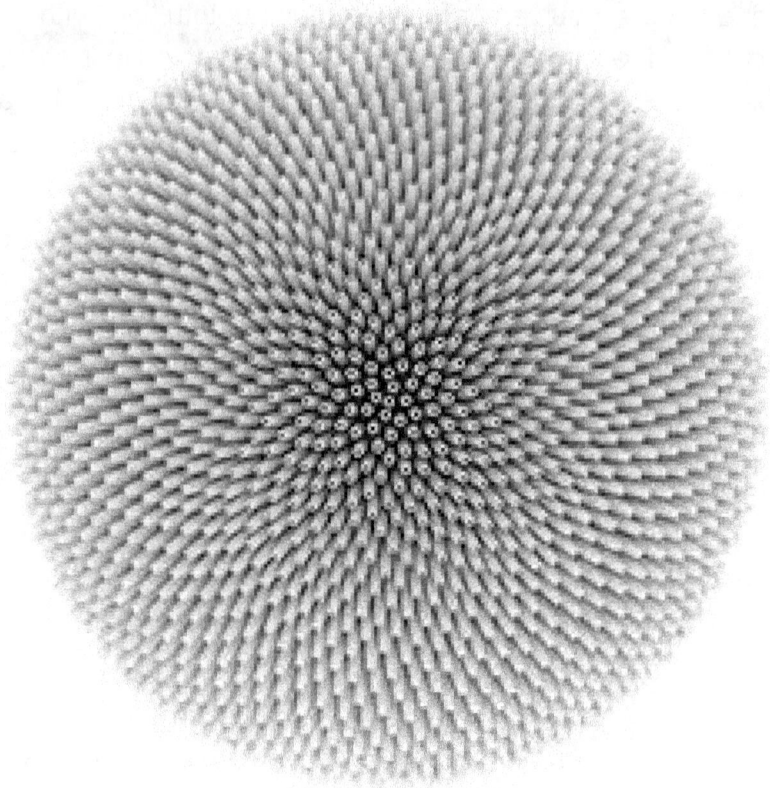

In this manual, you can find other examples of practices and uses of your intuition through questions, for which you will be able to practice listening to the answers that come to your mind, while measuring and by learning to know the emotions that accompany them. Such as :

o 'What is now the best choice, or the best thing I can do?',

o 'Is my certainty well founded?',

o 'I feel an uncomfortable emotion in relation to this solution. Is it incomplete? Is there a better solution? '.

o 'Is the value of my past day, good?' 'Do I make enough progress?',

o 'Is this friendly, loving or professional relationship good for me?', 'Do I have an opportunity to improve it?'.


As well as examples of perception facilitating intuition, such as:

o 'My breathing filled my body with life, deep down and strengthens my confidence',

o 'It is now time for me, to relax or rest, listen or contemplate?',

o 'I have to give time to time, so that things can evolve'.

## 086 - GUIDE to multiply gestures

Multiply the gestures that give happiness to strangers or intimates (you will find some examples on the following pages that will give you ideas. But, by paying attention to this kind of activity, you will find many other opportunities, during your days). You will easily observe that by these gestures you will be happier.

What would you have done instead of those moments of happiness? Probably you would have pursued your path, perhaps even unconsciously, inert or mechanical, rather than in a conscious, living and human way.

With the butterfly effect[30] each of our gestures, even the smallest one, generates a cascade of effects. A positive gesture produces a cascade of the same nature, the receiving person is inclined to give in turn. Small streams make great rivers. The lives of the donor and the recipient are transformed. Consider an additional positive gesture made by millions, or billions of people and the cascades of effects of these gestures, one arrives at a huge sum that creates a real difference[31].

---

[30] The flutter of a butterfly's wings in Brazil can cause a tornado in Texas. In relation to the first law of the Chaos Theory: very high sensitivity to the initial conditions, minor differences in the initial conditions lead to totally different results.
[31] With the globalization, we will, soon, be able to establish and to recognize a first international day of positivism that will have enormous repercussions.

It is also likely, that with this mechanism, someone, from this group that you initiated with your simple little gesture, will give you a gift of happiness in return, which promotes your next positive gesture by continuing to fuel this dynamic of change.

Perhaps you have already heard: 'When you make a positive gesture for someone you do it for yourself'? After verifying that this is confirmed with the Chaos Theory, we can see that quantum physics also confirms this assertion by demonstrating that the Universe is a single and entire energy field.

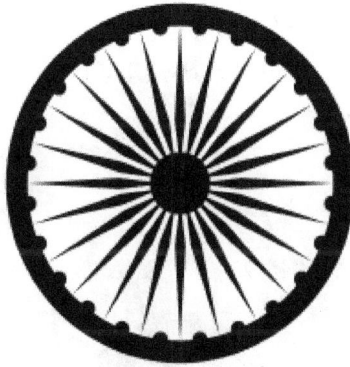

The opportunities to make better use of your time and your life by making gifts of happiness are many. Here are 4 examples :

## 1.  <u>Help to find the way</u>

By becoming more conscious, more alive and more attentive, during your travels, you will see more people who seem lost, or looking for directions on a map, in a place you know very well.

So, with confidence, generously offer your help to these people.

In most cases, the persons will be grateful. Others, will respond to your offer, with fear or even being unpleasant. Ask yourself, if these answers reflect your own lack of confidence, do not be affected, but be satisfied with this better knowledge of yourself and with the positive value of your intention; improves its accuracy and alignment, and continue to put it into practice.

Rather than a simple fleeting and punctual exercise you will have advantage to include this practice in your habits.

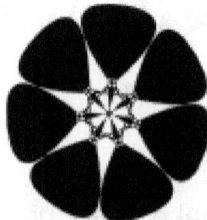

## 2. Blood donation

It turns out, that there is usually, a shortage in blood banks.

Giving blood requires a simple effort, which saves the lives of the victims of accidents.

If you have never given your blood, do it. You will then experience the pleasure of meeting devoted people and doing a good deed.

Probably even, will you have the good desire to renew this gift.

But no matter the probability of renewal, for you will find, already in this first gift, many satisfactions; And, thanks to a very large number of people making a first donation, the blood shortage will be of ancient history.

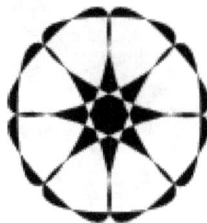

## 3.  Call a relative

Probably, you have not spoken, for a long time, to such lovely parent or lovely friend.

This exercise consists in calling him now, even without any particular reason, other than the pleasure of sharing, with love, availability, listening, and without embarrassment because of the time elapsed since your last discussion.

In passing, you will notice the pleasure of your interlocutor, first, when receiving your call, then, at this precise moment, when you say that you just call to say hello.

At the moment of saying good-bye, you will cultivate the art of leaving a conversation, without melancholy, and with the infallible ingredient of love.

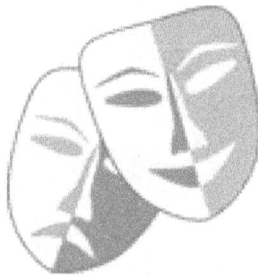

## 4. **Thank generously**

The words "thank you" have something like magical. When the thanks are done with a sincere feeling of gratitude, they bring a shared happiness. It is rewarding to seize the opportunities to say, "thank you".

It is likely, that in some cases, you would have the opportunity to say thank you, and yet, out of habit, you do not do it. As for example, to say thank you, to a bus driver who brought you to your destination; To say thank you to someone, who keeps a door from closing on you; To say thanks to a car driver who leaves you the priority to move on; Or, to say thank you, to a policeman who controls your papers (if it is not abused); Or, to any other official or trader, who does his job serving you.

Thankfulness, produces the same happiness cascade mechanism, as previously seen, generated by gift-giving.

♦

This exercise is for you, to increase the number of your thanks during the day. Have fun watching the people reactions when receiving your thanks, and the sparkle in their eyes in response to your sincerity. Renews this amusement frequently, and thus, takes the habit of enjoying yourself and living happily.

## 087 - GUIDE to play with the sacred geometry

We realized observing, calculating and taking measurements, that living organisms and matter, were constructed harmoniously, respecting constant forms and proportions.

We observed the same, in fractal convolutions, both limited and infinite, of elemental matter in motion; the structure of atoms; parts of the human body; minerals, animals, and plants; the form of tornadoes and typhoons, galaxies, and the cosmos; the mathematical representations of, the Universe and the Multiverse.

Sacred geometry represents these proportions and forms, and the development of matter from the beginning (big bang) of our universe represented in the center of the geometries. It is a point on which to focus one's attention and meditation. The whole, from periphery to center, representing the Universe.

We find the sacred geometry, from ancient Egypt. It was used by philosophers and mathematicians (including Plato and Pythagoras). It is very much to be found in art, (for instance, used by Nicolas Poussin and Leonardo da Vinci), and in architecture (including pyramids and many religious monuments), in many symbols, in all civilizations, and on all continents.

Sacred geometry, sometimes, has, sometime, a reputation of occult science, and magical practice. It is certainly rich, and one could study it for years, while continuing to understand new things, but, it is, by no means, an occult science or a magical practice. It is the representation of life and its development. It also contains many philosophical, cosmic, mathematical, and spiritual dimensions, if you are interested in studying them.

♦

Contemplating, sketching and coloring representations of sacred geometry, are very simple and enjoyable exercises, that bring to each and every one of us the same benefits as those that will be listed for the mandalas in the following exercise.

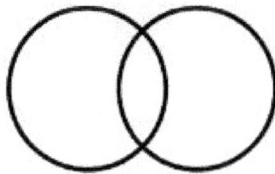

## 👀 Exercise 80 : Drawing or coloring

## 1. Drawing or coloring mandala

Mandala, is a Sanskrit term, meaning "circle". Mandalas are structured graphic representations, built around a central point, that have great aesthetic value and great symbolic values.

The uses of mandalas, consist either in drawing, contemplating or meditating. Some practices are famous, such as sand designs, in Tibetan practice, that are extremely sophisticated and aesthetic, taking days to be completed, to finally be scattered by the wind, in recognition of impermanence.

We find the same principles of the mandalas, in the rosettes, present in almost every cultures.
Mandalas are also used today in botany and permaculture to design gardens and vegetable gardens.

♦

Drawing, coloring and contemplating mandalas, or rosettes, is a relaxing exercise, which also allows a refocusing, which is especially useful, after life challenges.

Geometric and mathematical structures, proportions, perspectives and kinetics of the mandalas naturally favor our balance, concentration, creativity, efficiency, memory, intuition and discovery of solutions to our questions.

These exercises of drawing, coloring and passive contemplation of mandala, are likewise beneficial to your children, who taste even more easily their playful aspect, and spend a good, relaxing and instructive moment, especially building the balance of the two hemispheres of their brains. This same ludic aspect, which also brings to the adult, the value of retrieved innocence.

◆

You will find, in the following pages, the seed of life, and, the tree of life, search them on the Internet, then print them, take colored pencils and have fun coloring. You can also, highlight certain forms, or groups of form (petals or circles). Or even have fun, joining points, to form and then color triangles or stars. You can give these same instructions to your children, before leaving them free to explore their creativity and imagination.

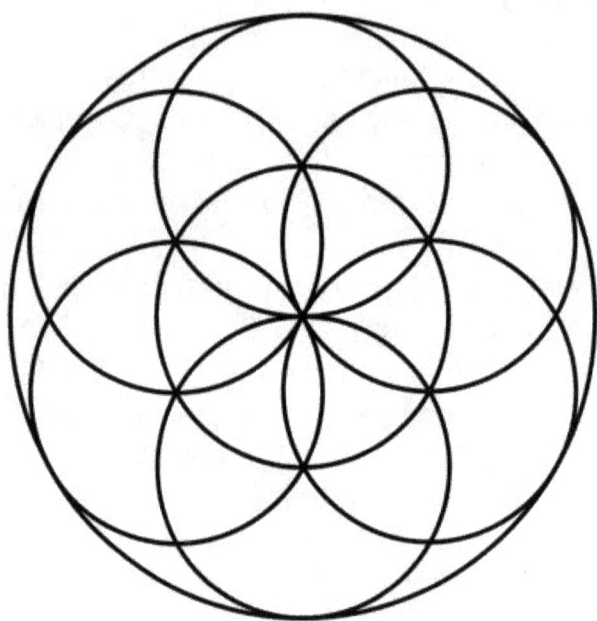

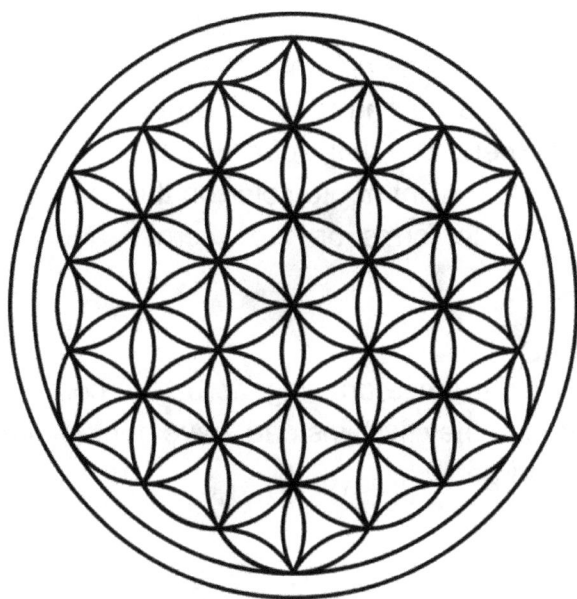

## 2. Draw or coloring geometry

You will find below and on the following page, the flower of life, and the cube metatron. Take colored pencils and have fun coloring them. The richness of shapes here is still very great, and you can still have fun to highlight with your pencil and to color, petals, circles, squares, rectangles, diamonds and stars. If you want not to color on this manual you can easily find these forms on the internet, and print them bigger.

Do not consider these drawings to be too complicated for your children, they will instead have fun, express their creativity and get rich.

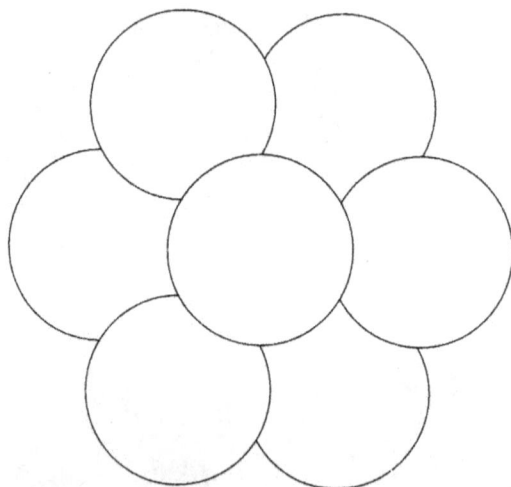

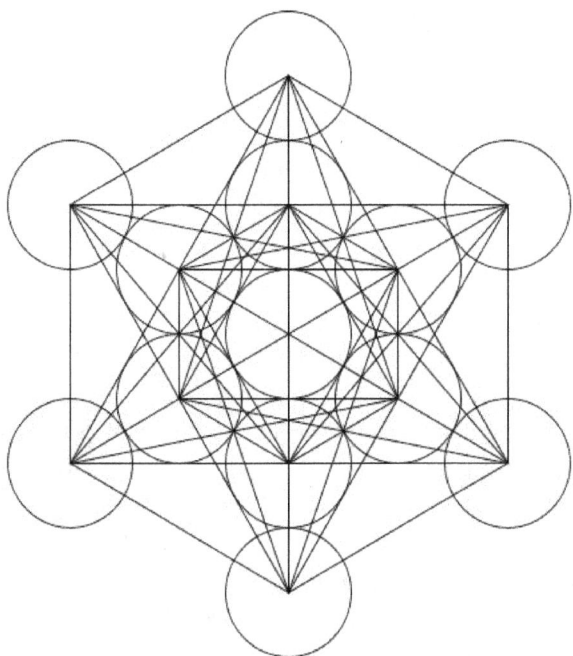

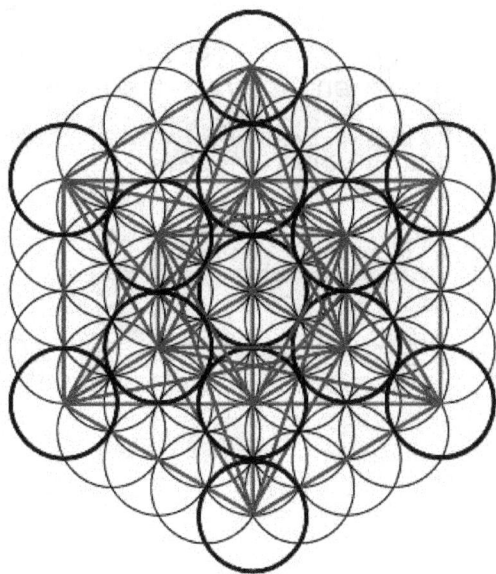

## 088 - GUIDE to keep updated

As changes are getting faster, it is increasingly important to keep us informed. We will give preference to the many positive information, avoiding or only flying over inconsistent bad news, and avoiding being exposed to the incessant repetitions of the latter.

Let us take advantage of our growing access to the whole of knowledge. Let us take advantage of variations in nuances in different cultures and traditions, in order to refine our understanding, of fundamentally identical concepts.

Let us commit ourselves to the adoption and application of practices that we believe in, are which are better than those we are currently experiencing. Let us be patient, persevering, and constant.

By taking advantage of the cultural wealth within our reach, our differences disappear and cease to be obstacles o our evolution. The poor and the rich, the black and the white, the woman and the man, are succeeding, after much struggle, to integrate their equities.

Knowledge, modernity and the sum of our individual improvements are materializing our ideals.

Read, watch videos, discuss about the good reasoned things that progress brings and about the good things that are going to happen soon. As, they will soon, greatly change our individual commitments and our ways of life.

## ๏๏ Exercise 81 : Every day

Every day, in the management of your time, make sure that you have learned something new by reading a book, an article, citations, having a discussion, looking for new things, new activities, Meeting new people, etc.

You will also be able, to include the memory of these new things learned during the day, when you review the positive things that happened during your day and which you are grateful for. You will often be amazed, to see how many good things have happened to you and which you have accomplished during the day. You will also be amazed, reviewing what you learned in a single day.

◆

*'If I had one hour to solve a problem, I would spend 55 minutes thinking about the problem and 5 minutes thinking about the solutions'*

*'The only thing you need to know is the location of the library'*

Albert Einstein

◆

*'Is better to know some of the questions than all the answers'.*

J. Thurber

## Interesting topics

Interesting topics are numerous. And we have the chance, with the internet, to have access to information on all subjects.

Here is a list of sample topics (you can also create and regularly update your own list of topics you would like to have more information about).

The exercise consists in choosing one subject, then another, which interests you in this list, and to get informed:

o Super high-speed Internet, soon hundreds of times faster than today. While, we are just beginning to use the internet, that will take a much bigger place in our lives, in the next few years.
o Artificial intelligence. What is it ? Why is it dangerous? What ethics should we establish? What are the prospects?
  Do we realize, for instance, that it will allow drones' autonomy, so as to be able to land anywhere and in all atmospheric conditions?
o The spectacular dance of Venus, showing the drawing of a flower by the course of Venus and the Earth.
o The model of the solar system, which we still learn at school, with the planets that revolve around the sun, is false (as in other times it was taught that the earth was flat). It does not consider the speed of the path of the solar system in space (70,000 km / hour). In reality, the planets rotate around the sun following a helical movement.
  (It can be noted here that despite the teachers' efforts, the school curriculum contains many errors, due to the slow updating of the programs)

- Nanotechnology and its many applications, particularly in medicine, also in many other fields (including food, cosmetics, clothing, energy, furnishings, equipment, environment (depollution), waste reduction, etc.).
- The pyramids, which are found all over the world and which constitute one of the greatest phenomena on a planetary scale. Special ordered locations drawing networks on entire planet, mysteries of construction, attributed properties, knowledge of astronomy contained in their constructions.
- The bee dance, giving to the hive, information for pollen harvesting (direction, distance and quantity of pollen allowing to define the number of bees having to go to the place of harvest).
- The Fibonacci suite. Description. Where is it found in nature, the arts, our anatomy?
- The disappeared civilizations, and their technological advances, proved by the archaeological discoveries. Here again, what one learns in school is false, especially the dating of the first civilization.
- Sacred geometry. Description. Where is it found in nature? In archeology? In art? In anatomy?
- Crop Circles. Photos showing their rich diversities. Pleasure of the eyes and mysteries (Non-conclusive attempts to reproduce the phenomenon, interpretation, etc.).
- The fractal structure of elementary particles, fractal objects in nature, cosmic spiral.
- Investments in renewable energies. Constant evolution.
- The Hyperloop train (actually under construction). 1200km / h. Such speeds greatly alter our notion of globalization.
- Electric cars and smart cars, in a few years they will be the only ones.
- How the 3D printer is changing our lives (innovation, production, consumption, medicine, etc.).

o Water desalination techniques, rainwater and air water harvesting, progress and prospects.
o What will be the (huge) place for robots in our lives? What systems are envisaged to adapt to reduced need for man to work (minimum wage is much praised)?
o What will be the (enormous) place of drones in our lives? (Agriculture, media, humanitarian assistance, environment, transport, medicine, etc.).
o The quantum computer. The information processed faster than the speed of light. The solution discovery prospects it offers.
o Project-based work. Announced as the mode of operation of tomorrow. We will have to get used to this new mode of work in short terms.

For some of the subjects listed above, you could deepen your knowledge but you will be able to simply watch, for a few minutes, with amazement, a video on U-Tube (It is the case for example for : The helical model of the solar system , The dance of Venus, The specificities of the pyramids, The sacred geometry in nature, The crop circles, The disappeared civilizations).

Other subjects are more technical, more specialized and require more concentration. For those, it will be good that you acquire a basic knowledge, as they will greatly change our lifestyles in the next few years (this is the case for: super high-speed internet, artificial intelligence, nano-technology, Robotics, 3D printer, renewable energies and "free" energies, and water desalination techniques).
The subject of the quantum computer, although it is the subject of much research, and although significant progress can be made at any time, seems more futuristic. However, it can become operational, at any time, and it will also, in an extraordinary way, change the course of mankind.

The subject of the evolution of the way we work, for a mode of operation "by project", is special. In the sense that, on the one hand, we are all concerned, and on the other hand the search for information on the subject is more difficult and would require more effort from you.

This evolution of the mode of work, is a projection, based on the study of the current evolution of the working mode of work. We are all concerned because it will change our lifestyles. Some of us are more concerned than others, such as young people who have to choose their career paths, or who are already engaged in the workforce, at the time of life when energy is at its maximum, and allows the choice of the best methodologies, or such as the older ones, who remember how to tap into the same vital energy, to fully live their lives by making the necessary adaptations. Some of us, however, are less concerned (such as craftsmen, liberal professions and civil servants), but this change in the way work, will still influence their ways of life, their ways of working and their tools.

Working "by project" means, that the duration and location of the employment contract corresponds to the duration of the project.

Many parameters are defined before the start of the project: for example, duration, budget, actors, subcontractors, objectives, risks and solutions to mitigate, results, resources, plan of action, mechanisms for monitoring progress, means of control, environmental impact and sustainability.

It is a mode of operation that allows a greater motivation of the actors, and that eliminates the routine lassitude of the work identical for a lifetime. This mode of operation itself will evolve considerably over the next few years, becoming more and more functional (simple to use and allowing for better and faster results) and allowing the inclusion of new parameters.

What can we do now?

It is enough for us, to think how to put in place our lives, our projects, and our choices of the world in which we wish to live in. As for the means to achieve this, we have just seen a list of several of the progress and discoveries, that will greatly help us, to which are added many other advances that are not listed, and the many to come. The progress we are making in our energy transition (clean energy, in large quantities and at a lower cost of production, making energy available and almost free of charge) will help to optimize further progress. Energy being life, we can choose, pushing the limits, the life we want to live.

We, that is, all men. There is a lot of work to do, for all of us. The amount of human beings on earth, is mistakenly called "overpopulation"; Population's number is not a problem, because comfort, automatically reduces the birth rate. And we have enough resources, to be able to comfortably accommodate a much larger number of people than we can never reach, it is just a matter of management. So, the people involved are all human beings, and this is an essential reality to understand and to integrate.

Let us begin, then, to reflect together, on this type world in which we desire to live. The comfort, we can have, we have enough resources to produce this comfort in the respect of the environment. Wars motivated today by the conquest of oil and gas fields and their transport routes, of course, we no longer need them. Health, we know how to optimize it and we are moving forward with giant steps to cure the incidents. The only course to be taken, is the intention to do things at best. Happiness, we begin to understand how to enable it; And we are already pleased to be engaged in this rich process.

We will also have the ideas and the means to adapt to climate change.

Maybe, do not you feel concerned by all these current advances, believing they cannot change your way of life, either thinking that you will see, in time, when it is happening, or that it is not even certain that these progresses will take place.

Undeceive yourself, you are quite concerned. These progresses are part of an unstoppable ongoing development. They are fast. And they will influence your choices. In the new world, your way of life will be very different, in only, a dozen years.

Developing your curiosity, will allow you to live these developments, to participate and also to see the opportunities, in the best conditions. Your life will be more interesting and happier; And you will have, more and more, good reasons to love yourself.

◆

*'The man who has not the habit of reading is imprisoned in his immediate world, in respect to time and space. His life falls into a set routine; he is limited to contact and conversation with a few friends and acquaintances, and he sees only what happens in his immediate neighborhood.'*

*'There are no books in this world that everybody must read, but only books that a person must read at a certain time in a given place under given circumstances and at a given period of his life'*

Lin Yutang

◆

*'There is no friend as loyal as a book.'*

Ernest Hemingway

## 089 - GUIDE to read

This guide may not be for you. Especially, since you are, currently, reading, and that you may, usually know the happiness of reading.

Reading, it is the most effective way to be informed. Thanks to it, we record and understand a lot more information, for example, compare to watching a video (although some photos are worth a thousand words). It deserves, therefore, a privileged place in our choices of activities.

Reading is traveling, in other worlds, surfing on new ideas. This is learning. It is stimulating the mind and preventing it from becoming numb and aging; While, for example, watching television, is a passive activity, that does not stimulate the mind.

Read helps reducing stress, and helps stopping obsessive thoughts, and finding solutions to problems that are important to us.
Read allows us to develop our analytical capacity.
Read allows us to enrich our vocabulary, our conversations and our writing.
Reading improves our ability to concentrate.
Read helps to better understand others and thus offers social and professional benefits.
Read develops imagination and creativity.

Many readers testify, that this or that book has changed their lives

It is possible that you read very little or not at all.

If this is the case, it is highly in your interest, to manage your time differently, making choices of your activities to include reading, then, to read regularly. If, for instance, you are starting the process of reducing your time spent watching television, reading will very well furnish your newly freed time.

You can then take the resolution: to read at least one page a day.
This is an interesting trick, that will allow you easily to harvest the benefits of reading. You shall, strive to respect this resolution.

It is possible, that after some time, you will develop a taste for reading and you will wish to read more. You can then decide to read for at least 10 minutes each day, and later move to 15 minutes and gradually increase. You will be surprised to find that, like many, captivated by the contents of a particular book, you have not been able to stop before it is finished.

◆

If you read before sleeping, it is better, to spend a better night, and a better tomorrow, that you read pleasant things.

*'Great books help you understand, and they help you feel understood.'*

John Green

◆

*'A great book should leave you with many experiences, and slightly exhausted at the end. You live several lives while reading.'*

William Styron

## 090 - GUIDE to be curious

Nobody could imagine, 10 years ago, what the world would be like today. The changes today, are faster than they were 10 years ago, and they continue to accelerate. No one can claim to know, how his world will be, after 10 years. It will be very different from today's.

There are many very encouraging signs that animate our curiosity and our reflective efforts to show themselves at their best.

Until today, our young societies, have been barbaric. Some have dominated, despised, chained, tortured, exterminated, murdered, deceived, exploited, robbed and corrupted others. However, we have developed ideas, we made and we are making our revolutions, we declare our rights, we learn to know them, we demand them, we communicate, we cooperate and our living conditions improve. Already we have made great progress. We shall be able to understand, and apply, that the interests of all pass through the interests of each; We will find the appropriate mechanisms to respect this principle.

Thanks to our curiosity, human relations will continue to improve. Our curiosity has already made us discover amazing things, that we were far from imagining. With what we have already discovered, we can be optimistic. This optimism will be reinforced with the future discoveries that we are not yet able to imagine today.

I have copied the entire Universal Declaration of Human Rights into the Annex, because it is good that we know our rights. And they have the merit of existing. You will notice, with surprise and interest, that none of the 30 articles is still fully respected. And you will notice, that each article gives us rights of value to be respected, to solve the problems we are encountering.

(Note: Legislation usually takes many years after legalization, before being satisfactorily respected. As other examples, we can observe the 'recent' laws prohibiting racial and gender discriminations on hiring, and the reality that is, still, very different. But these laws, too, have demanded great effort to get legalized, they have the great merit to exist, and they are making humanity evolving a lot).

⚖

*'Anyone asking a question may be considered a fool. Whoever does not ask for it is sure to remain so'*

Confucius

## 091 - GUIDE to remain opened and objective

The bicycle was invented in 1817.
When the first ones appeared in our countryside, some villagers were panic-stricken, and started running and shouting 'The devil is kidnapping such a man!'

At that time, and especially in the countryside, there was no access to information; The cheap press, therefore affordable for a larger number, will not appear until the end of the nineteenth century.

These villagers probably believed to this diabolical vision throughout their lives. Perhaps they also conveyed this belief to their children. Perhaps entire villages shuddered at the thought of this man struggling with the demon, and with the fright of being themselves suddenly carried away by the flames. Then, the explanation of the simplicity of the bicycle, arrived. Yet the refractory spirits have remained for many years, continuing to believe and suffer, that at every moment, they could tip into the eternal agony of their crepitating skins.

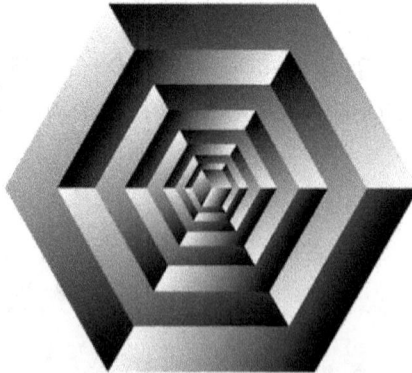

The beliefs and values we share with our parents and communities become our identities, certainties, and sometimes even reasons for living. It is then natural that we can resist new developments, which change our habits, our identities and our comforts.

But the days when our environment remained the same for centuries is gone. And because of the rapid and multiple changes we are experiencing in our day, we become more aware that everything changes except change, and many more have the freedom, the capacity and the love to act for even more changes.

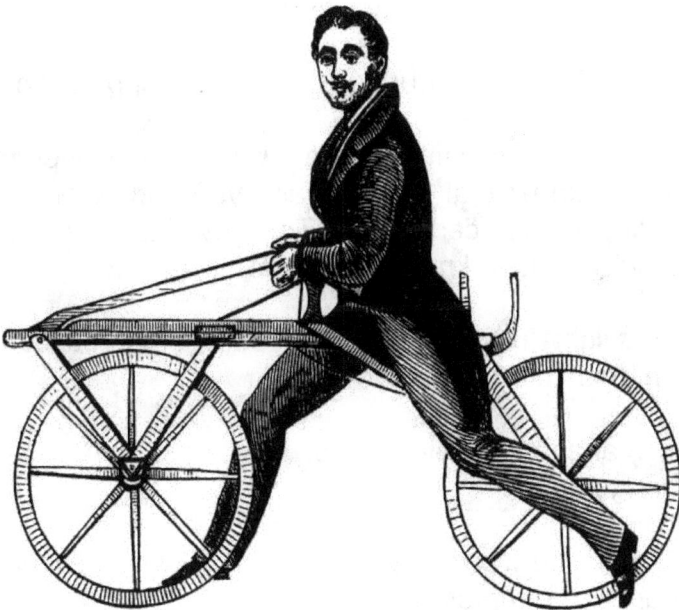

It is good to cultivate an open and critical mind.

o  To expand our horizons.

o  To explore and measure the origins and limits of our beliefs,

o  To listen to our opponents, with substantial attention. And to reflect on the origins of their ideas.

o  To imagine and activate innovations,

o  To seize opportunities,

o  To have better relationships with others. To be also more appreciated.

o  To be free to become stronger by adopting with serenity the many benefits of our errors, the first of which is our desire and then our resolution not to repeat them.

o  To be more stable during happy or unhappy changes.

o  To know that it is impossible for us to know everything. And to know that there is always information that is lacking to our certainties. To know that the ultimate knowledge is to know that we do not know.

o  To be light, free, confident, amused, contented, curious, dynamic, tolerant, and loving.

o  To manage to maintain our happiness, whatever the changes.

o  To gain the freedom to experiment, which is our only chance to understand.

Each of us, become stronger every day to exercise these abilities. This flexibility, awareness, curiosity and skill are the new characteristics of the human personality. It is neither astonishing nor disputable, but the simple reality that one can rejoice (without apnea).

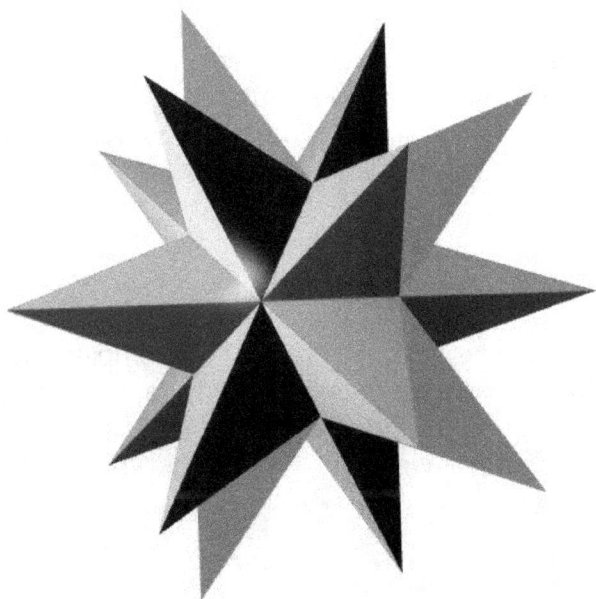

## 092 - GUIDE to learn another language

I worked and lived several years in Azerbaijan. The inhabitants of this country are saying, that when one knows how to speak another language, one has gained an additional personality.

Learning a language, gives us a vision of another culture, gives us access to other information. Moreover, the roots, origins, subtleties and stories of the words convey, in a language, specific and amusing ideas. In particular, it is interesting to note that each language includes words that cannot be translated, and others that are difficult to translate. When one knows another language, one realizes that the paths of ideas are different, from one language to another, enriching the thinking.

Nowadays, it has become a big advantage, and often a necessity, to speak fluently one or even two other languages. In particular, due to a 10-year advance in the United States in some areas, and the complementary and innovative information available only in English in these areas. And, because each culture, has interesting peculiarities, that we can only attain by knowing the language.

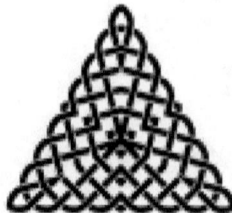

Moreover, international interactions are increasing sharply with the globalization. And this trend, is going to be accentuated greatly, in the years to come.

Speaking another language, offers opportunities to converse with new people, a better appreciation of literature, songs or movies (so much more enjoyable to watch a movie in the original version, to appreciate better the acting). Learning another language, helps to activate and develop our mind, keep it alert and prevent it from aging.

Learning a new language develops our ability, necessary in the modern world, to be more effective in managing multiple and varied tasks. It also allows, to open our minds to new cultures, understandings and acceptances. This allows us to change our selfish focus, and to open doors to the world.

Knowing another language also increases opportunities to travel and the benefits when traveling. It can even give us opportunities to spend long periods of our lives, in other countries.

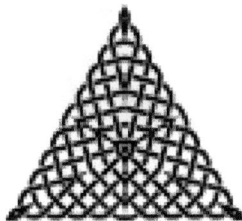

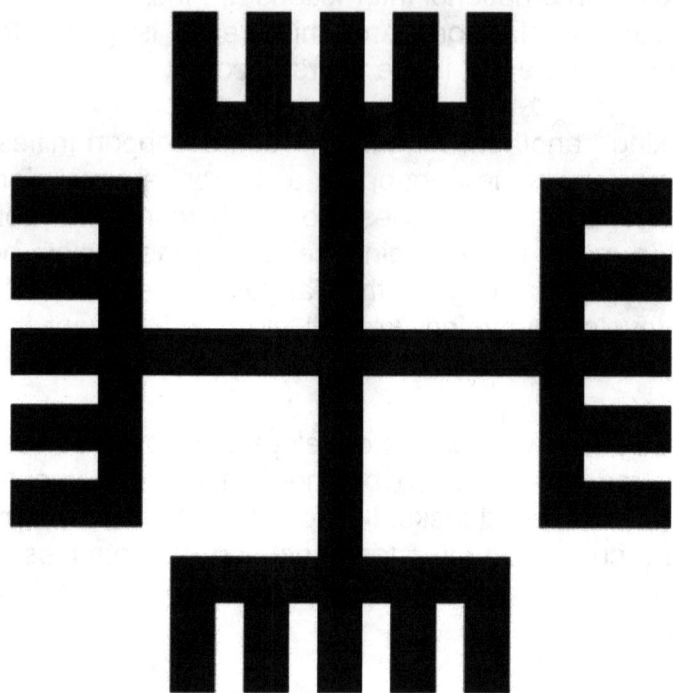

**Read in other language**

I have been confronted with the language barrier. Starting to work for International Non-Governmental Humanitarian Organizations (INGOs), I had to speak, read and write reports exclusively using English, while I had only the low level of English acquired at school.
It was not easy. But, I could see that I was making enormous progress through reading, and that this was the best technique of learning a language.

This exercise is for you to practice reading in English (or in another language studied).

o   Select an article in English on a topic that interests you. You can also select the lyrics of a song you like, or browse through a magazine.

o   Now read the article, without worrying about not understanding a lot of words. Continue your reading.

o   Renew the exercise regularly. Little by little you will understand the general and then more precise meaning of these articles. You will taste the words, the sounds and the grammatical constructions. And finally, you will realise having made big progress.

## 093 - GUIDE to slow down

Our actions are getting faster and faster.

Every day, we do more and more things, we receive more and more information, and we live faster and faster.

For example, studies in sociology, show that we walk in the street, at a higher and higher speed, over time. Our parents, our grandparents, were already living at a much lower speed. And, our children live faster than us. These same differences in speed, appear from one country to another, and even from one region to another in the same country; Even if, everywhere, rhythms are accelerating.

This is part of our evolution. This is a good thing, because we have the capacity to do so, because our lives are becoming richer in events, knowledge and experiences, and all this makes us happier.

However, it is also becoming more and more important, that, we develop our ability to slow down, in order to allow ourselves, at certain moments, to digest, process or filter information, to pause in the tumult of our thoughts, and, to access the power of our subconscious. Also, to remember the sweetness and plenitude of life, when it is simple, and not so furnished. Then, to return to the action, with our potentials bonified, with a restored efficiency, and, with the ability to cultivate a deserved satisfaction.

## 👀 Exercise 82 : The meditative walk

This technique can be practiced, for a few minutes, or for several hours, (begin with 10 minutes). The best place to practice, is in nature, in a forest, by a river, in a park, or on a terrace. But you can practice this technique in your apartment, even if it is small one.

o You are going to walk in slow-motion (like in a slow-motion movie). Gently and slowly putting your foot down at each step, and slowly rolling your steps. If you make other gestures, such as turning your head, or taking something in your pocket, do it also in slow motion.

o Think about breathing (at best, conscious breathing).

o Hold your attention on your gestures, on your balance and on your breath, and retrieve it when it gets lost. Consequently, you become free, not to think.

o Preferably, walking barefoot or with soft shoes.

o Preferably, do not listen to music during the practice. This will contribute to the calmness of your body and your thoughts. But if you feel happier listening to it, or if the music facilitates your introspection, you can also do it, but you will benefit, nevertheless, to practice also, at other time, the exercise without music.

Practice the meditative walk several times before going on to the next exercises to familiarize yourself with slowness, gesture and balance.

## ☻☻ Exercise 83 : The 3 points walk

The 3 points walk, is a technique offering many benefits.
It is a very easy technique, that is within everyone's reach.
Whatever your beliefs, your age and your personality, its
practice will be pleasant and very beneficial to you.

This technique is useful for improving well-being.
It produces sensations at specific points of the body, and
the specific benefits that correspond to it. Therefore, it also
makes us benefit from, a better feeling of the body, in its
entirety.
It allows us to have a stronger anchorage of our feet on the
ground (fundamental, comfortable and necessary stability),
to improve our balance, to improve the circulation of energy
in our body, to increase our consciousness , to move more
easily, more easily and more gracefully, to correct the
misalignments of our joints, then to carry out the work
(including wearing heavy objects) more easily and by
reducing the risks to hurt us, to correct our posture, to be
more decisive, to have greater self-confidence, and to be
more efficient in our actions.

The 3 points walk also allows us to calm down, to relax, to
breathe consciously, and to taste reality (here and now).

During this practice, we enjoy the feeling of new sensations
of multiple points and multiple mechanics of our body. We
then have the desire to explore, to know better and to
improve these new sensations; For example, our
equilibrium is at first uncertain, it rapidly improves, and it
improves continuously; As another example, we realize

that we usually walk with the back curled, or with a misalignment of the hips, knees or ankles, and we are happy with these new sensations and little by little, we enjoy the corrections we are making; Finally, as a third example, we correct the alignment of the spine, shoulders and head.

The practice is so easy and so enjoyable, that we enjoy repeating it. It allows to print the multipoint schema in our memory. The reproduction of this pattern is then done, as well when we are animated by the desire to practice the exercise formally, as, gradually, automatically. And we reap the benefits of the 3 points walk every time we walk. And as we walk every day, we practice and harvest every day.

The formal 3 points walk, like the meditative walk is done in slow motion. The practice in slow motion makes it possible to record the feeling that follows the visualization of the 3 points. Then, it becomes possible to practice this technique during faster walks. We can thus enhance our days of conscious feelings that have a playful character, and, above all, provide us with a general well-being (including a greater balance) through this physical feeling.

By practicing this technique, we are going to do a work on all the points of support of the foot on the ground. In particular, we will work the two points of the kidneys.

## The point of the kidneys

is, under each foot, in the middle of the arch of the foot, at the point of intersection of the mount of the thumb and the mount of the other toes. The point of the kidneys is the starting point of the meridian of the kidney, which then circulates under the arch of the foot, then inside the leg, reaches the pubis, then crosses the abdominal region, passing through the median axis, up to the sternoclavicular region.

After feeling our feet on the ground, and after feeling this point of the kidneys, we will work on two other points, corresponding to, the point of the sacral chakra and to the point of the crown chakra. (Some characteristics are recalled here, in order to facilitate the practice of the exercise). By extension we work on the whole body.

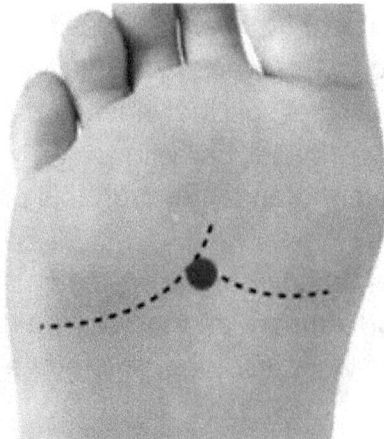

## The sacral chakra

located three fingers under the navel, is the center of gravity of the body, playing a biomechanical role particularly important. Thus, the focus on this point, during the exercise, will give us a superior balance. Moreover, this attention contributes to the improvement of the mobilities and the alignments of all the articulations of the body.

Recall that from an energy point of view the sacral chakra is the main source of energy for the whole body.

## The crown chakra

located at the top of the skull, is the upper point of the median axis of our body. From a biomechanical point of view, focusing on this point, during the 3 points walk, allows us to straighten up, lengthen ourselves and thus continue the alignment of our entire body. In this technique, it also symbolizes the mind, the consciousness. He also has a celestial symbolism, which can make us say, that this practice allows us to have, feet on the ground and head in the clouds.

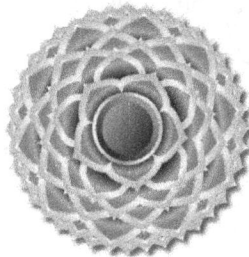

Before practicing the exercise, begin by making several deep pressures on the point of the kidneys, as well as massages, with the thumb of your hand, in order to feel it and to spot it. Exert these pressures on your two plantar vaults, during the time you judge necessary for the good feeling of your two points of the kidneys. Also, to optimize their feelings, pressures and massages, on the point of the sacred chakra, and on the point of the crown chakra.

When walking, focus your attention successively on the following points:

o By placing your right foot on the floor, visualize and feel the point of support of your heel on the ground.

o Then, visualize and feel the point of the kidneys.

o Visualize and feel, the numerous points of support of your foot on the ground, located on the mount of the thumb, on the mount of the other toes and on each of your toes.

o Continue focusing your attention on the sacred chakra.

o Continue, focusing your attention on the crown chakra.

o Now, placing your left foot on the ground, continue on the same support points as those described above for the right foot.

o Continue, with the sacred chakra, and with the crown chakra. And so on, start again with the right foot.

Search for the alignment of your knee, ankle and foot. Also work your balance throughout the exercise.

Begin by practicing the simple technique 3 points walk. Then once you're comfortable, if you want, you can practice the options :


## **Option 1** :

For some time, practice, having an exclusive focus, on the role of blood pumping of the sole of the feet winding during walking. And, by extension, have a focus on the blood circulation of your entire body (this will be especially beneficial to people with circulatory problems, such as heavy legs sensations). You will visualize the physiological direction of the blood circulation : from your heels to your toes, continuing the ascent of the anterior face of your body, then descending the posterior face of your body.


## **Option 2** :

Visualize the energy of the earth, starting from its center, and going up to cross the point of the kidneys, go up along the meridian of the kidneys, cross the sacred chakra, continue to the crown chakra.

Then, we see the path of the earth's energy into the cosmos. And finally, visualize, in this same column of energy, the flow of cosmic energy penetrating your body through the crown chakra, crossing your body along the median axis, passing the sacral chakra, rejoining the point of the kidneys, crossing the earth, to its center.

## 👀 Exercise 84 : The 10 points walk

The 10 points walk has features and benefits comparable to those of the 3 points walk. Again, this technique benefits the triangular dynamic body-mind-action. This technique has also specific advantages.

### The specific advantages of are:

o You will learn to know, to locate and to feel, your 2 sacroiliac joints. You will also be able to feel the touch of these two joints.

The sacroiliac joints are the joints between the sacrum and the two iliac bones. These joints form the connection, between the spine and the pelvis, therefore, between the column and the legs. (See drawing on next page).

The pains in the lower back often have their origins in these joints, and are often due to a lack of flexibility of these joints.

This technique will allow you to work this flexibility; And, to locate the origin of many pains, to relieve them (by using the techniques of pain relief, contained in this manual).

o You are going to learn to locate, 2 other very important energy points, which are the heights of your iliac bones.

You will perceive, the sophisticated work of your pelvis, during the walk. (See drawing on next page)

This knowledge will allow you to improve the balance and the horizontality of your pelvis, as well as your balance, to harmonize your walk, and to correct any imbalances and disharmonies causing pain.

(Outside of the 10-point walk, it will also be interesting, to exert pressure, on these 2 points.)

o 6 points of contact, on the muscles, on either side of your spine, will allow you to feel the great work of these muscles at every step of your walk.
These muscles work much. It is interesting to know them and to realize how much they are working when you walk. This will allow you, to harmonize the functions of these muscles, to harmonize your walk, your postures and all your movements.

It will be also, an opportunity to perform a massage of these 6 points, to know them better, and to relieve frequent pains in this area.

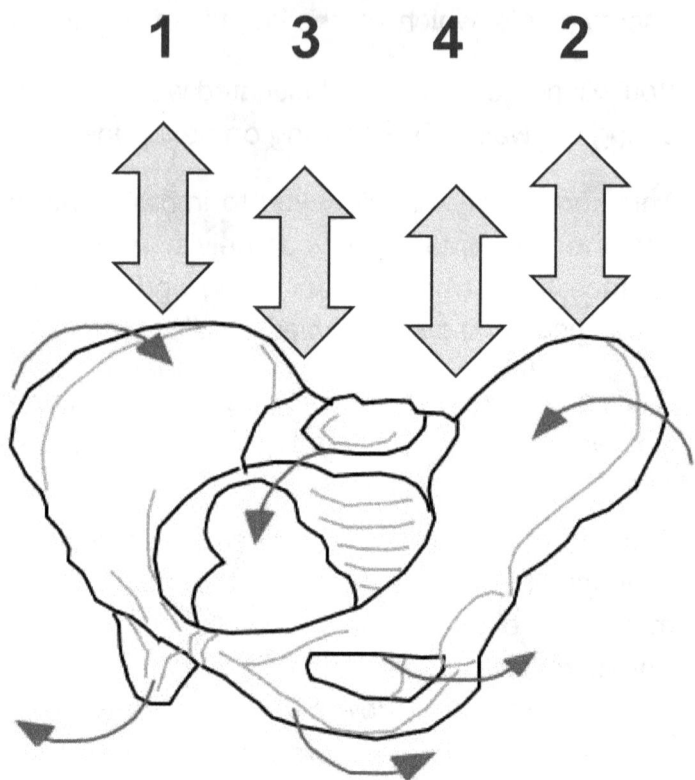

**1  3  4  2**

(Source drawing UVMaF)

**The 10 points walk, step by step:**

o  Place your hands on your hips.

   Place your two thumbs at the tops of your two iliac crests (positions 1 and 2 on the diagram).

   In preparation for the exercise, take some time to pressure these important points, to feel them well.

   During the 10 points Walk, you will press the two points, exactly at the tops of the iliac crests.

o  Place your two index fingers at the junctions of the two sacroiliac joints (positions 3 and 4 in the diagram).

   These junctions are like gorges, between two mountains. During the walk, you will feel these mountains waving.

o  Place your other three fingers in both hands naturally on the muscular columns on either side of your spine.

Perform your walk, feeling and exploring, all the sensations that have been described.

After practicing this technique for some time, you will add, a careful unfolding of the foot (see, The meditative march).

**Note 1:**

In case you are overweight, you will not be able to feel precisely the heights of your iliac crests or the gorges of your sacroiliac joints, and maybe even, with difficulty the muscles on both sides of your spine. For the hips are privileged places for the accumulation of fat.

You shall still practice the technique, all the same, applying strong pressure with your fingers to get closer to the feelings of these points.

As you lose your overweight, you will have the joy of discovering these points more and more, massaging them, performing excitations on them, and perceiving their work and movements with precision.

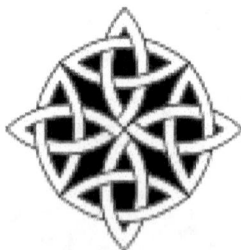

**Note 2:**

Observe, when you walk, or when you run, if there is a lateral angle, between your feet and your legs. If you have "duck" feet turned outward. Or, if they are turned inwards.

These deviations can create tensions and muscle pain, as well as arthrosis of the knees and hips.

With The 10 points Walk, and with the careful feeling of the unfolding of your foot, you can correct this angular deviation. (If after some time you cannot make this correction, it may be impossible to correct, because bone malformation, or you may need orthopedic insoles, consult a Podiatrist or an Orthopedic to make sure.)

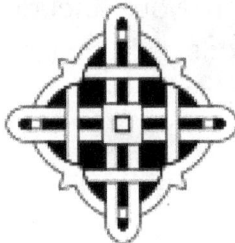

## 👁👁 Exercise 85 : The freed pelvis

It is common, to lack flexibility in the lumbar vertebrae (lower back), sacroiliac joints, and multidirectional pelvic tilt movements (see diagram in the previous exercise). These lacks flexibility, are at the origin of the frequent pains in these areas of the body.

These consequences are as follows:

- Your movements are limited;
- Blocks are forming, then they generate disturbances and pains.

As these consequences affect all of us, and as it is very easy, with this technique, to avoid them, it is worth recalling their repercussions on the triangular dynamics of body-thought-action: these genes, pain, and physical limitations, as the others do, reverberate on your thoughts and on your actions. The practice of this technique, improving your joint flexibility, eliminating disturbances, pain and limitations, will improve your well-being and your mobility, and, it will have a positive impact on your thoughts and actions, by suppressing bad moods, and making you more dynamic, enterprising and resistant.

You will find the description of the technique, step by step on the following pages. Do not be frightened by this description which could, a priori, appear to you complicated. A simple and small effort will be necessary, but once you have understood the movements to be carried out, the duration of the practice of this exercise will be of 1 minute only.

It will then be beneficial for you to get into the habit of regularly practicing this exercise, taking advantage of a pose in the middle of your work, waiting for the arrival of the bus or the subway, or including it in a series of other exercises.

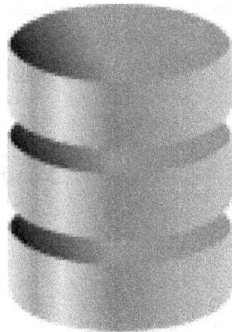

**Technique of the freed pelvis, step by step:**

o  Stand upright with legs slightly apart. Keep your legs straight. Bend your knees slightly, comfortably and in a natural way.
   During the first practices of the exercise, your movements will be of small amplitudes. These amplitudes will increase during the practices. During the practice, each movement will be repeated 5 times, gradually adding the amplitude to your movements, up to the maximum.

o  Place your fingers on the same 10 points as in the previous exercise (The 10 points Walk). And during the practice, in the first place, feel the work of your sacroiliac, lumbar, pelvis joints and your femur heads turning in your pelvis; later on, feel the work of your knees and your ankles; And finally, the position of your spine and the feeling of your whole body.

o  Movement 1a: Lean your body to the right, pointing your hips to the left, with a regular movement (without yank), counting "1".

o  Movement 1b: Lean your body to the left, pointing your hips to the right.

   Repeat 1a and 1b, counting "2", then counting to "5".

- Movement 2a: Toggle your body back, pointing your hips forward, counting "1".

- Movement 2b: Tilt your body forward, pointing your hips backwards.

  Repeat 2a and 2b, counting to "5".

- Movement 3a: Keeping the body straight, tilts your hips forward (the genitals pointing forward), the curvature being at the lumbar and sacroiliac joints.

- Movement 3b: Tilts your hips backwards (your buttocks pointing backwards).

  Repeat 3a and 3b, counting to "5".

- Movement 4a: Perform 5 rotations clockwise, forming a circle, increasingly wider, with your hips (combination of the 6 previous steps).

- Movement 4b: In the same way, makes 5 rotations, in a counterclockwise direction.

This previous exercise is effective in itself.

Once you are used to his practice, you can, optionally, add a coordination with your breathing:

Remember that your breath will lead your movement.

- o <u>Movement 1a</u> : Inspire by leaning your body to the right, and breath-out by bringing your body upright.

- o <u>Movement 1b</u> : Breath-in by leaning your body to the left, and breath-out by bringing your body upright.

- o <u>Movement 2a</u> : Breath-in by tilting your body back, and breath-out by bringing your body upright.

- o <u>Movement 2b</u> : Breath-in by rocking your body forward, and breath-out by bringing your body upright.

o Movement 3a : Breath-in by tilting your hips forward, and breath-out by bringing your body upright.

o Movement 3b : Breath-in by tilting your hips backwards, and breath-out by bringing your body upright.

o Movement 4a : Breath-in by making a semicircle, from the front position to the rear position, breath-out in the semicircle from the rear position to the front position.

o Movement 4b : Breath-in and breath-out in the same way as in movement 4a.

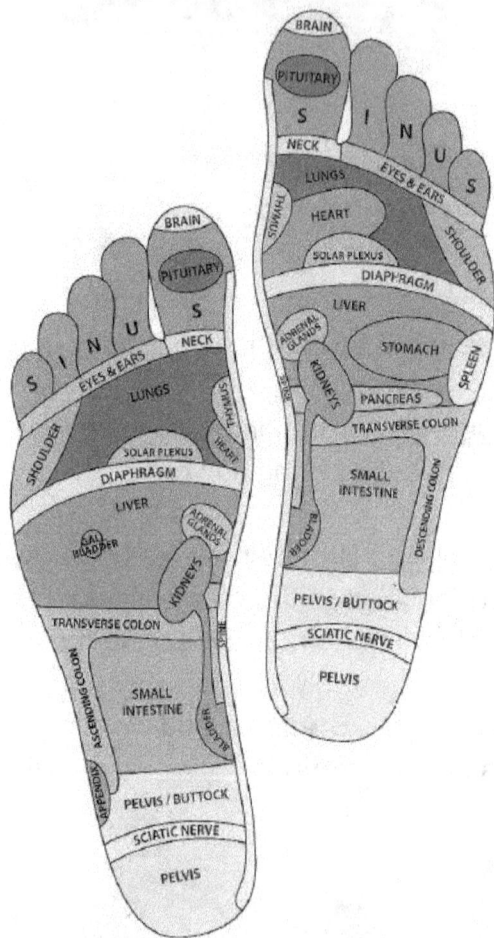

## ◉◉ Exercise 86 : The pebble walk

When it happens to you to feel under your foot, a stone that slipped into your shoe, considers this event as an opportunity.

On the soles of the feet are hundreds of energy points, which correspond to the anatomy and physiology of the human body.

o Consider, precisely, the point where you feel the pebble, corresponding to an energy rebalancing, that your body needs.

o Walk, for some time, exploring this point, in depth.

o Remove the stone, when the pain becomes intense, and may cause inflammation that turns into a bleb.

o If you have the opportunity later, continue pressing and massage, on this point, with your thumbs. Considering, that it will allow this energy rebalancing to continue

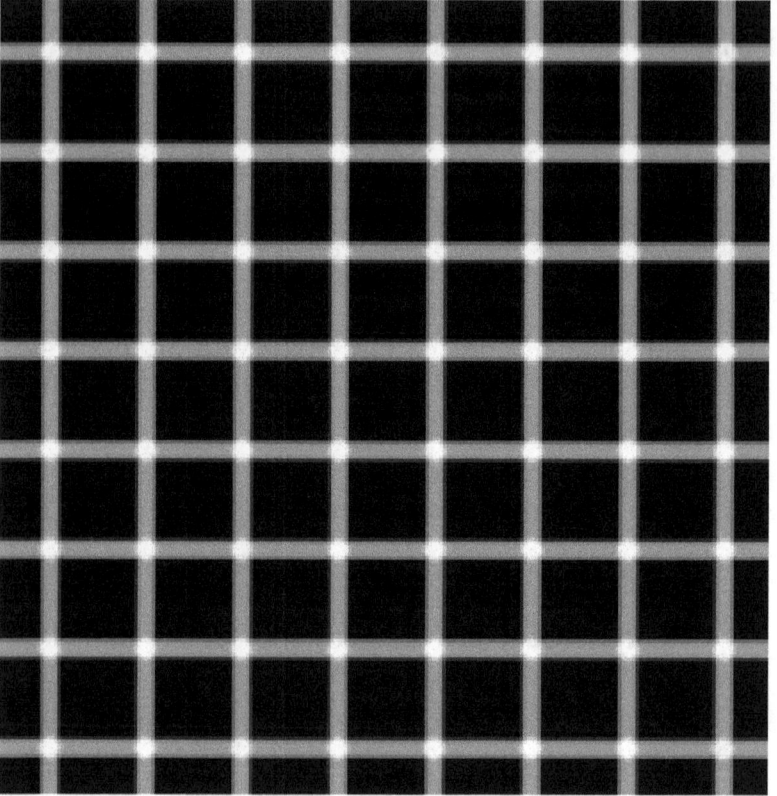

32

---

[32] Optic illusion : watch the black spots appearing.

## ◉◉ Exercise 87 : Breathing from heels

This practice is multi-millennial. It is found in the Tao Te King written (600 BC) by Lao Tzu, the wise founder of Taoism. It had even been recommended by the famous Chinese wise man and philosopher Chuang Tzu (4th century BC).

It consists in walking, by imagining the inspiration entering through the heel, filling the whole body, then coming out, through the mouth.

It is a technique that gives breathing its full value as a synonym of life.

This technique also makes it possible to correct the straightness of the vertebral column.

This practice can be carried out at any walking speed. During, for example, a brisk walk, inhaling and exhaling will be lasting ten steps each.

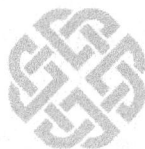

## ◕◕ Exercice 88 : Slower actions

We must not confuse speed and precipitation.
Precipitation affects the quality of the result, and sometimes causes errors, nuisances or accidents.

We can perform our activities in full awareness and with maximum efficiency, while doing them at the right speed. The possible feeling of wasted time when we slow down certain activities is a mistake; moreover, mindfulness allows us to optimize the coordination of our activities and allows us to avoid the loss of time caused by forgetfulness, errors, accidents and missed opportunities.

o   **Eating slower**

The fault of eating too fast is a reality for many of us.

This frequent reality is like the other one, seen at the beginning of this manual, which many of us do not drink enough, knowing that we are daily wrong, that this causes us problems (Digestive disorders, sensations of heaviness, bloating, nausea and constipation, disorders that greatly affect our mood and joie de vivre, without our knowing that these are the causes of our lack of energy and our black thoughts) and nevertheless knowing that it is easy and beneficial to correct for better habits.

Digestion begins with chewing, which allows the grinding of food and the integration of salivary gland secretions (degradation of starch).

In addition, the sensation of satiety is related to time, and eating more slowly, it can be satisfied by having eaten less and thus having a better control of our weight. By keeping foods long enough in our mouth, we allow a lot more information, delivered by the taste buds, to reach the brain. This allows nutrients to be extracted more efficiently from each food. Moreover, their integration with blood begins under the tongue. When you eat too quickly all these functions are used insufficiently.

It is important that at each meal you remember, eat more slowly, chew sufficiently, and maintain a relationship with the food.

## o **Moving slower**

The faster the driving, the greater, the risk of accident, the fuel consumption, the pollution and the stress. So many reasons, to convince us to slow down.
Driving too fast, is simply a bad habit, that can be corrected, but cannot be justified by being in a hurry, because the time gained on a trip is negligible. And in case of an accident the loss of time, the loss of money and eventually the loss of life, are important. Being in a hurry is a stressor. It is bad for your health. It increases the risks to make mistakes; And, it goes against the priority you give to your happiness.

In a much happier way, you will be able to make these moments spent by car (even if you are stuck in traffic jams), privileged moments, where you will cultivate the sensation of happiness, the availability and the freedom to practice exercises of this manual.

## ☻☻ Exercise 89 : Making choices

If you watch yourself running, look for better planning and better management of your activities.

Look at the activities you can shorten or eliminate.
Here, too, is the need to know how to say 'no' that we have observed previously.

In particular, some recreational activities, are big time eaters.

For other leisure and other activities, you have an initial impression, that they are necessary. Observe them, and judge if your time would not be better used; To walk, calm, serene and happy rather than to run, irritated, anxious and discontented; And to live with happiness and efficiency chosen activities, rather than live optional activities, with the frustration of not having enough time to properly perform your favorite activities. Greater freedom also gives you opportunities to discover new activities.

♦

*'Smile, breathe and goes slowly'*          T.H. Hanh

## ☻☻ Exercise 90 : A Sunday without watch

Make the choice, that such Sunday, will be a 'day without watch'.

Spend your day, in complete freedom, total relaxation, and without considering the time that passes. If you live in family, or in group, warn others of your decision.

Take advantage of this opportunity to reflect on the hilarious side of the expression 'I do not have time'.

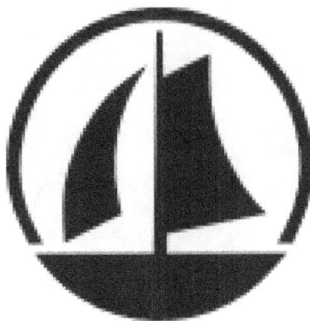

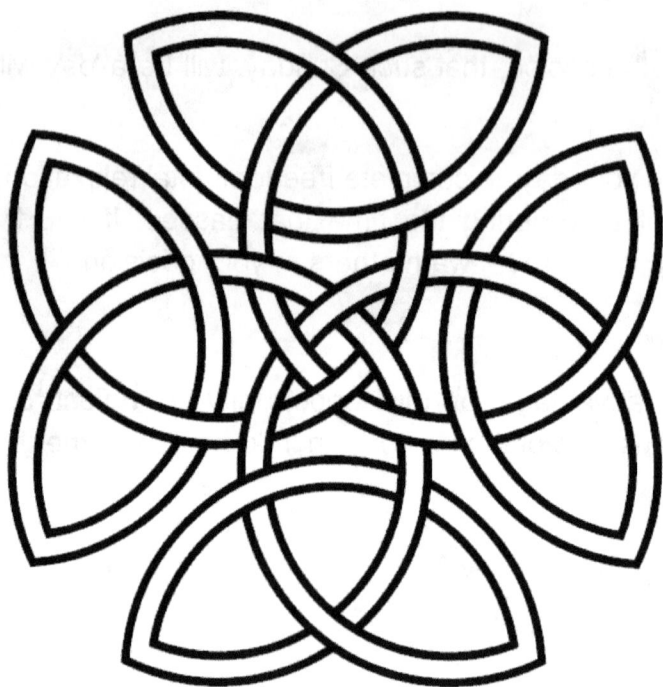

It took me time to realize I was far happier, focusing on spending all my time doing what I love to do, and loving all the things I had to do.

## 094 - GUIDE to make disaster preparedness

It may be surprised for you, to see this guide appearing in the quest for happiness. It appears, because we will undergo, in the coming years, frequent natural disasters and unknown magnitudes so far. There will be floods, heat waves, cold waves, long extreme cold, droughts, tidal waves, and cyclones. They will have an impact on the lives of all of us. And it is preferable to be prepared, mentally, according to our specific ways of life, and as far as possible. Not to be then, overly surprised and devastated. The quest for happiness also includes seeking to avoid or overcome misfortune.

This will not change the love you have for your newborn baby, nor your ability to take pleasure in making deep inhalations.

Disaster preparedness is a topic I know, having worked in this sector for several years. The debate between the responsibility of man in climate change and other reasons does not interest me. What is certain, and despite very positive progress, is that man has enormously polluted the planet. And there are disturbing black spots in the degradation of our environment. This is inadmissible, and we must multiply our efforts to totally stop polluting and to make it a priority. What is also certain, since several decades is that natural disasters are progressing in quantity an in intensity. And that is going to continue.

At the time, I was living in Bangladesh, one of the cyclones, among many, affected seven million people. This number of victim, for a single disaster was amazing and unprecedented. A few years later, at a meeting with a colleague, working in the same sector, I quoted this figure. My colleague told me that the previous year, 60 million people had been affected by a drought in Pakistan.

Future natural disasters will cause enormous losses. Future direct victims, if they currently have the chance to enjoy comfort, will be the most vulnerable, when they lose it. And we will have to assist them so that they can quickly become useful again.

It is important to know and take it into account in our various planning this multiplication of disaster, to prepare for it and to adapt to it. It is well known that disaster preparedness save at least five times its cost by limiting losses. It is important that in any planning, we analyze the potential risks from natural disasters.

We have good logistics, and the means to prepare ourselves, then to adapt. It is better to anticipate than to be forced after suffering.

The experiences of large-scale disasters will shake our indecisions and strengthen our convictions. And, a new wave of awareness, will further energize our evolution.

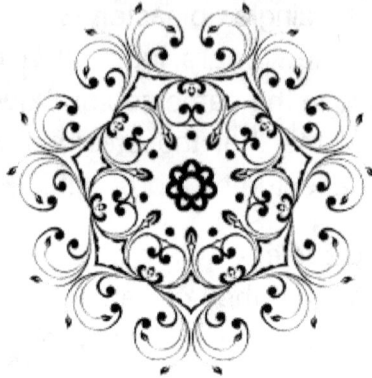

'Temperament lies behind mood; behind will, lies the fate of character. Then behind both, the influence of family the tyranny of culture; and finally, the power of climate and environment; and we are free, only to the extent we rise above these'

John Burroughs

## 095 - GUIDE to remain flexible to change

Love and happiness live perfectly well, in the worst situations.

Of course, we do not want to be among those who live in the worst situations. However, these situations are, for all of us, part of the life. And if we have the comfort of not remaining, for a long time, in the worst situations, we witness it, and we hear, for example, more and more often, about the extraordinary possibility of extinction human race.

Today we are walking along the edge of the razor with the chance to switch to a possible world of happiness and justice for all, and the risk of sinking with the current system.

This current system, which, at first, has made us greatly evolve, is proving, now, to not respect human being and his environment.

This agonizing system, which, by definition, can only function by creating budget deficit, debt, unemployment, poverty, and the destruction of our habitat. For the driving force which governs our societies is the speculation of profit, the biggest possible and the quickest possible, even if it does not profit us in the long term by creating our misfortune and our destruction. This system, which proves us not to be the system we want to continue to use.

That's our story. We have lived the beliefs of superiority over each other, the law of the strongest, and imperialism. These beliefs, which remain powerful and governing, define our programs of propaganda and education. It is not a question here of condemning one or the other, beyond the legal system we have developed, which allows us, for example, to judge and condemn war criminals and crooks. Nor is it a matter of engaging in an anarchic, bloody and destructive revolution.

Because, fortunately, driven to introspection, following our growing knowledge of the disastrous and self-destructive effects of our system, through our instinct to survive and love, we become a majority to want to change our system. We have developed the means and the ability to do so. We are numerous. We have good know-how. Nature is generous, and it will remain our habitat, if we stop destroying it. Because we are unhappy, we want change, we are the ones who operate the system, more and more of us are making individual and collective changes, our system is evolving greatly. We will continue to make it evolve, even making the profit necessary for its functioning, because there is much to do and work for everyone. But this time, profit will not abuse or harm anyone. It will no longer cause negative effects or destruction. The reasonable margin will remain with which all parties involved in the action or transaction are satisfied. A margin that allows to evolve durably.

In addition to our evolving notion of profit, the volume of volunteering and volunteering to help the weakest of us is also increasing. And, even though our motivation comes from our compassion, we benefit individually and collectively from defeated weaknesses and gained strengths.

It is an equation that can only have a positive result. The costs of the old system and its transformation will mark the beginning of our history. You have to get used to it. Be ready and continue to commit to great change and for great opportunities. These extraordinary changes are underway. They are visible around us, just look, sit in the running train, participate, relax and have a good time.

It is thus highly probable that our access to knowledge allows us to correct the unnatural interference of egoism. Because of this greater probability of our progression towards a golden age, we can legitimately be happy and stay the course with confidence. We can even stay the course in case of incidents of course or detours.

□

*'I think therefore I am'*

Descartes

Let us realize the value of the change of our being.

Let us realize that, at every moment, we are becoming a different person.

For every moment happens an event, which, even if it is small, is an important agent of change.

Like the displacement of a beat of a butterfly wing, is at the origin of a chain of events that includes a hurricane. As a simple thought transforms us into a different person.

And as a brief silence does the same.

♦

Some of us are saying that today the amount of information is too great, that the train goes too fast, or not enough, that they are afraid and that they cannot adapt.

They are mistaken.
For they forget that it has been very easy for us in recent decades, to change a lot by increasing our capacity to absorb a huge amount of information, and by increasing our means and our capacity to act.

When we lived in our villages, the landscape of the hill opposite was the only one we saw throughout our lives. And throughout our lives we met only a few dozen of our neighbors. Today, during a single one-day drive, we see millions of different landscapes, and tens of thousands of people. Our new set is made up of galaxies, we can also visualize the microscopic and the infinitely small.

Everyone, as much as we are, and wherever we are, we are changing, improving our knowledge and our capacities, progressing for a better, sometimes by making detours.

Our changes are progressing exponentially, energizing each other.

It is very interesting and encouraging to realize the amount of change this represent.

Being comfortable, familiar and in love with the new person we become during the change, is very important. This comfort facilitates the stability in the state of this new person and in the following one.

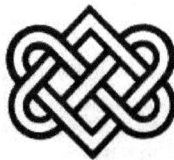

The exercises in this manual help you to perceive your inner happiness, and help you build your outer happiness. They are making you stronger and they are supporting you in your adaptation and in your participation to the negative and positive changes to come. While remaining confident, strong, balanced and active, even in difficult times, knowing that individually and globally our evolution is clearly positive.

We have seen changes in our being by doing the exercises in this manual:

- We were somebody not breathing well, we now know how to breathe deeply. We were not eating well; our best nutrition makes us happier.

- We were someone feeling bad and who was unhappy when he was alone, and who left the bitterness directing our well-being, our thoughts and our actions. We are now feeling good, and we appreciate, as much, being alone, and being accompanied, for we have discovered and experienced happiness by being alone, which was formerly unknown or refuted. This is, now, making us happy, in the three components of our triangular dynamic.

- We were someone spending a lot of time stressed by memories of the past, regrets, suffering caused by an accident, a loss, a crime or an old disappointment, and by expectations, jealousies, cravings. We use, now better our life time in the present.

- We could easily laze, we are now enjoying the happiness of the action.

- We have also increased our ability to change to the extraordinary of tomorrow.

The change process remains a difficult process, as we move from a situation we know, to a situation we do not know. We are weighed down by the weight of a distant past, while being exalted by the progress observed in the near past. We have constraints in the present, while having many opportunities and the happiness to exist. And we face the unknown of the future.

Today, you have three priorities, which will enable you to experience changes in the best conditions:

--1. To nourish your desire to be happy, remembering to make the impulses of chosen actions.

--2. To observe, that we are, obviously, experiencing great and rapid changes.

--3. To observe, the dominant sense of the current of change. To find out that it is positive.

It will be useful for you to imagine your happy future. Once you begin to have an image of the happy person you want to become, you will start practicing the habit of putting yourself in the shoes of that person and being comfortable with it. In the beginning, you will not recognize yourself in this new skin. It will seem to be a theater actor playing a role. There will be a lag between the person you were and the person you are becoming. This shift will make you feel like being a spectator at the same time as being actor of the play. It will be a pleasant sensation, but because it will be a new one, you will have to get used to it, until you eliminate the lag, and you become the happy owner of your new skin. Knowing this process of mutation will allow you, thereafter, with ease, to change costumes, shoes and roles to continue exploring new happy characters.

And once you know the changes you have to make to become that happy person, you will have to get used to the happiness of performing and then multiplying the actions that contribute to that goal.

This method applies to the objective of being happy, in general, whatever the circumstances. This method also applies to all your specific goals, whether they are part of your goals to be happy in your body, in your head, or in your actions (private and professional).

According to these specific objectives, the efforts, in many cases, are proportional to the importance of the changes you want to achieve. Often also, important changes can be rapid, following a single decision.

If, the image of this new happy person is clear, work your well-being and your concentration on the three priorities mentioned above.

If, on the contrary, you are now walking in the fog of questions: When will I get there? What should I become? What should I do to get there? Then, work also your well-being. Because today, no matter what are the answers to questions When? What and How?
As, becoming stronger and more attentive, by addressing the three priorities above, you will have, at the right times, the answers to these three logistical questions, and you will

observe steady progress in your discovery of these answers. And in the meantime, you will already have reached your primary goal, to be happy.

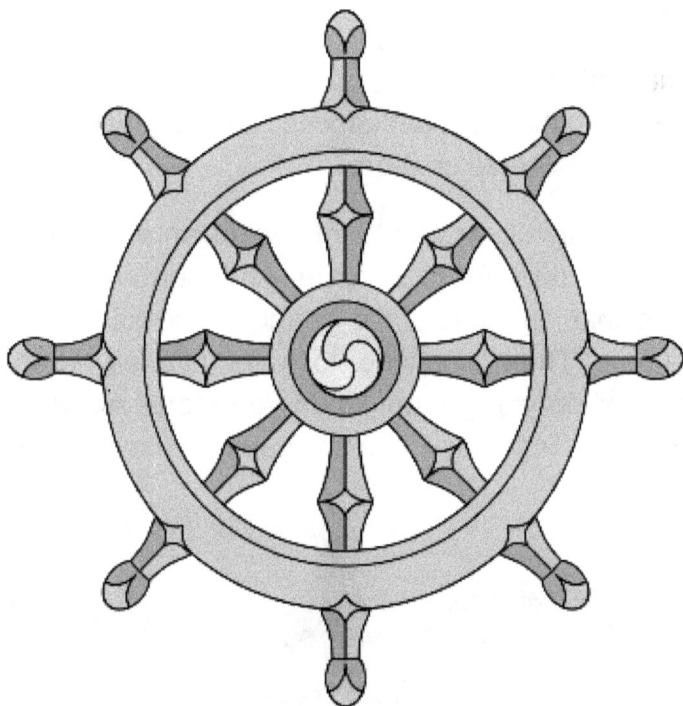

It is clear, that we are having a hard time changing our habits because they define our identity. Yet, our inability to change our bad habits can be particularly incoherent when habits are easy to change, and their consequences are particularly difficult.

To illustrate this, let's take the example of many of us suffering from gastric acidity:

These people know very well that eating lighter, which is a small behavioral change, would help them avoid suffering. Yet, they prefer to exchange daily, a few short minutes of emotional and identity comfort that are similar to bulimia, against many long hours of suffering and insomnia.

We must strive to be reasonable in order to change the causes and their consequences. Starting with our bad habits the easiest to change.

Observe yourself. Accept to love yourself, and to become the person you want to become. And, performs the initial impulse that engenders the change process in order to achieve it. Then, continue to love yourself when you relapse, when you get up, when you progress, when you are different, and when you are happy to have reached a stable result.

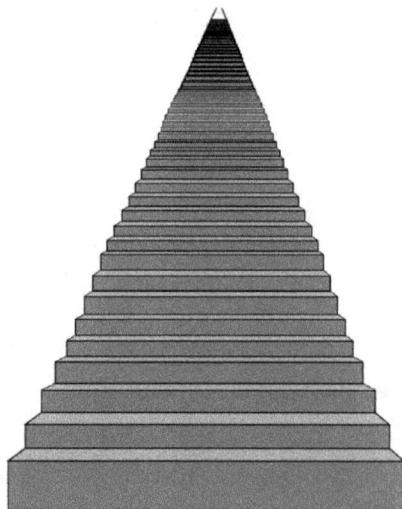

## 096 - GUIDE to let chance to inaction

In our universal functioning in dualities, each thing has its duality, complementary but not opposed. The dualities come together to form a dynamic system.

The duality of action is inaction. We can realize the role of inaction in achieving the result, and the advantage, as well as the need, to respect, both, the role of action and of the role of inaction. Allowing events to arrive, at the right moments, realizing that they always do, and that it cannot be otherwise, because it is the reality.

We can and must be able to relax, comfortably, serenely and confidently, in the deep void of the inaction, and then return to action more efficiently.
We also gain patience by understanding that our time of inaction is necessary to achieve the result we are seeking, and by recognizing the time necessary for the maturity of the results of our actions and of those of the other actors.

Perceiving the role of inaction is particularly useful in these times, of emptiness, or, on the contrary, when we are very active and overwhelmed by the responsibilities and sensation of necessity to act even more; We can then step back, gain confidence and expand field of view, and then return, more effectively, to action. We then correct, our tendency, for many cultural and also psychic, identification with our action, and we transform it into an identification with the couple action-inaction. We correct our tendencies, pretentious, erroneous and pernicious, to identify ourselves with the result of our action, and, on the opposite, to believe that action is not necessary.

In the same way that we have become a spectator of our thought, we amuse ourselves at the spectacle of our action and our inaction.

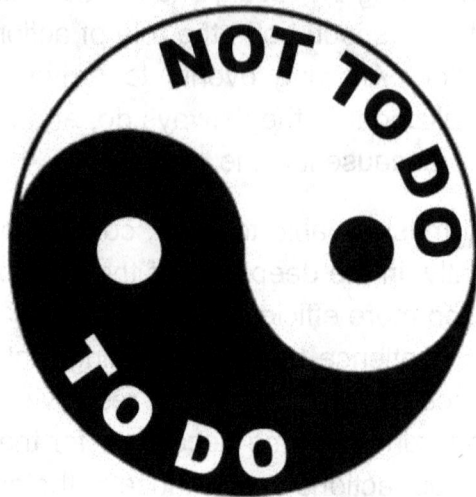

On the other hand, and optionally, by relaxing and allowing the participation of inaction, by understanding the capacity and effectiveness of inaction, and, by letting things happen, we are also more inclined to perceive another paradox: that in doing, we are not those who do. Facilitated access to this new perception is welcomed. For it is not an easy perception, without taking the necessary distance. And, when it is realized, it fills us with well-being and serenity, without, however, making us renounce the action.

What is free will?

Clearly, at every moment, we believe to have the choice of our thoughts, our sensations, our emotions and our actions. However, when one observes our lives, can we decently claim, that it is our free choices and decisions that have led us here?

Our free will, is certainly responsible for a great part of the unfolding of our actions. And, if we do not choose to act, the action will not be done or not done well. But, if our free will was responsible for the totality of our actions, then our actions would be done extremely well, or, from the respectable domain of the absolute, free from dualities. This does not correspond to the human condition. Human reality is also dependent on circumstances, external events, interactions, accidents, errors and impulses more powerful than our will and those of others.

It is good to have the illusion that we are driving our lives. It is good to realize that this is an illusion.

Another interpretation of our free will is, our freedom to respond to events, in a positive or negative way, feeling love and vital strength rather than fear and despair, to think about the past and the future or to live in the present moment; to regret or value the mistakes of the past; to cultivate the thought or emptiness of the mind; etc.

Our lives are like rivers, we swim in a flood of events. It is good to swim in the direction of the current, looking for serenity when the current makes us cross beautiful landscapes and also when it leads us through steep lands. Smiling, and being particularly happy to swim and to watch the events happening.

## 097 - GUIDE to manage Positive-Negative

Our future system, whatever positive it may become, will always work in positive-negative duality.

However, we are increasing our ability and our consistency to be aware of the reality. We are appreciating negativity differently. We become grateful for the benefits that it brings us, including that to exist and to evolve. And we learn to relativize our negative reactions to events.

Thus, much of our negativity becomes positive by returning to normality. It is absorbed by reality in its center creating a spin movement favorable to the development of the positive.

While, our consciousness of negativity changes and our negativity diminishes, our awareness of the positive and our positivism increase. These increases contribute to the acceleration of the dynamic system of positive transformation.


And ... we're happier. Hurray !

This is one of the Positive-Negative dynamic systems. We have seen another Positive-Negative dynamic system, with our good and bad choices that influence the Body-Head-Action triangular dynamics.

We have glimpsed the dynamic system of the good, and, the dynamic system of evil. Good and evil, is another subject that is of great concern to us. However, it is not necessary, and even desirable, to be so concerned. For, it is simple to observe, good and evil, from an exclusively dynamic point of view: the positive cascade generated by a positive event, and the negative cascade generated by a negative event.

Good and evil, keeps a disturbing side. For good, can be, really good. And evil, can be, really bad. However, from the strictly dynamic point of view, that has just been stated, it is easy for us, to generate positive impulses and to enjoy positive cascades, as it is easy, to avoid impulses negative, and to interrupt the negative, incoherent and stronger than will cascades.

By only wondering about these dynamics, in addition to nicely progress, we also benefit, from removing the worrying side kept by, the concept of good and evil. And finally, we regain control of our free will.

## 098 - GUIDE to be AND not to be

The same dynamic system of dualities, answers Hamlet's question, the of Shakespeare hero, 'To be or not to be? That is the question by, 'To be AND not to be that is the answer '.

By discovering the synergy of the parts of this other duality, we realize the role of the second part of our nature. This allows us to correct the pretension, the possible discomfort, and the handicap of the imbalance of identification more important to one or the other of the parts, which can not be conceived without the other.

Our perception of being, is, tangible and natural. And it is important that we are strong and comfortable in it.
On the other hand, the sensation of 'not being' is by definition intangible and subtle. To perceive our non-being, we must identify and explore it. We identify it, at times, when we realize we are only a spectator of our existence. We also explore it in the silence, during contemplation, when we are submerged by happiness, or during meditation.

Our understanding of non-being is, by nature, limited and ephemeral. It is also precious, for a small quantity produces a great effect on our being. On the other hand, the absolute nature of the union of dualities we must accept not being able to understand. But no matter, we have no need to understand it.

The need, as mentioned above, for solid ground anchoring, takes on, fully, its importance here. It includes a fully lived life, with a maximum awareness of being.

The solid anchoring in the earth gives us stability. This stability is necessary for, on the one hand, not to have to protect ourselves from our fears, by ignoring, without even realizing it, the brilliant and timeless brilliance of our non-being when we see it, on the other hand, not be unbalanced when you are conscious of seeing it. In return, when it is seen, this shine enhances the experience of our being, including its stability.

Let us note, that the equations of quantum physics demonstrate here again, to have established a bridge between metaphysics and physics, and between non-being and being. When they compare the universe to a film. The universe exists at the moment of the photo and does not exist between the photos. The succession of photos gives the sensation of the movement. A movement in which, once again, it is difficult to perceive, but possible to explore, the instant between the two photographs, which belongs to non-being.

It is difficult to understand that both we are and we are not. However, we must think about it. And use techniques (including those of this manual) that allow us to approach this dimension as much spiritual as real. A reality, which is very useful to us to use as energy axis, maximizing our mastery of its understanding, its feelings, and the balance and dynamics of its halves. A firm anchorage in the being, the ability to float in the ocean of non-being, knowing that the rope connects us, constantly at the anchor.

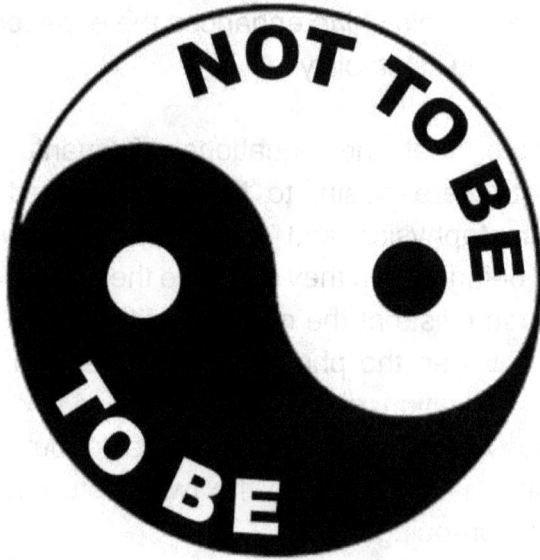

I know that I am and that I am not.

I cannot know what I am not.

I cannot either know what I am,
Because I am what I am and what I
am not.

I am very satisfied to be what I am,
and to be able to perceive the interlaced
dynamics between the dualities, to be
happy in my body, in my head and in
my actions.

To be and not to be, is our complete definition. The perception of not being is really advantageous to search (through thinking and understanding, conception, meditation and control of thought). Doing so, we integrate the not being to the being, and the being to the not being. This search is basically challenging as our being is strongly determined to exist, defining its existence with what we possess and with what we do; it also rejects the concept of not being, seeing it as a threat to its existence, not understanding that the existence is incomplete without the integration of both being and not being.

The same apply to the universe, with its marvelous beauty. We are marveled by the infinity of the scale and the beauty of its being, often missing that we can similarly and equally be marveled by the infinity of the scale and beauty of its not being.
The result of integrating being and not being is definitely more marvelous, beautiful and comfortable. We enjoy the feeling of being complete, understanding that we were suffering because of being incomplete.

As we saw other synergies, there are synergies between being and not being. Cultivating the qualities of one enhance the qualities of the other. But again, this require the initial impulse of the effort to conceive the not being to allow changing our incomplete believe of what is to be. You shall remain comfortable now, as you always do the best you are able to do now; but whatever is your current level of understanding of being and not being, the impulse is to your advantage.

Again, no judgment, each one of us is doing now the best that he is able to do, depending on each one his history. Just to realize that the frequent feeling of being in absence of the feeling of not being does not serve us and brings us fears and disappointments. Similarly, some are making the opposite exclusive cult of not being; for instance, the persons met in the streets of Katmandu, without clothes, never taking a bath, never cutting their hairs and spending hours meditating; or this Zoroastrian in a cabin chaining himself and contemplating a flame till death. The latest are maybe happy? It is impossible to say when it is not our own experience.

Although the concept of not being can initially seems difficult to conceive, there is the very comforting fact that it is confirmed by quantum physique. Therefore, we can approach this concept on a materialistic point of view. Not even need, at the basis of the concept, to have mystical or philosophical considerations. No need to even consider the concept of consciousness. In that way, the concept of not being appears finally to be very simple, accessible and liberating. Being cannot be without not being, as much as black cannot be without white. This concept brings us a very powerful and not arguable (therefore not doubtful) stability.

By conceiving the reality of being and not being, we expand our reality. Conceiving our not being brings us comfort, softening the pressions brought by our challenges, our struggle, our pretentions, our failures, our fears and our obsessions. After we are giving some focus on the integration of this concept, we are becoming a richer and more able person.

Not being is not a reality in itself, alone as much as being is not a reality in itself alone. Because one cannot be without the other. As it is a proven simple fact, it cannot be said that not being is an illusion as much as it cannot be said that being is an illusion.

This is a very simple reality whatever are our believes. There is no mystery in that concept, just a perception that is enriching our being. Exercising our focus is opening doors and is changing our perspective, whether we don't believe in anything, or we are atheists, or materialistic, or mystic or whatever is our current perception. Passing these doors, each one of us will, empowered, freely continue its own path. The sum of individual added powers and the sum of individual change process, without the restriction of limiting believes, are seriously, significantly and with synergies enhancing the change processes at collective levels.

Again, to mention that the reality of being and not being became clear with the quantum physic; to mention that the diffusion of knowledge is getting facilitated by the knowledge revolution; therefore, to realize that we are now the actors of a big and global revolution. Again, mentioning that the world is actually changing a lot and is going to change further in the coming years. The previsions of big changes are worth to repeat, to allow us to become open to changes. Do not worry, what will be will be, and get comfortable being and not being.

While this reality is proven by the quantum physic, it is interesting to underline that the concept of not being is approached by mysticism and philosophy since millenniums, and more recently by the researches on consciousness, but sometime under-evaluating the being.

## ☯☯ Exercise 91 : Remove the pressure of fears

One interesting application of our definition "being and not being" is to release the obsessions we can have regarding identifications to one character.

This exercise can be made with all identifications that are pressuring us.

But, as an example, let's take the most common obsessive identification to the character having such fear.
Realizing that our definition is also not being, therefore not being this character having such fear, the obsessive pressure is naturally released, and we are stopping the sterile repetition of the uncomfortable thought.

## 099 - GUIDE to understand the Unity

We find the concept of Unity, also called the Whole, in mystical and philosophical texts, for centuries. Mystics use this concept, not to describe God, which is not descriptive, but to generate sensations, in a deliciously poetic way, as in Sufi poetry, in innumerable other literatures, of all times and on all continents, or in contemplations of representations rich in symbols, such as rosettes, labyrinths, calligraphies, yantras and others.

From the beginning of the last century, quantum physics describes the universe as a Unity. Quantum mechanics observes the connections between all the particles of the Universe, under the names 'entanglement'. These equations are validated, in an experiment, in which a photon is separated in two. The halves are placed in two laboratories, several kilometers apart (their separation of thousands or billions of kilometers would produce the same result), then an excitation is carried out on one of the halves, the same reaction is then observed, on the other half. In a subsequent experiment, in addition to showing the tangling of matter, it also shows the relativity of time: the second half of the photon reacts before the excitation on the first. Let us take another example of an event in the Universe, the Big Bang. The quantum entanglement of matter shows us that there is a link between all the elementary particles, coming from the big bang[33], even

---

[33] The big bang was, $10^{-43}$ seconds after time zero, much smaller ($10^{-35}$ meter) than the nucleus size of an atom ($10^{-15}$ meter).

distant tens of billions of light years. We are not only made up of dust of stars, we are also intimately linked to all the stars of the universe.

In the same vein, Einstein translates the cosmological principle that man does not occupy a privileged position in the homogeneous and isotropic universe, that is to say, similar to himself, whatever the place. This absence of a privileged position, in an infinite universal matrix, helps us to relativize our being. It also shows us that being, although very palpable, is not as obvious and tangible as it appears. These cosmological considerations support us in our realization of belonging to a universal matrix, the quality of relationships between individuals, and the quality of relationships between individuals and their environment. They also, give us a perspective on the definition of our being: To be and not to be.

Nowadays, the theory most recognized by mathematicians, and by physicists, is that of the multiverse, infinite and entangled. This theory is, by definition, also described as a Unity.
The many hours of these experts' great reflection, and the speed of calculation of the new equations, by the supercomputers, to understand the infinite, can only add the infinite again to the equation already containing the infinite. And here we are talking about the big infinity, and the small infinity (found in the structure of the elementary particles, therefore in ourselves).

Apart from making ourselves full of admiration, such dimensions are impossible for us to conceive. And this is even more so, when looking at 'before' the big bang, which conditions for us the existence of time and space. Or, when nothing prevents us from thinking that there is an infinity of big bang.

Albert Einstein, one of the pillars of Quantum Physics, made known the famous equation $E = MC^2$.
Where E is Energy, M is the mass of matter, and C is the velocity of light (multiplied by itself ($C^2$)).
C = 300,000,000 meters per second,
(7 times the turn of the earth in 1 second).
$C^2$ = 300,000,000 x 300,000,000
= 90,000,000,000,000,000

This equation has taught us that matter is energy. It has caused a turning point in our history.

Which led Einstein to say:
'Matter is solidified energy',
'Everything is energy ", and,
'Our separation from each other is an optical illusion'

Which led Max Planck to say:
'All matter originates and exists only by virtue of a force... We must assume behind this force the existence of a conscious and intelligent Mind. This Mind is the matrix of all matter' [34]

---

[34] See the very beautiful representation of the Universe by the researchers of the Max Plank Institute:
https://www.youtube.com/watch?v=UC5pDPY5Nz4

And, which led Nikola Tesla to say:

*'We are whirling through endless space, with and inconceivable speed, all around everything is spinning, everything is moving, everywhere there is energy. There must be some way of availing ourselves of this energy more directly. Then, with the light obtained from the medium, with the power derived from it, with every form of energy obtained without effort, from the store forever inexhaustible, humanity will advance with giant strides. The mere contemplation of these magnificent possibilities expands our minds, strengthens our hopes and fills our hearts with supreme delight.'*

♦

$E = MC^2$, thus, calculates the amount of energy contained in a quantity of matter. As we have seen that the value of $C^2$ is enormous. The amount of energy contained in the matter is confirmed as being enormous. Even that contained in a quantity of matter of the size of an atom. It is the principle of the dangerous, and yet replaceable, nuclear energy production that breaks the atoms (fission) to extract the energy.

♦

And, which led Richard Feynman to say:

'In a cubic meter of space there is enough energy to boil all the water of the oceans'

---

## 👀 Exercise 92 : Your vibrational body

The analogy, between our physical body and our vibrational body, has already been made in the '050 - Guide to remain standstill', where are evoked the vibrations of high frequency, when one feels good, and the vibrations of low frequency, when one feels bad.

Seeing in the preceding pages that everything, including our body, is energy; and since energy is a vibration, we perceive that the analogy between the physical body and our vibratory body is not an extravagance, but another form of our reality.

Overloaded meals, aggression, warfare on TV, annoyance or dissatisfaction are all stress that feeds our low-frequency vibrations.

While, pleasant sensations, laughter, joys, positive thoughts, and positive actions fuel our high frequency vibrations.

We begin to recognize, thanks to medical statistics, the effects of stress and the effects of happiness on our health. It is a dynamic, action-reaction between our body and thought, which we can use to our advantage.

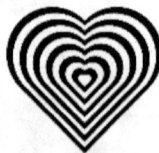

With our emotions, we navigate between these low vibrations to these high vibrations. The ones balancing the others. The serenity, and our most fluid circulation of energy, lie at the point of equilibrium between these low vibrations and these high vibrations. It is at this point that our greatest happiness lies.

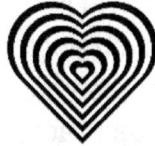

We optimize these benefits of the balance of our vibrational body in three ways:

o   By reducing, the number, duration and intensity of our low vibration states;

o   By increasing the same for our high vibration states;

o   By cultivating, through the silence (thoughts, sounds, and movements of the body), and in meditation, with the knowledge and the feeling at this point of equilibrium between high and low vibrations.

## 100 - GUIDE to remember

It is easy for us to recognize and appreciate the advantages and benefits of this or that idea, practice, project, concept, activity or resolution, and that we soon forget. In particular, after an interruption in practice, for one reason or another, it is often difficult to repeat it.

Every teaching and technique requires a practice to achieve results. And the more the practice is repeated, the better the results. When it is interrupted, they wilt.
This process is neither worrying nor tedious. You will taste, that, pleasure and happiness are within the practice, giving you the desire to continue practicing.

With regard to the techniques transmitted in this manual, and in order to avoid oblivion, you will benefit from establishing routines. And also, to use all the possible opportunities to practice the techniques (like on the bus or any other means of transport, in your car while waiting at the traffic light, in a waiting room, in a waiting time , during your walk, doing a domestic task, washing your teeth, etc.). Seeking, more and more, to feel alive every moment.

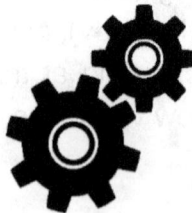

You will certainly agree, it is better to live in this way, being alive, being conscious, rather than the days passing, without really realizing it, or suffering.

Do not formalize yourself on the best ceremonial or the best conditions to practice. As in silence, in solitude, sitting, standing or lying down. If the results can be better under the best conditions, any practice produces a result. And any benefit is good to take. The ceremonial and the conditions that are best for you now, and which make you easy to practice, are the best.

We sometimes forget that we are alive.
We forget to love.
One forgets what would be better to do and one continues to do what would better to stop.
We forget impermanence. We forget to hope.
We forget to stay in touch with family or friends.
We forget so many things, the remembrance of which would make us more happy and whose sum would make us very happy.

For now, let us take, here, the decision to be happy, then to remember to add progressively and fortunately, supports and experience to our decision.

You will not be able to adopt a new behavior until you have perceived by practicing it that it makes you happier than the old. Gradually, you will exercise your freedom of choice, more and more, and better and better, to use your time (or rather your present), your life, your body, your thoughts and your actions, in the best possible ways . And the choices that have just been quoted, will be complicit, in order to allow you to prolong your decision.

You will have only one constraint: to remember; because right after the start of the new behavior you have chosen, you feel the joy of living it. These changes will thus easily become new habits. The constraint of memory will disappear because these new behaviors will have become your new nature.

For other behavioral changes, the joie de vivre that follows at the start-up will be very palpable and addictive, but you will need more effort to remember to renew this joie de vivre, to make it your new nature, and to forget the addiction of the behaviors that define your personality less happy.

Begin with the practice that you like the most, then add new practices, always by following your preferences. Practice regularly, best daily.

These greater difficulties of change, which require more effort, are, however, happy and welcome, as are all difficulties. Because it is thanks to them that we can taste, their contraries, the joy of life and freedom.

All our lives we will forget and we will have to remember, as for example of this famous apnea, which furnishes our lives in times of stress. Forgetting to breathe is the duality of breathing. Forgetting is the duality of remembering. Only the existences of these dynamics can allow us to feel the immense joy of breathing.

All the practices of this manual, deserve not to be forgotten.

And for each of them, it is desirable to measure our reactions, in order to understand, how pleasant it is to practice them, how much they bring us well-being, and how easy it is to forget to practice them, before to have, to our greatest benefit, integrated our new personality.

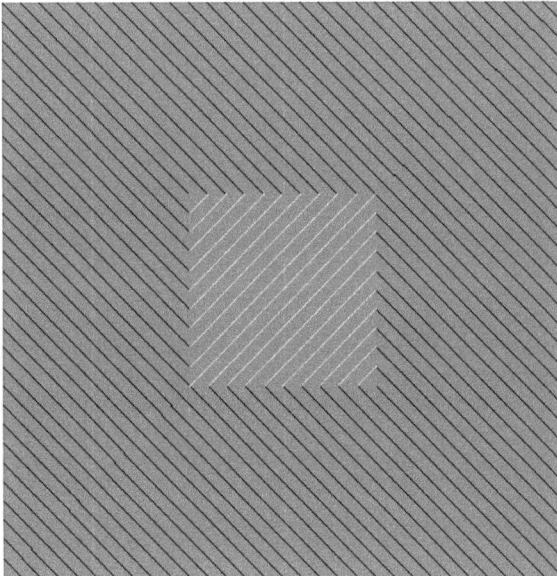

Reflections are not good, without practice and without feeling. It is fundamental to have a pyramid, body-thought-action, balanced.

Only practice allows us to recognize in what dualities we find ourselves. Without practice, we are likely to misunderstand and even to be carried away, without really realizing it, in a negative cascade more powerful than our will. Practice allows us to privilege, in these dynamics of dualities, those we prefer. And it enables the legitimacy and illegitimacy of unhappy dualities to be lived, better, faster, and gradually at the speed of a flash.

Let us remember, the words of Einstein :

**'Nothing happens before something moves'**

So let us remember to practice, choose, live, breathe and be happy! Let us seek to attain a permanent state alive and conscious.

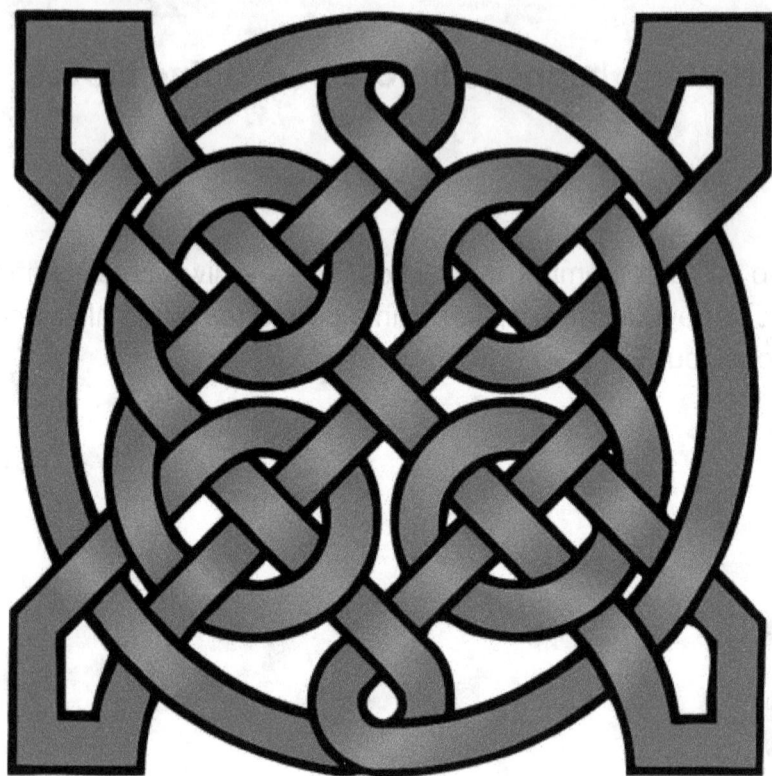

## 3.4.  COMMON DENOMINATOR

The common denominator is the practice of meditation.

Meditation has an important role in this manual, because it is the common denominator for building happiness in your body, in your head and in your actions. It allows, for example, to reduce the obsession of overeating, tension and health problems. It helps improve thoughts, mood, stress and effectiveness, and many other benefits.

And the growing popularity of meditation, with its benefits for the body-thought-action triangular dynamic (enhance, energize and amplify it), significantly contributes, to the great positive changes that are observed today, and to the construction of a better world.

Meditation is also a common denominator for all cultures, today, in history, and on all continents. A common denominator for which we easily have everybody singing from the same hymn sheet.
This growing popularity can be observed on all continents, and more and more often, mass meditations are appearing, whose effects on reduction of violence and criminality are measured.

As globalization allows us to consider the massive perspectives of positivism days on a planetary scale, the massive prospects from the practice of meditation can, reasonably and joyfully, be considered. This is easy, enjoyable and life changing.

We hear more and more about meditation. You've certainly heard of it, maybe even, with the birth of a desire to try.

Meditation is increasingly practiced, individually, in clubs, centers, businesses, and even in schools (in several countries, particularly in Quebec, where it is now part of the curriculum. We measure positive effects on children's concentration, performance and attitudes). It is thus, easily predictable, that the increase in the number of practitioners will be significant in the coming years. It is likely, that you will become one of them.

People who practice meditation are happy to do so. On one hand, it is the most effective method to relax. On the other hand, practitioners appreciate, quickly, its many other advantages (listed on the following pages).

Maybe you are already a regular or occasional practitioner. Perhaps you have already said that you would like to meditate. Or maybe you think that meditation is not for you, at this time of your life.

Its many advantages, and its simplicity to practice, are within the reach of everyone.

My experiences of the meditation are manifold, in the practice of martial art[35], in the practice of other teachings[36], in the integration of concepts such as the silence, the Unity, the All and the Absolute, and in my personal research.

Yet my experience has not, so far, consisted in several hours' meditations. But rather in the simple and easy integration of meditation in my daily activities. And I was able with this method to taste its advantages.

It is this simple method, which I want to share with you here, so that you can easily, now, benefit of its advantages.

Everyone experiences transient meditative states. Mainly in times related to breathing. Because breathing is the basis of meditation and more specifically conscious breathing. These meditative states, which we naturally live are, for example, the moments when one is filled with happiness, feelings and ecstatic emotions; also, the moments when we enjoy filling our lungs with a good air of forest, sea or mountain.

If at that moment there is a beautiful sunset and an entirely orange sky, then visual contemplation adds to the contemplation of the breath. If there is the sound of wind, birds or waves, then auditory contemplation is part of the

---

[35] Viet Vo Dao: 14 years of practice with Master André Gazure, and regular personal practice.
[36] Including 2 years of practice of the Pranayama (Yoga Respiration - "Art of Living" Sri Sri Ravi Shankar), Shamanism, Yoga, Buddhism, etc.

game. You will agree, that in these moments, thought is neither vagabond nor tormented. And if a thought of a problem arises, it flies with the wind, and it is quickly forgotten.

Some people are mistaking thinking that meditation is a state of unconsciousness. Meditation, on the contrary, seeks a state of maximum consciousness. In the state of maximum consciousness of meditation, one is conscious that one thinks and one succeeds in suspending one's thought. So, we are not only identified with our thinking, but we are a thinking being able to observe his thought. It may even happen that people sometimes say to themselves, sometimes with amusement, sometimes with astonishment, 'Well, I am now thinking of this or that.'

With conscious breathing our mind focuses on the air that comes and goes during our inspirations and expirations. This concentration of our attention has many advantages. One of the advantages is that at the moment when our thought or our attention is concentrated on the breathing it cannot wander in the memories of the past, in the imaginations of the future or in the next room. More than to manage your thought, you will no longer allow your thoughts to control you.

In addition, breathing can easily be identified with life, on the one hand, the essence of life that penetrates our body, and on the other hand, the breathing that allows us to live.

Meditation is a practice that is accessible to everyone because it is simple, easy, it does not require any particular belief, and it does not contradict any belief

Conscious breathing can be self-sufficient, it may remain the sole meditation technique you will be using, while getting all benefits of meditation.

If you want to vary the pleasures, there are many other techniques that can be used. These techniques do not require any particular beliefs either, but only require the use of visualization. Visualization is our mental capacity to represent an object, an action, a sound, a sensation, a situation or an emotion. It is necessary to know, that the cerebral activity is the same, during the visualization of an action, as, when the action is actually performed. As a result, visualization is a technique, which is now, for example, used by top athletes and contributes to the precision and the feeling[37] of the required movements. The practice of visualization technique, therefore, will only require from you, a freedom and an open mind to let your imagination travel. Even if you are skeptical, you still can make the experiences, then to judge the results. You will find further in this guide, examples of meditation techniques, using a lot of visualization and imagination. I recommend, you play the game, by practicing these exercises, to give free rein to your imagination, without shame, without a priori and without reluctance, but with curiosity.

You can also find numerous and varied guided meditations on U-Tube, made with a lot of talent. I encourage you to explore them. You will then find those that suit you. You will be able to notice, that often these videos recommend you renew the experiment, and affirm that after only one week

---

[37] Proprioception

of daily practice of one hour (average duration of a guided meditation), you will be able to clearly feel new sensations. I can testify that this statement is correct. These sensations being new, it will be the first time you feel them; they will delight you, and they will engender transformations of your being that you will appreciate.

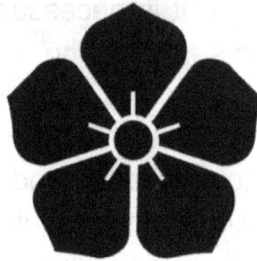

Someone asked to Buddha:

*'What have you gained from meditation?'*

He replied:

*'Nothing! However, let me tell you what I lost : anger, anxiety, depression, insecurity, fear of old age and death'*

♦

*'If you have time to breathe you have time to meditate. You breathe when you walk. You breathe when you stand. You breathe when you lie down'*

Ajahn Amaro

*'Meditation is not something that should be done in a position at a particular time. It is an awareness and an attitude that must persist through the day'*

A. Swami

♦

*'One conscious breath in and out is a meditation'*

Eckhart Tolle

♦

*'The things that trouble our spirits are within us already. In meditation, we must face them, accept them, and set them aside one by one.'*

*C.L. Bennett*

♦

'The whole of meditation practice can be essentialized into these 3 crucial points: Bring your mind home. Release. And relax!'

Sogyal Rinpoche

♦

'If you mind is empty, it is always ready for anything; it is open to everything.  In the beginner's mind there are many possibilities, in the expert's mind there are few.'

Shunryu Suzuki

♦

*'Meditating on the problem of the day, or even on one's personal problems, is the last thing the normal individual desires to do'*

Henry Miller

## Meditation brings many advantages:

- This is the best way to relax.
- Allows you to suspend and slow down your thoughts, even if initially, your mind is agitated.
- Decreases, to eliminate, depressive tendencies, anxiety, and stress.
- Decreases irritability, confusion and moodiness. Enables better management of emotions, till equilibria of your emotional body.
- Increases intuition, analytical ability and creativity.
- Improves the ability to make good decisions and to avoid mistakes.
- Increases connection with reality. Strengthens the anchoring of the feet on the ground, balance and stability.
- Allows for a clearer, alert and helpful thinking. Increases efficiency.
- Develops the ability, quicker and faster, to return to positive thinking and to restore smiles.
- Increases self-confidence.
- Improves all interpersonal relationships.
- Increases the ability to love others and oneself.
- Is more effective than sleep to rest.
- Improves the quality and effectiveness of sleep.
- Helps to stay younger in body and mind, increases vitality and longevity in good health.
- Lower blood pressure. Reduces muscle tension and pain (including chronical pains).
- Increases serotonin secretion. Strengthens the immune system.

- Facilitates personal development.
- Helps people in spiritual quest.
- Generates functional, as well as structural, transformations of the brain.
- Improves memory.
- Decreases tendencies to forget.

Completed studies, already confirmed the above, and ongoing ones, point to many other benefits, particularly in the areas of physical health and mental health.

There are many techniques of meditation. We have already seen the conscious breathing and the meditative walk, so easy to practice and to integrate into our daily gestures. Many other exercises in this manual, in which our attention is focused, also reflect meditation practices. There are many others, original, attractive and varied, offering their sensations, their benefits and their specific practical integrations.

100 techniques are proposed now. The multiplicity and the variety allow to satisfy your curiosity, to discover new sensations and to gain new capacities; but your main goal is to practice daily, during your entire life. You will achieve this goal more easily, using a technique, during days or weeks, that you particularly appreciate. Then, moving on to another technique.

## 👀 Exercise 93 : Sweeping the floor

We have seen that it is possible and desirable, on the one hand to seize every opportunity to meditate, and on the other hand to seek to live in full awareness 24/7.

Each of our activities can be done in full awareness, fully focused on the activity itself. By living this way, we are happy.

Your first step on the floor, when you get out of bed, is so mindful, when you take your breakfast, when you wash your teeth, when you take your shower, in your car or other transport, and so on. You will start by choosing a specific activity. Then, you will take the habit of living this activity in full consciousness. Then you will practice mindfulness for another activity, and so on.

To facilitate this practice and this lifestyle, here are some tips to follow:

o Before starting an activity, do 3 long, deep and conscious breaths.

o Concentrate on the present moment, fully aware of your environment and the sensations of your 5 senses, without remembering the past and without projections in the future (if not, at the end of the activity to best coordinate the following activities).

o Be aware, in the present moment, and focused on each move, during the entire duration of the activity.

## ☯☯ Exercise 94 : Accept the reality

We have seen the benefits of accepting reality. Acceptance is not resignation, which can overwhelm us and be charged with negative energy. The acceptance of reality is rich in the positive energy of truth.

Yet, even if we believe in the benefits of accepting reality, our mind continues to play tricks on us. Regrets and fears continue to swirl in our heads, fill our insomnia and make us uncomfortable.

The practice of this meditation allows us to relieve and eliminate these disorders, to see things as they are and not as we want them to be.

o Slowly and deeply inhale through the nose, paying close attention to the air passing through your nostrils and filling your lungs.

   Observe your thoughts and emotions without judgment. Like if you were an independent observer.

o Exhale slowly and deeply through the mouth.

o Put an alarm on your phone to tell you when your practice, at least 10 minutes, is over.

If your troubles are not dispelled, continue for an additional period, until you feel good. After that, you can continue as long as you want.

## ☻☻ Exercise 95 : Meditation of the food

Very often, we eat in a robotic way, without thinking about what we do, a bit like an obligation, or as emotional comfort; without thinking of what we eat; and without being grateful for the chance we have of eating what we eat.

If we have sensations, they are limited to taste. If, for example, we eat a vegetable, we do not really consider the vegetable, only its taste. Certainly, at best, we are gourmets, and we take a great pleasure with this range of tastes. But we do not consider, for example, that the vegetable has been a seed, and that it has grown in the ground or on a branch, that it has bathed with the energy of the sun's rays and the drops of rain. We, as the only one in the world, do not consider the farmer who took care of the plant, nor the other actors who allowed the vegetable to arrive on our plate.

When we eat, being aware of what we are doing is also better for our digestion. In addition, by being conscious and grateful, we gain a greater benefit from the nutritional value of food; and we can eat less, which is very helpful, to feel better, and to solve an overweight problem.

The meditation on the story of food, is a technique in which, you will have a great consideration that you are eating and for the food that you are eating. What is its story? You will look and appreciate its forms, its colors, its textures, its perfume. Thoughts for the actors (farmers, transporters, merchants and others) will break your loneliness and isolation, and make you feel the (sometimes distant) space between you, the different actors and the different phases of production of this food. As such, you will feel belonging to this space. Practicing this technique will give you new benchmarks. It will be good for your physical and mental health, and for your existential feeling.

For a food, this practice consists in viewing its path from production to the nutritional and taste benefits it brings to you.

Let's do with an example (bread), an exercise that will make you practice this technique and that will give you ideas to imagine your own stories with other foods. Practice this technique before starting a meal, so that your appetite is a good actor. The first time you practice this technique choose a meal where you will be alone and quiet. Keep the manual near you so you can read it while you are doing the exercise or practice it with a loved one who will read the text for you.

(Note that the meditation of the food below contains many details, which will allow you to see, how much it is possible to travel extensively using this technique. Of course, it is not conceivable to apply as much details at each of your meals. The process is to choose an appropriate time when you are free and available to practice this detailed meditation in its entirety, and then it will be easy for you to quickly reproduce the principle of this technique at each of your meals.)

At each step, explore the sensations that the practice of instructions gives you.

- o Take a piece of bread between your fingers. Begin by expressing gratitude for the chance to be able to eat it. You feel the soft texture of its crumb, and the hard texture of its crust. You can imagine the crispy.
  You approach the bread of your face and fill you with the delicious smell of fresh bread.

- o You now, carry the piece of bread to your mouth. And you begin to eat it, being aware that it is bread that you eat. You feel the sensations on your teeth, on your tongue and on your lips. You feel the first flavors and you explore them.

- o You are now, thinking of the seed (of wheat or other) from which your piece of bread is made. You see it planted in the ground. You see it germinating, the first white root that digs the earth and sinks. The green stem beginning to rise to the sky, emerging from the earth and beginning to develop its first leaves. The first leaves that unfold, like a cocoon that turns into a butterfly.

- o You now feel, the light and heat of the sun nourishing the first leaves. The rain refreshing them. The wind that making the stems to dance. The cobs are growing.

- o You now see, an entire field of wheat cobs. Their waves formed by the wind. Their brilliant colors lighted by the sun.

- Now, the agricultural machine, harvesting them. The farmer driving the machine, putting the grain in bags and carrying them. Ground grain and white flour. The baker who works the dough. The dough rising and then cooked in the oven. The breads just out of the oven, then transported into the store.

- Your visit to the store, then return home. You are now in front of your plate tasting the flavors of the bread.

- When swallowing, you feel the benefits of vitamins, minerals and all other good constituents.

- You are feeling the power of the sun. You even see the sun at the doors of infinity of space.

- You now find on your plate one of the seeds that covered the crust of your bread. You take it between your fingers and roll it. You pay attention to your sensation when touching this seed. Then you move this sensation to feel it in all the cells of your body. You're playing for a while with this feeling.
  Then you put the seed in your mouth and make it crack between your teeth. The taste of the seed is particular. You pay attention to this taste. Then you move this sensation to feel it in each cell of your body. You're playing for a while with this feeling.

- By eating this seed, you have finished your piece of bread. You made a great trip and you felt nice sensations. You are happy and grateful.

Now that you have understood this technique, you can practice it again, choosing other foods for which you will imagine and view their stories. You can, for example, choose exotic fruits (e.g. bananas, oranges) that will take you on African, Asian and South American lands. Their rich and intense tastes will allow you to let fly lyrically your imagination. After this first practice by being alone, you can practice this exercise in a restaurant or being accompanied. You can then practice short and fast practices by following the same principles.

♦

This practice is very effective. From the first practice, your relationship with food will change. A mechanism of meditative feeling about the history and origin of your food, and the actors involved, will be printed in your memory. This feeling will accompany you when you eat. Sometimes you will notice its presence, it will make you smile and make you happy. The formal repetition of this practice, or even simple conscious regular nutrition, will improve the benefits you will derive from it. The increase in moments of consciousness and presence, and the reduction of moments of absence, will enable you to live your life more fully. The priority you have given to happiness, will allow you to privilege these moments of happiness.

Other benefits of this technique are numerous:

- Your sensations of Unity and your integration in Unity are amplified,

- Your sensation of the interactions between the constituents of Unity is amplified,

- The amplitudes of your taste, your smell and your touch are amplified,

- Your benefit from the vital energy of food is increased.

- Your digestion is improved.

- At times when you focus your attention on your life, specifically on the conscious action of eating, your obsessive thoughts are forgotten. The result is a reduction in stress and an increase in joie de vivre. A presence exchanged against an absence.

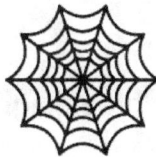

*'Everyone eats and drinks yet only few appreciate the taste of food'*

Confucius

## 👀 Exercise 96 : The mindful digestion

(Duration: 7 minutes)
The practice of this exercise requires the improvement of abilities, gained during the practices of the exercises of the manual, relaxation, breathing, feeling of the energy currents, feeling of the body, the silence of the thought, and concentration.

Exercise benefits the whole body.
And because of the great influences of digestion and the digestive system, it also improves the quality of your thinking, your emotions and your actions.

This technique demonstrates perfectly, the effects of body sensations in the triangular dynamics body-thought-action (which exist for all bodily sensations).

Concentrate, <u>exclusively</u>, on the bodily sensations given by the practice of the exercise.

♦

Sit comfortably, lying down. And relax.

Inhale deeply, 3 times, exhaling slowly and calmly.

(Each step: 2 minutes.)

o Concentrate on your breathing, with the desire to slow it down. By relaxing, the depth and rhythm of your breathing will decrease naturally. Be free, sometimes to take deeper inspirations, if you feel the need. Feel the air in your lungs.

   Throughout the exercise, you will maintain this calm and slowed breathing.

o Feel your stomach enlarged after the meal.

Breathe especially with the rib cage.

From now on, and during the rest of the exercise, you will maintain the feeling of a slight tone of the muscles of your abdominal belt.
Moderately inflates the belly at the inspiration.

o Keep your breath calm and slow and feel the delicate touch of your diaphragm on your stomach. Concentrate on this touch.

It is a delicate sensation, which is entirely new to you. Before you did this exercise, you never felt it. This is the culminating moment of this exercise, enjoy and savor it.

Finish the exercise by relaxing for 30 seconds.

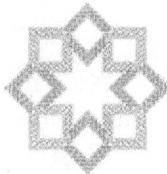

Note: Once you become familiar with the feeling of your stomach, you will be able the measure different feeling after different diets. This will be very useful to better, explore, discover, manage, enjoy, and react to, the sensations given by fasting, delight, hunger, satiety, food overload, favorable diets to your well-being, vivacity, and happiness, disturbing diets, and intuitive desires.

## 👀 Exercise 97 : Becoming breathing

Who are we ?

We define ourselves in many conventional ways. We will, also, benefit from defining ourselves as being our breathing. Or, as the air we breathe. The air, which is life penetrating our body. The air, we breathe full lungs. The air, that we also breathe with our heart. The air, that oxygenates all the cells of our body. The air that raises our rib cage, which lowers our diaphragm and our stomach. The air that swells our belly and makes us feel our abdominal belt, our kidneys and our bladder.

We define ourselves in many conventional ways. The sensation of becoming breathing is a culmination of self-knowledge. It is a sensation that we are not used to.

**Technic 1**

During your meditation practices, think of concentrating a few moments on this feeling, to learn to know it.

Do not worry if you do not feel anything. This is completely normal. The sensation is so delicate that, much more than in other exercises, it is necessary to learn to feel it, to recognize it and to assimilate it. And, as with any other exercise, repetitions of practice develop awareness of sensation. Thus, gradually, your feelings of identification with your breathing will be better, and you will be able to prolong it.

You can already imagine the depth of this existential definition. Until now you did not really know how to define yourself, between your palpable body, your worries tormenting you, your ideas, your job, your family, your hobbies and many other conventional ways. With this technique, you will feel being your breathing, simply air, between everything and nothing. Air, which is at the same time the essence of life, and which cannot resist the wind.

At the same time, you maximize your presence and the energy that makes you live, you identify with the essence of life, and you let them evaporate.

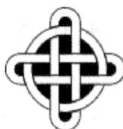

For this technique, as for all the others contained in this manual, you will find other methods to integrate them in your life. The sensations, and the feeling of their evolutions, will also be very specific to you. For you are their sole owner and their only Master, and because you are one.

## Technic 2

- o  Sit comfortably, relax and practice a few staged breaths.

- o  Visualize that the entire surface of the skin of your body is like the membrane of a fairground balloon.

- o  Visualize with inhale that the air is filling your body, and that your body is made of air up to the limits of your skin. And your body deflates on exhale.

- o  Stay with this visualization for a few minutes of inhale-exhale.

## ◉◉ Exercise 98 : Sri Yantra meditation

On the next page, you will find the Sri Yantra.

Sri Yantra is the most famous yantra. It is called the mother of the Yantra because all derive from it.

This is a Tantric meditation chart. The Sri Yantra is a graphic meditation support from the Hindu tradition, borrowed by Buddhism (called mandala), and by Taoism. The graphic in its central part is structured in a very sophisticated way, with figures of sacred geometry, series (4,5,9,43) of triangles, the sequence of Fibonacci, the gold number and the number Pi. The central part is surrounded by two crowns of (8 and 16) lotus flower petals, themselves surrounded by circles. The whole is contained in a square that has four doors. All these representations are very rich in deep symbolisms, to which the meditator identify, aiming at integrating them.

A total of 111 aspects are symbolized in Sri Yantra. The 2 crowns of lotus petals, with 4 crowns of triangles, and the central triangle, symbolize energy circuits that correspond to the 7 main chakras. The central point symbolizes the point of creation or the big bang, and the set represents the arrangement of matter from the big bang.

Sri Yantra is a representation of the macrocosm and the microcosm, a vision of a multitude of attributes, of totality and Unity, and an overview of the Absolute. It thus contains, all the potentialities of becoming.

Like the labyrinth, Sri Yantra symbolizes a pilgrimage, an initiatory journey for a better self-knowledge, with its different stages that lead to the center of the figure, and beyond that point, while maintaining an understanding of the whole.

The Fibonacci sequence found in the Sri Yantra is a fractal element of sacred geometry that is also found everywhere in the formation of matter, from the form of elementary particles to the shape of galaxies, and the measurements in the human body. The sequence of Fibonacci (of which you will find a graphical representation on the following page) is a sequence of integers in which each term is the sum of the two terms that precede it (Thus the first terms are: 0, 1, 1, 2, 3 , 5, 8, 13, 21, etc.). The Fibonacci sequence is found everywhere in nature, and in the most visible way for example in the sunflower, in shells, in pine cones, pineapples, cacti and cyclones. It is also found in the arts such as music, painting (e.g. Leonardo da Vinci's Mona Lisa), and in architecture.

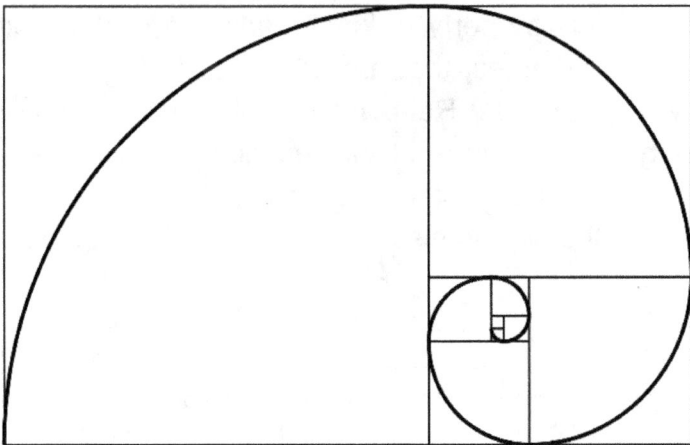

Write 'Sri Yantra' on your Internet browser. Then, you will find many Sri Yantra, multicolored, aesthetic and decorative. You can frame one, or place it as your computer or your cell phone background. Then to the aesthetic benefits are added the properties of the Sri Yantra acquired during furtive or prolonged glances. Again, here we perceive the interest of savoring the pleasure and the happiness of furnishing our lives with opportunities of contemplation and of conscience. In doing so, our happiness capital, our balance, our well-being and the quality of our reactions increase.

Note that Sri Yantra is very popular for its credited capacity to generate prosperity. It is useless to cultivate this superstitious belief, as all superstitious beliefs are useless to cultivate. However, prosperity is a logical consequence of a very real action of contemplation / meditation of Sri Yantra, and its effects.

The Sri Yantra meditation consists of fixing the central point while seeing the whole of Yantra. You will then see the shapes moving, this is normal, spectacular and pretty. It is thanks to this property of kinetic art, and to the multiple dancing geometries, that are attributed to Sri Yantra the following properties: Relaxation - Improved concentration capacity.-. Integrations of the feminine[38] and masculine aspects of being. (Intertwined as in the Yin-Yang). - . Balancing the two hemispheres of the brain. Expansion of consciousness.

---

[38] The equilateral triangle pointing downwards symbolizes the feminine aspect. The equilateral triangle pointing upwards the masculine aspect.

Continue (5 minutes at least) this practice. It is likely that you will appreciate this exercise and that you will want to do it more often and more time. You will benefit.

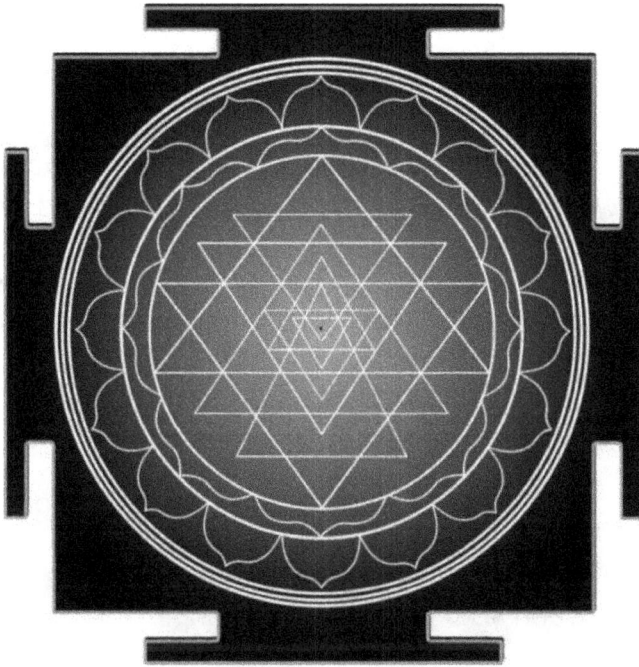

## 👀 Exercise 99 : During insomnia

o You must have a single intention: to get back to sleep.

o Do not consider any other alternative (such as reading, watching a movie, playing a game on your phone, thinking, etc.).

o Do not look at your watch. Would it be early in the night or soon before your planned waking time, it would make you think. And feeding your thinking, that's exactly what you want to avoid, because it might get carried away.

o If when you wake up you realize that your thought is already very active, do not worry, you will manage to interrupt it.

o The only thing you need to do is:

   ▪ Feeling your belly that rises to the inspiration. And,

   ▪ Feel the air coming out of your nostrils, or passing between your lips, when exhaling.

o According to your preferences, breath by the nose or by the mouth. The important thing is that you are comfortable.

o This focus, on your belly, nostrils or lips, will prevent other thoughts from interfering.

o Come back to this focus as soon as you start thinking.

o Continue this focus until you sleep.

## ◉◉ Exercise 100 : Gong meditation

Using the gong sound, during meditation sessions, offers several advantages:

- At the beginning of the session it allows us to place ourselves in a situation of meditation.

- Regular intervals of sound of the gong, during the session, indicate the time remaining to us, in the length of sitting we have decided.

- During the session, the deep vibrations of the sound vibrate our whole body, with the same advantages that we have seen in the practice of sound 'OM'.

- Listen to the sound of the gong from the beginning to the silence that follows.

- During the session, the sound of the gong brings us back to the focus on conscious breathing.

- Two or three sounds from the gong indicate the end of the session, without one having to worry about watching his watch.

To practice this exercise, you can find free gong timers on the internet.

Your initiation to the use of the gong sound, to return to a happy and efficient state of consciousness, will allow you getting used to take opportunity of other sounds for the same benefit during your day (even a noise pollution, such as siren of the car of our friends the fireman).

## ☯☯ Exercise 101 : Meditation in infinities

This meditation is a journey in the range of our three-dimensional knowledge (height, width, length). It is a journey into the known. Let us recall the dimensions of reality: day after day, we discover the confines of the cosmos, more and more distant. The size of the universe is now estimated at about 100 billion light-years (The speed of light is 300,000 km per second). A few years ago, we discovered the fascinating infinite fractal structure of elementary particles, moving and reproducing.

This meditation will therefore take place in this gigantic space " known and palpable ", in which we live, and, which lives in us. We will travel to the finite limits, and in passing we will wink at the unknown of the infinitely big and the infinitely small. But we will remain in this finished garden, whose size is very satisfactory.

Now, we will not ask ourselves the questions to which we have no conceivable answers (like the probable infinity of the number of universes, or the depth of the infinitely small).

The visualization of this space allows us to better know ourselves. This journey, like all travels, is also an opportunity to see new horizons, relax and interrupt our worrying thoughts.

You will be able to make this trip by reading the following lines. It would also be interesting, that one of your relatives can slowly read to you, this would allow you to close your eyes in order to travel more freely. If you are alone, close your eyes after reading each instruction, and immerge in each detail of its description.

**Step by step :**

o Consider the space where you are currently, for example, your bedroom. Consider precisely where you are, for example sitting on the floor or in an armchair or lying on your bed.

o Eyes closed, look at yourself, from above. You see yourself sitting on your chair or lying on your bed. Now your vision rises, and you see the whole room, then an aerial view of your house, then of your city, then of your region, then of your country. Now you see your whole continent. Your vision still rises, and you see the seas and oceans, and then the neighboring continents. Now you see the planet earth. Your vision continues to rise, and you pass by the moon. Now the earth and the moon become smaller and smaller, and you pass by the planets. You now see the whole solar system. Your vision continues to rise, and the solar system becomes smaller and smaller. You pass by the stars, then you see the whole galaxy. The galaxy becomes smaller and smaller. It seems to you to be in the middle of an immense empty space. Then you see another galaxy on your right. You continue to rise, and now there are billions of galaxies under your feet in the distance, which form like a starry sky.

o Now these stars have disappeared. You are comfortable, in the middle of an immense empty and silent space, you profit from this well-being.

o Then you start the reverse path.

Under your feet begin to appear stars. You pass by the same galaxies. Now, in the distance you see the Milky Way. You pass by the same stars. And you see the solar system in the distance. You pass by the side of the planets. You see the earth in the distance. The continents, the oceans and the seas are emerging. Then the continent where you live, your country, your region, your city and your house.

o You see the room where you are, and you sit on your chair. Your imagination no longer travels, and you feel great stability throughout your body.

o You now see the surface of your skin.

Your gaze passes through your skin, and you find yourself in the current of the red corpuscles of your blood. By identifying yourself with one of these red blood cells, you make an entire turn of your body. Your gaze now passes through the envelope of this red globule. You see more and more deeply, and you now see, in the distance, atoms. You're heading for an atom. You pass by the electrons in the direction of the nucleus of the atom. The sensation you feel when traveling is similar to the feeling of immensity you felt when traveling between the galaxies.

You penetrate into this nucleus,
you see even more deeply.
You see elementary particles. You approach one and you penetrate into its fractal structure.
You continue to penetrate inside this structure fractals, and you feel well in the midst of the convolutions in motion

o You now make the path in the opposite direction: the elementary particles, the atoms.
You cross the red blood cell envelope again, the other red blood cells, your skin.
You are comfortably sitting on your chair.

o Your second trip is over. You feel with happiness a great stability throughout your body. You have some time to savor, the memories of the two beautiful journeys you have just made, and your well-being and stability, in the midst of the immense spaces in which your imagination has just traveled.

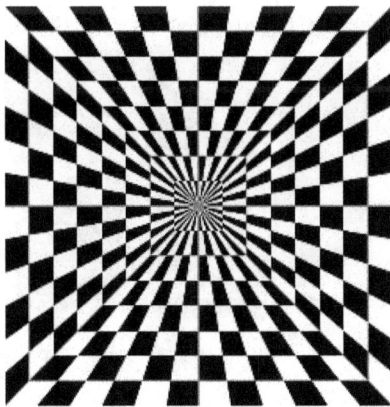

## 👀 Exercise 102 : Meditation of the rose

For this meditation get a rose, another flower, or, alternatively, a candle, to concentrate on its flame adapting the instructions bellow.

o Begin by taking three deep inspirations, followed by slow expirations. At the same time relax yourself completely.

o Contemplates the beauty of the flower, the curves of its petals, the changing reflections of its colors, its heart, etc.

o Penetrates deep into the heart of the flower.

o Comfortably, merges with the flower.

   Now your whole-body turn into the color of the flower. You are bathed in its purity. This purity penetrates to the hearts of each of your cells.

o Prolong as much as you can, this fusion with the beauty, purity and fragrance of the flower.

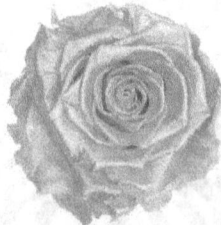

## 👁👁 Exercise 103 : Meditation of the blank screen

This technique can be practiced formally (with posture, relaxation and breathing) and for several minutes. But what makes it so useful is that it can be used anywhere and for a time as short as a few seconds. Therefore, you can practice this technique, at work between two tasks, when you have to stop your car because the fire has just turned red, etc.

So, you're turning off the left hemisphere of your brain. These short poses allow your brain to rest, to take a step back and to increase its ability to analyze and synthesize.

The method consists of visualizing and contemplating a white screen. Then your mind is empty of all other ideas and thoughts, and your emotions are calmed down.

(image : "image: Freepik.com")

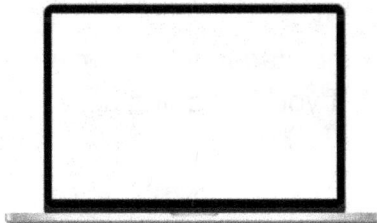

## 👀 Exercise 104 : 3 meditations love and empathy

### 1. Meditation Love 1

o Starts with three deep inhales.

o Simultaneously:

- Visualize a flow of pure love penetrating through your right forefinger, then climbs up your arm to reach your heart;

- Think, or pronounce, a long sound 'LO';

- And takes a long, continuous inhale.

o When you have reached the heart, simultaneously:

- Visualize this flow of love from your heart, to fill your whole body.

- Think, or pronounce, the sound 'VE'

- Exhale all along.

o Continue this meditation for five minutes, or for a longer period, if you feel doing so.

You have here, a very simple and powerful technique to give your attention to.

## 2. Meditation Love 2

o Starts with three deep inhales.

Practice each following step during at least 30 seconds:

o Feel a feeling of love in your heart.

o Extend this love to your whole body.

o Extend this love, and included in this field of love, a person you know and love.

o Include in this love a person you do not like.

o Now feel, at the same time, love in your heart, in all your body, including your friend and including your enemy.

o Now spread this love to the whole earth. Remain some time with this sensation, then extend this love to the whole universe.

## 3. Meditation Empathy

It's a meditation that you can practice every time you witness the pain or even a tragedy experienced by someone else. This person may be a relative, a loved one, a stranger or even that may be in the face of compassion for a large population that is experiencing a tragedy (misery, disaster or war situation).

If you believe in the power of love, you will easily appreciate this meditation. But you will have to be modest in believing in your power to change the event by sending your love; because this power cannot be absolute, otherwise the world would be very different.

If you are incredulous (believe only in what you see), this meditation will also be beneficial, possibly thanks to the unknown extent of the power of love, but directly by providing you with well-being; because the feelings of love and compassion will release the pressure of the sadness of your heart and your whole body. And, in cases where your action can be useful, you will be more able.

You can practice at any time of the day, anywhere, for a short time or for a long time. It may be the moment your gaze crosses an event, or when you settle in a more formal mediation situation for a longer time.

**Practice :**

o Visualize inhaling by the heart, absorbing in your heart the pain that you feel in compassion for the person or persons concerned.

o Visualize exhaling from the heart, sending the love of your heart to the person or persons concerned.

**Variant :**

Here is another technique that you can practice walking in the street or when you are in a place where there are many people.
You will introduce more love into your life.

o Inhale visualizing absorbing vital energy.

o Exhale visualizing sending love from your heart to the heart of a person you meet in your path. Then, do the same thing with another person, then another, and so on.

Do not have tender or sustained looks, stealthy glances will be enough, and they will avoid misunderstandings

## 👀 Exercise 105 : 21 other meditations chakra

While we gain energy benefits by doing exercises on the chakras, our focused concentration also corresponds to meditations. And in addition to the specific energy benefits, the benefits of meditation are also reaping.

By working on the chakras, it is possible that you feel something, like a tickle at the level of a chakra, or the well-being that work gives you. It is also possible that you feel nothing. It does not matter. What is important is to give importance to the exercises and to trust in their efficiencies.

It is good to remember that energy goes from chakra to chakra while circulating through the meridians, and that the main meridian is in the spine.

We have already seen some meditations on the chakras, which can be done, either with a little habit, in a quick and informal way, or, during long and formal meditations.

Here are 10 others:

## 1. Breathe inside the chakras

Stay some time imagining breathing inside each of the 7 chakras, starting with the root chakra and ending with the crown chakra.
If you wish, then return to breathe inside a specific chakra.

## 2. Méditation chakras and mantras

The practice of this exercise requires a little time, because you will spend about two minutes on each chakra.

And it is also possible that to this is added a quick cleaning of the chakras which is recommended before each practice.

It is also possible that your intuition, associated with a certain euphoria induced by the repetition, make you practice one of the mantras for a long time. Or, you can use this technique when you want to work on a specific chakra.

Each chakra is associated with a mantra, a sound, which stimulates the chakra.

The exercise consists in repeating the sound by focusing on the respective chakra and feeling the vibrations of the sound at the level of the chakra.

List of mantras:

- Root Chakra :          LAM
- Sacral Chakra :        VAM
- Solar Plexus :         RAM
- Heart Chakra :         YAM
- Throat Chakra :        HAM
- 3rd eye :              OM
- Crown Chakra :         HAM-SO

## 3.  Méditation chakras and mudras

Our body contains many energy channels; and many of them are on the hands and feet.

The practice of mudras is a practice of yoga of the fingers resulting from the Vedic tradition. It consists of finger positions that create energy flows and specific vibrations. These influence on the harmonization of our physical, psychological and psychic states.

There are many mudras. Here we will practice only the mudras associated with the 7 chakras. You will be able to practice these mudras alone by feeling your sensations for each mudra (at the level of the respective chakra and at the level of the fingers), or in association with other practices on the chakras (colors, sounds, rotations). And of course, when you want to work on a chakra to get its specific benefits, using the associated mudra position will make it easier. Mudras are very effective activation of chakras.

You can practice all these mudras during formal meditations, or practice a specific mudra informally, when you have the opportunity during the day.

Another common practice is to select a mudra, and practice it every day for 1 month, then move on to another mudra the following month. In addition to the advantage of fully benefiting from the energy currents of this mudra, this technique also allows you to memorize the mudras in a sustainable way.

Before each mudra, shake your hands several times.

- **Muladhara mudra**
  **associated to root chakra,**

  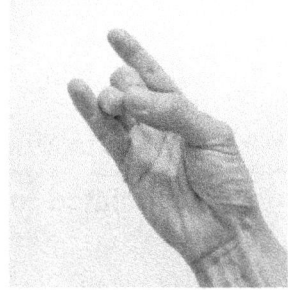

  Color : red,
  Sound : LAM


- **Shakti Mudra**
  **associated to sacral chakra**

  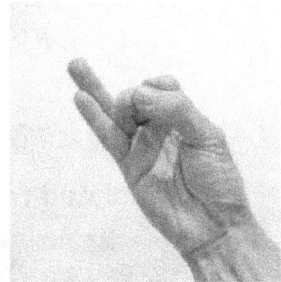

  Color : orange
  Sound : VAM


- **Rudra Mudra**
  **associated to solar plexus**

  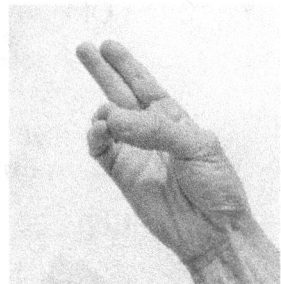

  Color : yellow
  Sound : RAM

- **Padma Mudra**
  **associated to heart chakra**

  Color : green
  Sound : YAM

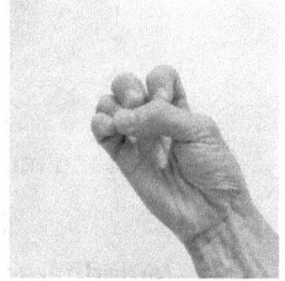

- **Granthita Mudra**
  **associated to throat chakra**

  Color : blue
  Sound : HAM

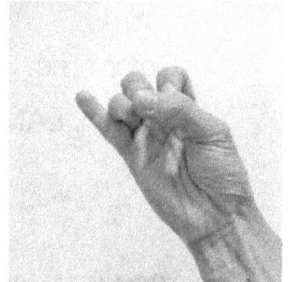

- **Chin Hasta or Gyan Mudra**
  **associated to 3rd eye**

  Couleur : indigo
  Son : OM

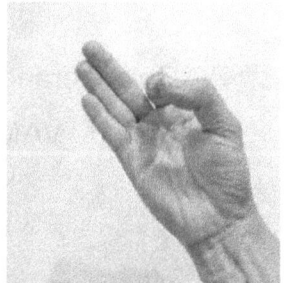

- **For crown chakra continue in the Chin Hasta Mudra**
  **position**
  Couleur : violet
  Son : HAM-SO

## 4. Spine Meditation

After sitting comfortably, having relaxed and having performed several staged breaths, this meditation consists of paying attention to the sensations (kinds of chills) that one feels in the spine during each inspiration and during of each expiration. And stay on this focus for the duration of the meditation (minimum 5 minutes, and more at will).
This is a subtle sensation, that will be challenging to feel; try a strong focus and repeat your try, but do not worry if you feel nothing.

## 5. Mentally singing OM

After sitting comfortably, relaxing, and having several staged breaths, this meditation consists of lingering on each chakra point (starting with the root chakra), and mentally chanting the OM mantra on this point.

## 6. Breathing and chakras

Makes the following visualizations on each of the 7 chakras, from the root chakra to the crown chakra.

○ Inhale through nose visualizing air flooding your chakra.

○ Exhale through nose visualizing air leaving your chakra.

○ Makes several inhale-exhale, on each chakra, before moving on to the next. And at each exhale visualize the color of the chakra you work in front of stronger and stronger. You can, if you prefer, not to visualize the colors, but for each chakra, a white light becoming more and more strong.

## 7. Chakras and elements

Each chakra is associated with an element, as follows :

- Root Chakra :          Earth
- Sacral Chakra :        Water
- Solar Plexus :         Fire
- Heart Chakra :         Air
- Throat Chakra :        Space
- 3rd eye :              Light
- Crown Chakra :         Bliss

It is best to perform this meditation formally (comfortable position, straight back and still position, relaxation of the whole body and staged breathing), to optimize the quality of visualization.

o  Start by focusing on your root chakra and visualize the earth element.

o  Then visualize that your chakra takes on the consistency of the earth element.

o  Visualize that this consistency widens around the chakra, and that little by little your body is transformed into the consistency of the earth element. This until your entire body is made up of this element.

o  Stay for a while with this visualization.

o  Continue, doing the same thing, for the sacred chakra and the water element.

o  And practice, going up, the other chakras, up to the crown chakra.

## 8. Chakras and organs

This meditation is practiced as the previous one, concentrating successively on each chakra, starting with the root chakra root ending the crown chakra.

But this time, you will visualize the organs associated with the chakras.

o   You will visualize positive energy filling each organ.

o   And also, you will visualize each organ being in perfect health and perfect working condition.


The organs and anatomy associated with the chakras are:

- Root chakra:       Large intestine, rectum and some functions of the kidneys

- Sacral Chakra: Kidney, bladder, ovaries, testes and the entire reproductive system

- Solar plexus:    Liver, gallbladder, stomach, spleen and small intestine.

- Heart Chakra:   Heart

- Throat chakra:  Throat and lungs

- Third eye:         Brain, eyes, nose

- Crown chakra:  For the whole body

## 9. The affirmations of the qualities of Chakras

Each chakra is associated with one or more qualities. You will benefit from memorizing these qualities, because they are important parts of the chakra's identity, and knowing these specific qualities helps to optimize them when working on the chakras:

- Root Chakra : The belonging to earth, The balance
- Sacral Chakra : Vitality, enthusiasm, creativity,
- Solare Plexus : Willpower, power, self-confidence
- Heart Chakra : Love, friendship, sociability
- Throat Chakra : Communication, self-confidence
- 3rd eye : clear ideas, intuition, creativity
- Crown Chakra : Decision making, realism

Until now, the technique of affirmations has not been addressed in this manual. It's a very powerful technique.

We are free to think what we want. And we are free to build the identity we desire. The use of the affirmations reinforces the characteristics that one asserts. The conscious repetition of affirmations imprints the subject affirmed in our subconscious and thus transforms our identity and our personality. One naturally becomes the person one claims to be.

You can do a meditation by going through all the chakras and incorporating some or every of the following statements. You can also practice a specific chakra according to your needs of the moment.

- **Root Chakra :**
  'I'm good, here and now' - 'Earth supports me'
  'I feel strongly rooted' - 'I'm safe'
  'I feel good in my body'

- **Sacral Chakra :**
  'I respect my needs' - 'I live well my sexuality'
  'I am: full of life, enthusiastic, creative, happy'
  'I respect my body and take care of it'

- **Solare Plexus :**
  'I love myself' - 'I respect my value'
  'I feel my power' - 'I make the best choices'

- **Heart Chakra :**
  'I am loved' - 'I love' - 'I am brave'
  'I allow myself to receive and to give love'
  'The power of love filled my body'
  'I forgive myself and I forgive others'
  'I am at peace'
  'I feel the connection with others and also with nature'

- **Throat Chakra :**
  'I express myself well, clearly and with confidence
  'What I write is clear, well-constructed and substantial'
  'I live following the flow of life'

- **3rd eye :**
  'My ideas are clear, well-constructed, and well argued',
  or 'I am clarifying, constructing and arguing my ideas'

- **Crown Chakra :**
  'I accept reality as it is, and I adapt, without being
  disturbed by my emotions' - 'I belong to the unity of the
  universe'

## 10.1 specific Chakra

At each chakra exercise, regardless of the technique used, energy flow is improved for each chakra. And consequently, specificities of each chakra are improved.

You can also insist on the work of a single chakra if you wish to improve a specific quality (for example: to relieve pain or to facilitate a healing you will insist on the work of the chakra which has the anatomical correspondence concerned; before making a speech, before taking an exam (even writing) or before making a presentation to an audience you will insist on the work of the throat chakra, etc.).

When you want to work a specific chakra, start (possibly with whole body relaxation and staged breathing) by working (even quickly) all the chakras to optimize the flow of energy. Then you can, for example, use one of the following two techniques, to which you can optionally add the use of mantras (sounds) and mudras:

### Technique 1:

Visualize a column of energy passing through your body, crossing the root chakra and crown chakra, and at the level of the chosen chakra you visualize this energy which diffuses the organ (s). While continuing to visualize the column of energy.

### Technique 2:

By practicing Exercise 46 Turn around the body, you stay on the chosen chakra and you visualize the energy that diffuses the organs.
So, you continue the rotation around the body, and each time you pass through the selected chakra, you linger.

## 11. Examples of pathologies

Here is a list of pathologies that can be relieved and whose healing is facilitated by practicing the chakras:

- **Root Chakra :**

    Addictions, Addictive Behavior, Ankle problems, Anorexia, Backaches, Blood diseases, Bones, Cold feet, Constipation, Colitis, Depression, Diarrhea, Eczema, Frequent urination, Gambling, Glaucoma, Hemorrhoids, Hips, Hypertension, Impotence, Itching, Kidney stones, Knee problems, Leg cramps, Menstrual Problems, Money addiction, Migraines, Obesity, Pain at base of spine, Piles, Prostate cancer, Rectal cancer, Spine problem, Sciatica, Skin problems, Stomach problems, Swollen Ankle, Weak legs, Weight problems.

- **Sacral Chakra :**

    Addiction to junk food, Alcohol, Backache, Bedwetting, Bladder, Creative Blocks, Cystitis, Fear, Fertility, Fibroid, Miscarriages, Fibroids, Frigidity, Hips, Impotency, Irritable Bowel, Kidney problems, Menstrual Problems, Muscle Spasms, Ovarian Cysts, Over-eating, Pre-menstrual Syndrome, Prostates Disease, Stomach problems, Testicular Disease, Uterine Fibroids, Vomiting, Womb problem.

- **Solare Plexus :**

  Abdominal cramps, Acidity, Anorexia, Bulimia, Chronic tiredness, Diabetes, Digestive problems, Eating disorder, Fear, Food Allergies, Gastritis, Gall bladder problems, Gall stones, Heartburn, Hepatitis, Jaundice, Kidney problems, Less immunity, Liver problem, Pancreatitis, Peptic Ulcer, Smoking, Stomach problems, Shingles, Ulcers, Vomiting.

- **Heart Chakra :**

  Allergies, Asthma, Blood circulation, Breast Cancer, Bronchitis, Chest Congestion, Circulation problems, Cough, Fatigue, Heart Diseases, High Blood pressure, Hyperventilation, Immunity, Influenza, Lungs, Nail biting, Pain in lower arms/hands, Pneumonia, Respiratory problem, Shortness of breath, Sleep disorders, Smoking, Tremor.

- **Throat Chakra :**

  Asthma, Bronchitis, Colds, Cough, Ear Infections, Fear, Hearing Problems, Hay fever, Hoarseness, Laryngitis, Lost Voice, Mental confusion, Mouth Ulcers, Pain in upper arm, Sore Throat, Stammer, Stiff neck, Teeth/Gums, Thyroid Problem, Tinnitus, Tonsils, Too much talking, Upper digestive tract, Vomiting, Whooping cough.

- **3rd eye :**

  Allergies, Amnesia, Anxiety, Blood circulation to head, Blindness, Brain Tumor, Cataracts, Cancers, Chronic tiredness, Crossed eyes, Deafness, Dizziness, Drugs, Dyslexia, ENT, Ear-ache, Fainting spells, Glaucoma, Growth issues, Headaches, High blood pressure, Hormonal imbalance, Insomnia, Left eye problem, Long-sight, Migraine, Nervousness, Nervous Breakdowns, Scalp problems Short-sightedness, Sinus Problems, Sty, Tension, Tension Headaches, Tiredness, Tremor, Visual effects, Vomiting.

- **Crown Chakra :**

  Alzheimer, Amnesia, Bone disorders, Cancers, Depression, Dizziness, Epilepsy, Fear, Headache, Immune system, Insomnia, Learning difficulties, Migraine, Multiple Sclerosis, Multiple personality syndrome, Nervous system disorders, Neurosis, Paralysis, Parkinson's Disease, Psychosis, Right-eye problem, Schizophrenia, Senile Dementia, Tiredness, Tremor, Vomiting.

## 12. Energy flow

- Inhale by visualizing flow of energy going down spine.
- Exhale by visualizing the energy flow that goes up the spine.
- Makes thirty inhale-exhale

## 13. <u>To the chakras are associated colors</u>,

because the Hertzian frequencies of the colors are in harmony with the frequencies of the chakras. You now know the colors associated with the chakras and it is not necessary to recall them here.

This meditation takes place during a walk in the nature. It consists in contemplating the colors found in nature which correspond to the colors associated with the chakras. For each color found in nature, take the time (as long as you want it to contemplate the color, harmonize it with the corresponding chakra, and then bathe all the chakras of that same color, and finally, do the same to bathe the whole body, for example: to contemplate the blue of the sky, the green of a tree, to contemplate the yellow, orange, red, indigo and purple flowers, butterflies or insects that are found, or any other color found in nature. If you find colored stones in nature, or if you have some at home, you can practice this meditation, and if possible, add the touch of stones to the contemplation of colors.

## 14. <u>Optimization with prana</u>

Our vital energy, also called prana, comes from nature, and mainly from air, water, food, and solar energy. Of course, better qualities of these elements bring us a vital energy of better quality. Hence the added interest of being in contact with nature, eating quality products and drinking good water. It is also an advantage to practice moments of meditation when we feed on energy sources (air, water, food and sun), visualizing that they nourish our chakras and our 7 subtle bodies.

## 15. The ball of energy

Sitting in a lotus position or cross-legged, place your hands facing each other.

o   Imagine that you hold in your hands a ball of energy the size of a handball ball. By moving your hands up and down and around this ball, you want to feel that energy (with a little practice you will be able to feel a ball of energy).

o   That you have already been able to feel this energy or not, imagine integrating this energy ball feeding your root chakra.

o   Place your hands again in front of one another to form a new energy ball, then integrate this ball into your sacred chakra.

o   So continue for next five chakras.

## 16. Healing hands

When during your day you experienced an event heavily loaded with negative energy (for example a meeting, the sight of an accident, a frustration or a failure), use your healing energy power:

o   Thinking about this event, place your right hand touching your sacred chakra and your left hand touching your crown chakra.

o   Move your hands a few inches away from these two points and visualize the healing power through your hands that erases the negative imprint of your body.

## 17. **The 7 subtle bodies**

Our energetic envelope is made up of 7 overlapping layers (like Russian dolls that fit together): the first body, the physical body vibrates at the lowest frequencies, or the slowest, and is the least dense, of all; Each next body vibrates at higher and higher frequencies, faster and less dense. These 7 layers are energetically connected to the 7 chakras, as follows:

1. The physical body: connected to the root chakra

2. The etheric body: connected to the sacral chakra

3. The astral body: connected to the solar plexus

4. The mental body: connected to the heart chakra

5. The causal body: connected to the throat chakra

6. The Buddhist Body: Connected to the 3rd Eye

7. The atmic body: connected to the coronal chakra

As the chakras are connected to each other and interact with each other. The 7 subtle bodies have also relationships with each other.
Many of our emotions and sensations have their origins in the 7 subtle bodies, following relationships with others and with our environment.
Meditating on the 7 subtle bodies will allow a greater knowledge of our being, a cleansing of the subtle bodies of debris caused by accidents of life, and a greater general well-being.

**Practice :**

o  Put yourself in good condition (comfortable position, relaxation, and staged breathing)

o  Start by focusing on the root chakra, visualize a column of energy from the earth that activates your root chakra. Then visualize this energy that radiates to fill your entire physical body (Depending on how you feel most comfortable, you can simply visualize energy, or a white color energy, or a red color energy) Imagine this energy cleansing your body and allowing it to work optimally, and do the same for the following chakras and subtle bodies).

o  Continuing to visualize this column of energy that enters your root chakra, visualizes this column continuing its path to the sacred chakra. And similarly, visualize that energy that fills your whole body, then fills your etheric body, cleans it and allows it to function optimally.

o  Continue for the following chakras and subtle bodies, maintaining the visualization of the energy column coming from the earth, crossing the chakras one after the other and filling the subtle bodies one after the other.

o  After practicing on the coronal chakra and on the atmic body, sometime remains to visualize the column of energy coming from the earth that unites with the column of energy coming from the sky, and this unified energy that nourishes your 7 chakras and your 7 subtle bodies.

Note: Visualization and imagination are powerful driving forces that allow us to reach new sensations. Whereas theory is the first step towards understanding, towards knowledge and towards the first sensations. Only practice allows us to explore these new sensations.

## 18. OM on chakras and subtle bodies

All sounds reach our subtle bodies. This meditation is done with the sound OM because it is a sound with powerful vibrations easy to feel.

We have seen the OM meditation on the chakras (Exercise 5 above), this new meditation is to perform again the practice described in this exercise 5, adding now, for each chakra, the extension of the OM sound to the subtle body which corresponds to the chakra worked.

When you work the root chakra, the vibrations of the OM sound fill your whole body. When you work the sacred chakra, visualize the OM sound vibrations that fill your whole physical body, then fill your whole etheric body. And so on.

## 19. Heart Chakra and subtle bodies

At the level of the heart chakra intersect the energetic lines forming respectively the 7 subtle bodies.
After a conditioning (position, relaxation, breathing), concentrate on the heart chakra by visualizing your physical body in its entirety. Then continue visualizing the other 6 energetic bodies.
Imagine feeling comfortable in each of the seven subtle bodies. And imagine that they work well.

During your first practices you will have few feelings; after several practices you will feel the need to linger on a particular point in one of the 7 bodies (in the same way that you have learned to feel and to pass the tensions in your physical body), then take the time to linger on this point until you feel that the discomfort has disappeared.

The 7 subtle bodies are part of your nature, so you do not take any chances to work a greater knowledge of these bodies. On the contrary, this better knowledge will bring you well-being and will serve you in many aspects of your life.

## 20. Subtle relaxation

o   Lie down on the floor, on a carpet or blanket, your arms on the ground and your palms up to the sky, seek the maximum comfort of your body so you can then stay still. If necessary, put a cushion under your neck. Close your eyes. Performs a hyper relaxation of your whole body. Breathe normally.

o   Feel your body become heavier with each exhale, for 20 exhales.

o   Now feel your body become lighter at each exhale, during 20 exhales.

o   Imagine that you see your body in a mirror in front of you, and detail every part, from head to toe.

o   Imagine that your body has become transparent, and you observe your organs (intestines, stomach, heart beating, lungs inflating and deflating, brain, etc.). They work perfectly well, and they become bright. This light extends and illuminates your whole body. You feel in perfect physical and mental health.

## 21. Work on densities

We can see how negative thoughts, stress and emotions are felt in the body. We have the 'tight heart'. We feel a lump in the belly. We are sweating. Our heart rate is increasing. We can even feel these thoughts, stress or emotions as oppressions in our entire body. We can even remain in these situations for a very long time, if we remain under the influence of these thoughts, stress or emotions. They can even become chronic. Our health, our balance and our ability to react are affected.

Perhaps you have never really realized these repercussions in your body. Whatever perceptions you have already felt, you see very well what is involved here. You also understand very easily these nuisances, and the advantage of remedying them.

We have seen many times that it is easy (if you are aware of it) to interrupt these thoughts and emotions, with a simple mental intention and with the help of conscious breathing. The following exercise will allow you to work in depth.

Practice this technique several times in a formal way (sitting position, back straight), in order to feel the sensations. Then you can also use this technique informally.

o The first thing to do is to dwell on the feeling of these symptoms (tensions at different levels of the body, oppressions and even pains mainly in the stomach and heart, chills and sweats, etc.).

To do this, keep your breath smothered, want to maintain these symptoms and explore them in depth (and the expression "in depth" is quite appropriate, because you can get to feel how much these symptoms are reflected in the depths of your tissues, your bones and your cells).

This better knowledge of the symptoms will facilitate their elimination.

In particular, you will be able to perceive that these symptoms, while being diffuse throughout your body, are also denser and stagnate in certain places (for example: your belly, your heart, the neck, the brain, one or more joints, one or more muscles).

o After feeling these stagnant densities, you will restore the flow of energy in your body by practicing Exercise 46: Turn around the body.

Keep turning around the body as you feel these densities dissipate and the fluid flow of energy in your body.

### ☺☺ Exercise 106 : Full moon meditation

It is beneficial to get in the habit of looking at the moon. As the days go by, she paces the time. She is always beautiful, and even more particularly the days of full moons.

**Practice :**

o   Sit comfortably, facing the moon, straight up your spine.

o   Practice hyper relaxation. (Exercise 21)

o   Practice stage breathing (Exercise 5).

o   At each inhale visualize the moonbeams passing through your body and filling it with light.

o   At each exhale relax your entire body.

Take every opportunity to go for a walk in the evenings of full moons (every 28 days). If you have time, contemplate this beautiful show, and practice the meditation of the full moon. If you do not have the time, you will benefit to visualize these rays of moon crossing your body made transparent.

**Variants:**

The following 3 variants have similarities to the full moon meditation. And these are also very interesting meditation topics:

1. As you have visualized the moonbeams that run through your body, you can, on a windy day, visualize the wind that runs through your body, during deep breaths.

2. And you will be able to visualize the rays of the sun crossing your body.

3. And finally, always practicing a conscious breath and savoring the joy of breathing, you will be able to visualize the dissolution of your energetic envelope in the vortex of total energy.

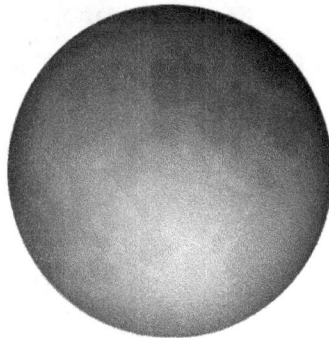

## ◉◉ Exercise 107 : 5 meditations Qi and Yin Yang

### 1. Méditation Qigong                    (10 minutes)

Qigong (literally: Qi = vital energy and Gong = culture) has roots in ancient Chinese culture dating back more than 4000 years. It is a holistic system of posture of the body and coordinated movements, breathing and meditation, used for the purpose of optimizing well-being, balance and health, performing spiritual research and practicing Martial Arts.

**Practice :**

o  Sit comfortably and position your spine straight.

o  Make a complete scan of the body in hyper relaxation. (See Exercise 23 on page 90)

o  Practice stage breathing.
   (See Exercise 5 on page 41)

o  Concentrate deeply on your sacral chakra. (Main center of vital energy = qi - See page 185)

o  Stay focused on your sacral chakra, and feel your vital energy flowing in and filling your whole body.

## 2. Meditation Qi                           (10 minutes)

- Standing upright, arms down the body, feet flat on the floor.

- Place the body weight on the front of the feet, automatically the body tilts slightly forward. Then, feel the Qi, vital energy, all over the front of the body: legs, pelvis, belly, torso, arms, neck and face.

  Stay 2 minutes in this position to cultivate the feeling of Qi.

- Place the body weight on the heels, automatically the body tilts slightly backwards. Then, feel the Qi, all over the posterior surface of the body

  Stay 2 minutes in this position to cultivate the feeling of Qi.

- Do the same on the right (2 minutes) and on the left (2 minutes).

- Stay upright for 2 minutes and feel the Qi all over the body surface.

Our being consists of two indivisible and complementary energy parts: Yin, also called feminine energy, which dominates our emotions, our intuitions, and our creativity; and Yang, also called masculine energy, which dominates our ability to analyze, plan and think.

Yin Yang meditations help to balance Yin and Yang. Thus, they contribute to improvements: well-being, health, balance, emotions, relationships, intuition, thoughts and efficiency. While an imbalance is the cause of the reverse effects.

All meditations improve this balance. Here are 3 techniques that specifically address this balance:

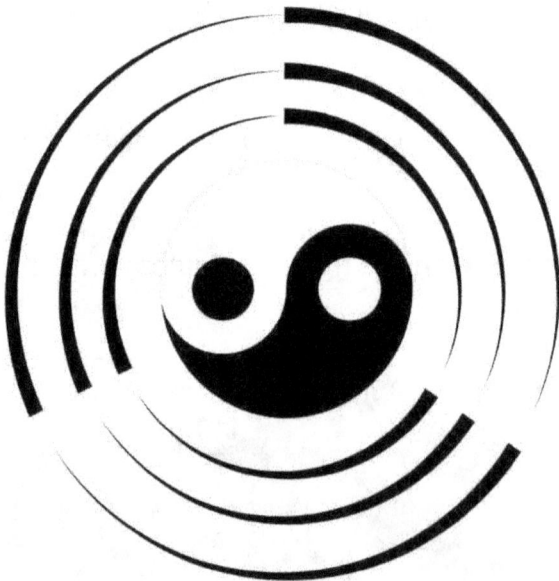

## 3.  Meditation Yin Yang - 1                    (10 minutes)

o  While sitting on the floor or on a chair (keeping your feet flat), close your eyes, relax your whole body, and practice a few minutes of stage breathing.

o  Concentrate on your heart chakra (in fact, focus on your entire thoracic region).

o  Inhale slowly and deeply, imagining sucking and storing in you, in the form of energies, all that you hope to get from life.

o  Exhale slowly and deeply, imagining releasing all these stored energies to the world.

o  Do twenty of these inhale-exhale.

o  Make one last relaxing inhale-exhale.

## 4. Meditation Yin Yang - 2          (10 minutes)

- In a sitting position, with your eyes closed, put yourself in condition (relaxation and stage breathing).

- Turns on Yin energy (water)

  This energy tends to stagnate (like stagnant water) in the lower part of the body.

  - Do a slow, deep inhale by visualizing filling your lower abdomen.
  - Do a slow and deep exhale visualizing expire in your legs to your feet.
  - Do 20 such inhale-exhale.

- Turns on Yang energy (light)

  This energy tends to stagnate in the upper body.

  - Do a slow, deep inhale by visualizing the air as light coming in through your crown chakra and filling your lungs generously.
  - Do a slow, deep exhale as you visualize this light fill the entire top of your body.
  - Do 20 such inhale-exhale.

- Mix the Yin and Yang energies

  - Inhale by visualizing the Yin energy rising from the bottom of your body, the Yang energy coming down from the top, and the 2 energies mixing.
  - Exhale by visualizing the 2 mixed energies filling your entire body.
  - Do 20 such inhale-exhale.

## 5. Meditation Yin Yang - 3                    (10 minutes)

o  In sitting position, with your eyes closed, put yourself in condition (relaxation and 1 series of stage breathing feeling your body is becoming heavier).

o  Do a series of 20 inhale-exhale :

   ▪ Visualize your inhales filling your body.

   ▪ At each exhale you become heavier and heavier (as if you were sinking into the ground). You feel more and more calm and at peace.

o  Do a series of 20 inhale-exhale :

   ▪ Visualize you inhale light, and you feel more and more filled with love, light and solar energy.

   ▪ At each exhale you become more and more lightweight (as if your body was going to fly away). You feel more and more calm and at peace.

o  Repeat these two series a second time, then a third time, in order to feel their contrasts.

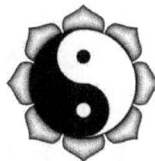

## 👀 Exercise 108 : Meditation Tantra

Tantrism is one of the oldest knowledges. It could be 5000 years old. It is interesting to note that Tantrism, like other knowledge, identifies, well before quantum physics, that everything is energy in the universe and that everything in the universe is interconnected (quantum entanglement).

One of the fundamental principles of Tantrism is that knowledge is acquired in experience. With Tantrism, one does not seek intellectual knowledge (why) but knowledge is acquired through experience and practice (how).

Tantric knowledge is very rich. It covers topics such as energy flows, the conscious, the subconscious, the ego and meditation. Tantra is not limited to sex and the quality of the union, as is popularly believed.

The Tantric meditation that follows uses a mystical concept of Tantrism that describes the body as being made of divine light. But, one can very well perform this meditation without having any mystic sensitivity, using the physical reality that everything is energy.

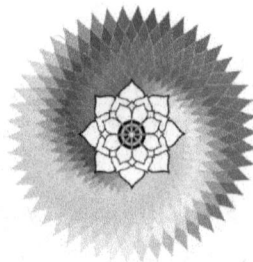

**Practice :**

o   Sit comfortably and position your spine straight.

o   Make a complete scan of the body in hyper relaxation.
    (See Exercise 23)

o   Practice stage breathing. (See Exercise 5)

o   Start by visualizing that your right foot is made of light.
    You will then continue the same all along your right leg.
    Then go to the left foot and go up detailing all parts of
    your body (as in hyper relaxation) to the top of your
    skull.
    Make this journey while inhaling and exhaling light.

o   Visualize your entire body being light and identifying
    with that light.

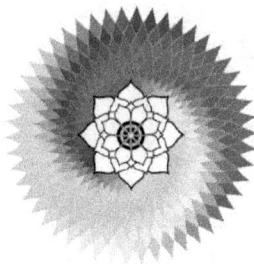

## ◉◉ Exercise 109 : Meditation Ham-Sa - So-Ham

This meditation simultaneously uses: breathing, two mantras and our coordinated identification with the breath and meanings of both mantras.

Ham-Sa and So-Ham are like the natural sounds of our breath. The syllables Ham and So corresponding to inhales. And the syllables Sa and Ham corresponding to exhales.

In Sanskrit, Ham-Sa means swan. The Ham-Sa mantra is symbolized by an immaculate white swan floating on the water, meaning purity.

So-Ham, means "I am". This mantra means our identification and our union with the purity of Ham-Sa.

सोहम्

39

---

[39] Soham mantra

**Practice :**

o   Make a complete scan of the body in hyper relaxation. (See Exercise 23)

o   Practice stage breathing. (See Exercise 5)

o   Then, by practicing the two mantras, you do not have to pay attention to your breathing; it changes naturally, slow or fast, superficial or deep, and from belly or from thorax or staged. It is important that the breath remains free and natural throughout the meditation.

   You take a short break between inhales and exhales.

o   According to your desires and your intuitions, and thinking about the meanings of the mantras, use freely, naturally and comfortably:

   ▪   Long series Ham-Sa (Inhale-Exhale),

   ▪   Long series So-Ham (Inhale-Exhale),

   ▪   Alternating Ham-Sa (Inhale-Exhale) and So-Ham (Inhale-Exhale).

## 👁👁 Exercise 110 : Extended heart meditation

This meditation will use the OM mantra and its vibrations, which we saw earlier in this manual, but here focusing only on the ribcage.

○ As you breathe out, say OM while feeling the vibrations of sound in your heart and throughout your ribcage.

○ By inspiring, feel those vibrations that continue and expand your heart.

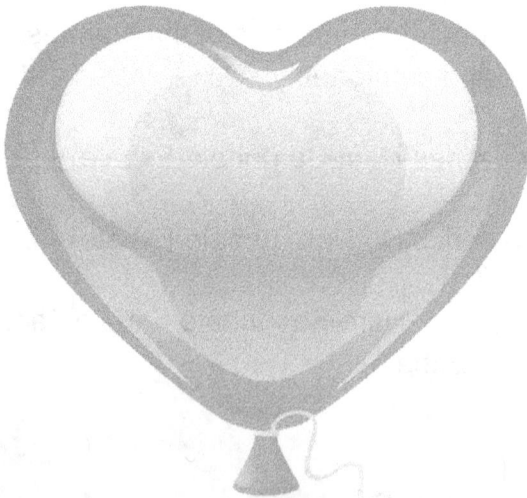

## ◉◉ Exercise 111 : Transfer meditation

o  Sit comfortably and position your spine straight.

o  Make a complete scan of the body in hyper relaxation.
   (See Exercise 21)

o  Practice stage breathing. (See Exercise 5). Then
   concentrate on the feeling of your breathing in the lower
   part of your lungs.

o  Place the palm of your hand in the center of your chest.
   Your attention is thus automatically transmitted to this
   place. And that will facilitate your meditation.

o  Visualize that it is no longer with the brain that you think,
   but it is with the heart. And observe the relief that this
   visualization gives you.

o  Continue for as long as you wish, keeping your
   concentration on both the breathing in the lower part of
   your lungs, and your heart being the organ of your
   thought.

You will have the opportunity to see that this technique will
help you in many other areas that immediate well-being.
Your intuition, your feelings, your emotions and your
decisions making will be improved.

## 👀 Exercise 112 : Meditate on the past day

You will therefore practice this meditation at the end of the day.

During the past day, events and encounters have had individually an emotional positive or negative charge. Few had a neutral emotional charge.

After conditioning and the usual relaxation, you will review, chronologically, from morning to night, the events and encounters of the day.

o Sit comfortably and position your spine straight.

o Make a complete scan of the body in hyper relaxation. (See Exercise 21)

o Practice stage breathing. (See Exercise 5)

o Practice about twenty inhale-exhale, feeling the happiness of the vital energy to the inhale and the comfort of the relaxation at the exhale.

o Continue this breathing with your concentration on the above points, for at least 10 minutes, including, every 5 breaths, thinking of an event of the day, represented only with words and with no other emotional feeling than the joy to breath, to relax and to exist.

## 👁👁 Exercise 113 : Funnel meditation

In this meditation, you will visualize two funnels. One with its wide-open part to the sky. The other with its wide-open part towards the ground. The two narrow parts meeting at the center of your torso.

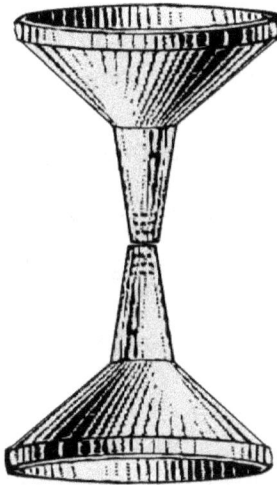

**Practice** (during at least 5 minutes)

o   When inhaling, visualize your inhale which widens, at the top of your skull, filling the sky.

o   When you exhale, visualize your relaxation which widens, at the lowest level of your body (which depends on your position: the tip of your sacrum in position of the lotus, your feet when you are sitting on a chair or in standing), filling the earth.

## 👀 Exercise 114 : Your identity as a meditator

o Make a complete scan of the body in hyper relaxation. (See Exercise 21)

o Practice stage breathing. (See Exercise 5).

o Now, observe yourself. Observe your well-being (happiness provided by breathing, a relaxed body, the thoughts and emotions that have become lighter).

o Integrate these observations as part of your identity.

o Affirms the choice to include this search for well-being in your daily life. And recognize your new identity of a person who meditates.

**Note:**

We have seen previously in this manual that getting into the skin of the character we want to become is the key to success. We have also seen that it is not easy, because we transform ourselves into a new person, a person we do not know. And even if we have a sincere desire to become this person, even if we know we will be happier, we need to get out of our pseudo comfort zone, and a part of us resist this change.

These are the same mechanisms that come here into play: we must make an effort to enter the skin of a meditator, in which we will feel very good, and that will offer us great benefits in many areas of our life (see advantages of the meditation).

## 👀 Exercise 115 : The bee buzz

We will see in the following exercise, 40 meditation exercises that you can do with your children. By doing these exercises with your children, it will also allow you to practice them. Knowing your children, you will know which other exercises in this manual you can practice with them. The following exercise is one that is attractive and beneficial for both adults and children. This technique is very effective to become calm and serene.

### Practice (5 minutes) :

o  Close your mouth but keep your teeth apart.
   Mouth your two ears with your index fingers.
   Place your elbows horizontally.

o  Inhale slowly and deeply through the nose.

o  Exhale slowly through the nose, while producing a continuous sound "bzzzzzzzzzzzzzzzzzzzzzzzzz". Focus your attention on the vibrations of this buzz in your head and in your chest.

## ◉◉ Exercise 116 : 40 meditations for children

You can introduce your child to meditation at the age of 3.

This will allow the child to recognize and then seek the feeling of calm. This will increase one's ability to concentrate. And this will allow him to learn how to recognize and control his emotions. Children who practice meditation are more successful in their studies; they also have greater respect towards others. They gain confidence and self-esteem. They improve their sleep and that promotes their good growth. Meditation allows children with hyperactivity tendency to reduce it.

Children gain with meditation the qualities that will serve them all their lives.

Since children have fewer barriers than adults and are also more interested in experimenting, it is easy to teach them meditation.

The duration of the sessions will be very short at the beginning: less than a minute. After a little practice, it will be possible to lengthen the duration of the sessions, up to 10 minutes. A guideline is a number of minutes equal to the age.

Your child must agree, and he must approach these sessions with joy. If he does not agree, you can try again later. You will leave your child a certain freedom in his practice, without submerging him with rules to observe and theories to understand; what is important is the benefit he will derive from his experience.

1. Standing in the lotus posture (sitting cross-legged) will be a game for your child. You can then guide him to stand with his back straight, hands clasped, and he avoids laughing for a few seconds.

2. Lying on your back, put both a cuddy toy on your bellies and invite your child to observe the cuddy toy going up and down with the breath.
   Then tell him to make the cuddy toy moving slower.

3. Tell your child to put his hand on his stomach to feel it coming up and down when he breathes.

4. Ask your child how is the time inside his body: Is there sun? Is it raining? Are there clouds?
   Do not make judgments about, or disqualify, the emotions your child expresses.

5. Tell your child to feel his breath, when he inhales and when he exhales. In another session you can let him count on his fingers up to 5 at the inhale, then 5 at the exhale.

6. Tell him that his breathing is like a cat that likes to hide and tells your child to watch his breathing so that she does not go into hiding.

7. Tell him to use finger meditation to regain his calm and serenity whenever he encounters a problem. This mediation consists in focusing on the touch, touching the thumb with the index finger, then with the other 3 fingers, and continue thus returning to thumb-index fingers.

8.  Give to your child the familiar image of balloon, telling him to inflate his belly like a balloon, then to exhale while making with his mouth the sound of the balloon deflating. (so he slowed his breath).

9.  Another familiar image for a child is that of candles being blown on a birthday cake. Tell your child to inhale deeply and slowly, and then breathe out quickly by imagining blowing out those birthday candles.

10. While standing, do the exercise together: arms on the sides, palms facing the sky, raise the arms by drawing a wide circle and inhaling all the way up. At the top, join the hands pointing to the sky and retain your breath for a short time. Lower the hands, in the middle of the body, placed one on the other while making a slow exhale all the way, until arriving at the bottom. At the bottom, retain the breath for a short moment, then continue with the next breath.

11. Tell your child to describe in detail, to his friend who is blind, everything he sees in this room or in this landscape.

12. The magic carpet: this technique is to practice with young children. It is an awareness of breathing and belly that swells with inspiration. It is also a privileged hug moment.
    Lying on your back, take your child on your stomach and tell him he is floating on a magic carpet.

13. Walk by holding your child's hand, asking him to keep his eyes closed and only listen to your instructions to take turns, go down a step, avoid an obstacle, etc.

14. Tell your child to notice and then listen to a sound (a singing bird, a barking dog, a ringing bell, a fan, etc.).

15. During a nature walk, tell your child that you will try to see animals. Then you will walk like tigers, without making noises, gently and slowly placing your feet on the ground.

16. Tell your child to close his eyes for 1 minute and record all the sounds he hears, then to give you a list.

17. Tell your child that he will observe the room or the landscape, and then, to close his eyes and describe in detail the objects, the colors and everything he remembers.

    By renewing the exercise, the following days, the child will have fun wanting to remember more and more things. And you can congratulate him every time he improves his performance. But you shall remain patient, and not censure.

18. If you have a Tibetan bowl, make it sing and invite your child to listen to the sound that gradually fades to silence. Then invite your child to listen to the silence. Also invite your child to feel the vibrations of sound that run through his body.

19. Lying on the grass on a summer day, invite your child to watch the passing clouds, which change size and disappear. Then, closing eyes, invite him to observe that he can do the same with his thoughts.

20. During a walk tell your child to find, and to observe, 10 small pebbles that he will use in a meditation. The pebbles will be stored in a box to be reused.
    Sitting cross-legged, tell your child to put the pile of pebbles on his left;
    To take one of the pebbles with the left hand and to inhale while observing the pebble;
    To pass the pebble to his right hand, holding his breath;
    And, to close his eyes, placing the pebble on his right, by making a slow and long exhale, by seeing the pebble in his memory (its color, its forms, its cavities);
    To continue like this with the next pebble.

21. While standing, closing eyes, tell your child to imagine being a tree, and that its roots are sinking, sinking and sinking deep into the ground;

    Now he raises his arms to the sky, his arms being like the branches of the tree that extend far and high, further and higher, to draw the rays of the sun.

22. This technique borrowed from sophrology will allow your child to channel his emotions: tell him to rub both hands until they get hot, then apply his hands on his face to feel the heat and linger on this sensation.

23. Two children of similar sizes sit cross-legged back to back, telling them to stay calm and without moving, and to concentrate on breathing at the same time.

24. Make a staging that will allow your child to imagine and better understand the management of thoughts: Put sand and water in a bottle, shake the bottle and explain that the thoughts in his head are like those grains of sand suspended in water; the meditation that allows the thoughts to calm down like the grains of sand are deposited at the bottom of the bottle.

    Point out to your child how deep breathing helps calm anxiety, and the benefit of using deep breathing before answering a question in class.

25. Young children like to imitate parents, so settle in to meditate and let your child imitate you.
    From time to time you will be able to guide him with one of the examples found on these pages, and even with other practices found in this manual.
    If they see you practicing meditation every day for a few minutes in the morning and evening, the adoption of this routine will be very natural for them.

26. Outside, on a windy day, with your child, close your eyes, spread your arms, feel the wind on your face and open your mouth making sounds changing with the wind.
    A rainy day, face turned to the sky, eyes closed, feel the rain on your faces.

27. In a dark room, light a candle, both of you about 1 meter away from the candle.
    For about 1-minute watch the flame, then tell your child that he will close his eyes and keep the image of the candle in memory.
    After about 1 minute, tell your child to open his eyes and observe the flame of the candle again.
    Repeat this way 4 or 5 times.

28. Sitting on the ground, eyes closed, tell your child to imagine what a person he loves is doing now (for example: his grandfather, his cousin, a friend, etc.), to imagine the place where this person is and what this person is thinking, his feelings.

29. Using a real metronome or metronome app on your phone tells your child to step one step at each sound of the metronome, then tells him to continue that way while you slow down the pace of the metronome.

30. While standing, tell your child to concentrate on his breathing (inhale - exhale).
    Then, while continuing to focus on his breathing, also focus on the point below his navel (sacral chakra). Spread the arms then balance on one leg, stay a little in balance maintaining both concentrations. One moment back in position on both legs, then move to balance on the other leg.

31. In this other exercise you will introduce your child to the exploration of his feelings.

Sitting on the ground, eyes closed, tell your child to imagine that he is at his school.

He meets his teacher, what does he feel?

How can he describe this feeling?

What does he feel in his belly when he has this feeling?

Then he meets his best friend, and you ask him the same questions.

Then, again the same 3 questions with another child that he does not like.

Then, the same 3 questions when meeting a child, he would like to know.

And finally, the same 3 questions to describe what he feels when he hears the ring at the end of class.

In doing this exercise, make no comment when hearing your child's responses (unless he describes someone hurting him).

32. Sitting, tell your child, that after closing his eyes, for 1 minute, every time a thought goes through his head, he will take out a small pebble from the box (see exercise 20 above) for the place in front of him.

Tell him when the minute has passed, count the pebbles, put them back in the box and repeat the same thing for another minute.

Then, the same exercise a third time.

At the end, point out to your child that there were fewer and fewer pebbles, because he paid attention to what he was thinking.

33. As children grow up, they often find it difficult to know the position of their bodies in space.

    Tell him to scan his body, from head to foot, in the same way as in the technique of hyper relaxation described in the manual, but here in order to feel the parts of the body: feel your right foot, go up along your leg and feel your right knee, ... etc., to turn the exercise into a very fun game for your child, tell him the story of the ant (which you can detail) who climbs on his foot, passes between his toes then on his ankle, which goes around his calf, tickles him behind the knee and then come on the kneecap, etc.

34. Moving the head under the heart helps to calm down. If he is angry, tell your child that you are going to do an exercise. And, legs apart, stay 30 seconds with hands flat on the floor.

35. The child intertwines his fingers under his chin and places his elbows horizontally (his arms are the wings of the dragon). He inhales, raising his elbows and his head. Eyes to heaven, he sounds 'ahhhh' imagining himself to be a dragon blowing flames. At the end of the exhale, he lowers his arms to the bottom. Then he starts to raise his elbows and head while inhaling. He begins again to do 10 breaths of the dragon.

36. Tell your child to jump up. After 1 minute, tell him to place his right hand on his heart, and feel the heartbeat and breathing.

37. Place yourself with your child in front of the wall, and three times in a row push the wall for 10 seconds.

38. While lying or sitting, with your eyes closed, you will tell a story to your child, work on his imagination and allow him to evacuate his stress.

Imagine that you are on a beach, the sun is shining. You hear the sound of the waves. Your feet feel a bit of warmth by touching the sand and then touching the water. You walk along the long beach. There is no one else. You look at seagulls that fly and disappear on the horizon. You do not think about anything. You're only happy to be in this beautiful place, ...

At the end of your story, tell your child that he has just had a nice walk and that he can imagine going back to this peaceful place at any time. May he now open his eyes and end the meditation with three deep breaths followed by slow exhales.

39. In a sitting position, tell your child to place his hands at the height of his eyes, palms forward. Then he will turn both hands inwards, going slow, as slowly as possible, trying to not perceive the movement of the hands.

Once he has finished turning and sees his palms, he starts again the other way. It will continue for 5 minutes.

Tell him to think about breathing. And, eventually, remind him if you see that he goes into apnea.

40. Lying on the floor, massage in the back with a tennis ball.
Roll a golf ball under a bare foot.

## 👀 Exercise 117 : The one minute meditation

Perhaps after reading or hearing about the benefits of meditation, you tell yourself that you should try, and yet you find an excuse not to do it, or you think you are not the kind of person who meditates. It is possible that you break the step later in your life. You have also, with this meditation that lasts 1 minute, the opportunity to experience now.

Perhaps you already practice meditation. And this meditation of 1 minute will be useful to you. Because you will have many opportunities, during the day, to practice it.

o   When sitting or lying down, close your eyes.

Decide that the next minute will be 1 minute of meditation.

You will inhale through your nose and exhale through your mouth.

o   Inhaling sense the freshness of the air filling your lungs.

o   By exhaling, relax your body and let go of your thoughts, your stress and your emotions.

Repeat 3 times: inhale - exhale.

o   Slowly open your eyes

## ◉◉ Exercise 118 : Fire breathing

You will gain a lot by regularly practicing this easy technique. And you will be able to feel this gain.
This is one of those techniques to include in your habits.

- o  Sit comfortably
  Position your hands in Gyan mudra. Close your eyes.
  Position your spine straight.
  The straightness of your column here is particularly important.
  Put the muscles of your lower abdomen in slight tension.

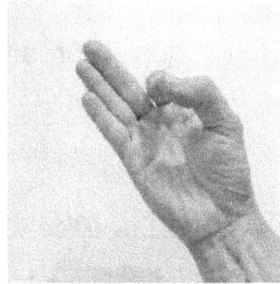

- o  Your inhales and exhales can be done either by the nose or by the mouth, as you prefer.

- o  A fundamental principle of this technique is that your inhales and exhales are equal in power and duration (you will not succeed at first, but with practice).

- o  Focus on your navel, which moves away from your spine to the inhale, and which approaches it at the exhale. Your diaphragm goes up and down.

- o  For 1 to 3 minutes perform inhales and exhales (2 to 3 per second). Rest 1 minute and do a second series, rest, then a third.

Contraindications: for the pregnant woman and the first 2 days of menstruation.

## 👀 Exercise 119 : 2 muscular breaths

This exercise, and the following, on originating from Yoga. Their practices allow to muscle and to have better sensations of the respiratory muscles; so they bring the benefits of better breathing. These exercises also have a quality of meditation because your attention is focused on a precise action.
Better quality breathing brings you more life energy and benefits all aspects of your life.

### 1.  Building muscles used when inhaling

o   Close your fist.

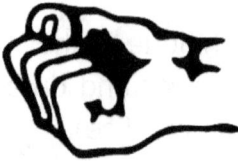

o   Put your mouth on your closed fist (thumb side), and inhale in force through the fist, controlling the resistance of your inhales by closing more or less your fist.

o   Exhale through the nose.

o   Do twenty inhales with a fist resistance, then 2 other sets of 20 inhales, increasing the resistance a little bit each time.

## 2. The sandbag breathing

This exercise will allow you to strengthen your diaphragm, to have better feelings of your diaphragm and to be more comfortable as well as more confident in the use of the very important diaphragmatic breathing.

This will benefit you, daily, with each of your breaths.

o Sit comfortably while lying on your back, with a small cushion to support your head and neck (this cushion should allow you to keep your neck in line with your spine).

Spread your arms and legs slightly, the palms of your hands open to the sky.

o Relax and do 3 inhale-exhale by inflating and deflating your belly like a balloon.

o Place a bag of sand (2 Kg to start) on your stomach, and up and down this bag with your breath. Place yourself in a relaxed and meditative situation, fixing your attention on your stomach that goes up and down.

o Starts with 5-minute sessions and progressively increases to 10-minute sessions. Similarly, increases very gradually the weight from 2 to 10 kg (if and when you feel doing so).

You will quickly see that you are much more comfortable with your diaphragmatic breathing.

## ☻☻ Exercise 120 : I do not need anything

This meditation is done in 3 periods :

○ **1. Put in condition**

- Sitting comfortably, straight and still  (1 min.)
- Relaxation of the whole body  (2 min.)
- Staged breathing  (2 min.)

○ **2. « I mobilize my thoughts and emotions»**

Now you will ask yourself series of questions.

- Each question is said, mentally, 3 times to inhales.
- At expiration, you mentally say the answer:

  "That's what ... answer to your question"

  Note: the same question can be repeated 3 times if you think you have other answers (that you will repeat 3 times each).

- Here are some examples of Question / Answer:

  ➢ Q : What do I think of myself?
  ➢ A : That's what I think of myself : …

- ➢ Q : What do I want ?
- ➢ A : That's what I want: …

- ➢ Q : What I miss ?
- ➢ A : That's what I miss : …

- ➢ Q : What is my ambition ?
- ➢ A : This is what I want : …

- ➢ Q : What do I like ?
- ➢ A : That's what I like : …

- ➢ Q : What is my resoluteness ?
- ➢ A : My resoluteness is to: …


- ○ **3.** You come back now to a calm and relaxed conscious breathing.

  And for 5 to 10 minutes, during long and deep breaths repeats, **"I do not need anything"**

  And you relax during long exhales. Feeling the fullness of breath and existence in the present moment, without thoughts or emotions.

## ☻☻ Exercise 121 : Meditation Tai Chi

This technique is very simple. This simplicity makes possible its immediate practice. In addition, like many other exercises in this manual, this simplicity makes it easy to practice anytime of the day and any place (for example informally: sitting at your desk, between two professional tasks). This simplicity does not reduce the richness of Tai Chi martial art. In addition, this exercise allows you to work on a fundamental principle of Tai chi: the coordination of breathing and movement.

It's a new opportunity for you to work on this coordination; remembering that breathing leads the movement; and by reminding you that you will benefit from adopting this mode of operation for your everyday actions.

- Sit in a lotus or suit. Straighten your spine by imagining a string attached to your head that pulls you up.

- Put both wrists on your knees, with your hands closed and your palms facing towards the sky.

- With one hand, coordinates the opening and closing of the fingers (star fingers and closed fist) with your inspiration and with your expiration. The deep inhales lead to the ample openings of the star. Exhales are simple and slow.

- The formal practice last at least 5 minutes. The unformal practice can last only 30 seconds.

## ☯☯ Exercise 122 : Meditation Yoga Sutra

o   Put yourself in condition: sitting comfortably, relaxation, staged breathing.

o   Continue to breathe consciously and comfortably. And explore, during inhales and exhales the sensations that you feel in your body.

o   Let inhales lead you to places in your body that are tense or sore.

    Note how your inhale does that very well.
    This new perception is a great interest of this meditation. Enjoy this new perception and its power of self-healing.

o   Stay for a while on each spot discovered, allowing your exhales to evacuate tensions and pains and contribute to your complete relaxation.

o   Then, let your next inhale take you to another place of your body.

## ☺☺ Exercise 123 : Meditation of the stairs

To be conscious is to be alive. The positive energy of life flowing in our veins. We tend to forget it, and to live, either in a robotic way, or bogged down in a molasses of problems.

We enjoy taking every opportunity to remember being alive. Going up and down the stairs is an opportunity we often meet. In addition to allowing us to be fully aware, the stairs also allow us to breathe and maintain our muscles and joints.

Already, one can often make the choice to use the staircase rather than the elevator or the electric staircase.

Here is the technique described step by step:

o By climbing the first step, concentrate on your inspiration that drives your movement; inspires through the nose.

o When climbing the second step, concentrate on your exhalation that drives your movement; expires through the mouth.

o Do the same thing down the stairs, one step after another.

You can practice this technique regardless of the speed of movement, adapting the speed of your breathing.

## ☻☻ Exercise 124: Meditation « LOVE » & « PEACE »

For this meditation, we will use the coordination of breathing and a mantra. The mantra that we will choose is either the word "LOVE" or the word "PEACE".

These two words are of course rich in meaning, but it is here their pronunciations that interest us because they are very well adapted to the practice of this meditation. Moreover, during this meditation, we will not have any mental or emotional focus on these words; only the coordinated dynamics of the breathing and the mental pronunciation of the mantra are important to us.

We will focus on breathing, which is the driver of the pronunciation.

Here is the practice, step by step, of this meditation, using the word "LOVE". You can, another time, do the same practice with the word "PEACE".

- o With a slow, deep chest inhale, imagine your inhale that sucks the word "LOVE". Feel the air on the outer walls of your lungs that inflate like a balloon.

- o With slow and deep exhale, imagine that your exhale propels the word "LOVE"

- o Continue for 5 to 20 minutes, or longer if you wish.

## 👀 Exercise 125 : Aikido breathing

Breathing is very important in our lives. Breath is life. Oxygen gives us energy. Oxygen purifies our body, our thoughts and our emotions. Thus, by learning to breathe better we improve all this, we become happier, more efficient and less subject to fatigue.

We have seen many techniques of conscious breathing and other techniques to increase the capacity of our lungs. The practices of these techniques and the sensations they give us are for us great benefits.

Before knowing these techniques and being able to reproduce these sensations, our breaths were shallow, we used mainly the upper part of our lungs; by practicing these techniques, we improve each of our breathing, about 30,000 per day.

We have also seen that breathing makes it easy to interrupt the sometimes-tumultuous flow of our thoughts and emotions. So, 30,000 times a day, our thoughts, emotions and actions are better qualities.

All of this makes breathing the foundation of meditation.

Here is another example:

**Practice :**

Imagine that your lungs are divided into 4 parts: top right, top left, bottom left and bottom right.

o Exhale slowly and deeply, until you empty your lungs.

o Inhale slowly,

- Focusing on filling the part of your lungs: top right.

- When you feel this part being filled, continue concentrating on filling the part of your lungs: top left.

- Following the same process, fill in the part: bottom left.

- Then the same: bottom right.

o Exhale slowly, focusing on the release of the air contained in each of these 4 parts, and moving in the opposite direction: bottom right, bottom left, top left, top left.

o Make 20 such inhale-exhale.

## ☻☻ Exercise 126 : Meditation for couple

As the name suggests, this meditation is done in couple (loving partners), provided that both are appreciative of the chakras.

The two are seating face to face.

o  Individually, they review their 7 chakras, including the symmetrical points of the 5 chakras on the posterior face of the body, and eventually feeling each of these 12 points successively in a circular motion in the anterior face-posterior.

o  After 5 minutes of this individual work, and if they agree to say that they are ready, they will begin the couple meditation.

o  Simultaneously the two people visualize a column of energy penetrating into their root chakras. Simultaneously, they visualize horizontal columns of energy traversing their next five aligned chakras.

o  They each visualize their vertical column of energy that runs through their crown chakras.

o  The couple remains 3 minutes visualizing these vertical and horizontal flows of energies.

o Now they individually view the 12 shared points as follows (It is not mandatory for the two persons to coordinate their visualizations) :

i) Root Chakra,

ii) Posterior Sacral Chakra aligned with the one of its partner.

iii) Same thing with posterior sacral, solar plexus, heart, throat, and third eye chakras.

iv) Crown chakra.

v) Both visualize their front third eye Chakra, then, their front throat, heart, solar, and sacred chakras.

vi) Now the couple visualize for three minutes this circulation of the 12 shared points, together, in a meditative energy communion.

## ☯☯ Exercise 127 : The Standstill Position

Throughout the day, and even throughout the night, a good position and a good feeling of our body, play an important role in our well-being and our happiness.

An optimal position is a position in which:

- Our vertebral column is in its best straightness, depending on the task in hand;

- Our bones are in the best alignment with our joints; The basin tilt is optimal;

- Our muscles and tendons have the best tension to perform our tasks with the greatest efficiency, supporting our skeleton and our organs. At rest, they maintain a minimalist and comfortable tone, which continues to support our skeleton and our organs in their optimal positions to prevent them from sagging;

- Our bodies are in the best rectitude for the best circulation of fluids, and without the pressures, caused by excessive tensions or looseness.

- The flow of energy in our body is optimal, through alignments and balances of, the energy channels, the meridians and the chakras.

We previously saw, the optimal position to sleep. An optimal position is also useful, when we are sitting, walking, wearing something heavy, and finally, in all our actions.

The good position of our body and its balance also greatly influence the correct position and balance of our thinking and our emotions.
The qualities of our body positions are reflected in the qualities of our body thoughts and emotions.

Here again, we have a perfect example of the synergy for happiness, with the optimization of balance and happiness in our body, influencing balances and happiness in our head and our actions.

The optimal positions of our body are studied in the practices of martial arts, yoga, sports and meditation. Because practitioners enjoy new pleasures, new feelings, new confidences and new perspectives, a wide leaning by doing, as they improve their positions.

The study of the optimal Standstill position is the most interesting of all. It corresponds to a silence of the body, without the reminders and distractions of the genes, the pains and the tensions. Our attention to the silence of the body, promotes the silence of thought, freed from the tumult of reflections, feelings and emotions.

Let us, now, see the effects of the Standstill position on our body and on our thought:

Effects on the Body :

- We increase our knowledge of the position of our body in the space. The importance of this knowledge has been mentioned several times in this manual. Our movements are more precise and more dynamic. We feel better in our body, in our postures and in our actions.

- We learn to recognize the position of our spine. And, we become capable of, keeping it in a straight position, and controlling it in all our movements.

- We can locate the tensions in our body, so we can relax them.

- We are able to recognize the muscles we need to keep us in the best position.

- We optimize the fluidity of energy in our body and consequently our vitality.

Effects on Thought :

By being motionless, the movements of our bodies do not distract the silence of our thought.

The silence of our body, in partnership with the silence of our thought, allows us to reach, greater depths of silence. Where, we discover, new beneficial levels of relaxation and serenity, and, out of which we discover new levels of vivacity, clarity of mind and perception of new thoughts.

The immobile position is thus rejoicing. Its practice, which will be described in the following pages, is useful to be done formally and in the most favorable position. We learn then, to approach the optimal point of balance of our body and our thought. We learn to know new levels of our mind.

Once recognized, the better balance and the new sensations, will be possible to find back, informally, at all times of the day, and whatever the circumstances of our lives. Consequently, our general well-being is improving significantly.

✶ ✶ ✶ ✶ ✶ ✶ ✶ ✶ ✶ ✶

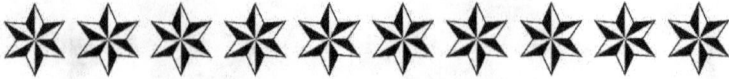

In the following pages, the practice of the still position will be described step by step. This practice could, as has been repeated several times in this manual, be like other techniques, practiced rather informally. In order to facilitate its use and the regularity of its practice.

However, now, you are going to experience the stimulating ceremonial ritual. Which we see the benefits and practice in this parenthesis.

This stimulus will make it possible to obtain more quickly the results of this practice of the still position. It could also be used to stimulate the results of other techniques seen in this manual.

Whatever the story of your life, you've already experienced the stimulus of ceremonial. For example, when you put on your best clothes to participate in an event.

In the example of martial arts, ceremonial allows, respect for oneself, respect for other students, and respect for the Master for his knowledge and for his teaching. Each one enters the tatami, saluting the place, in which he will give the best of himself, and be receptive to the improvement of his abilities.

At the moment when you wear your beautiful clothes, or your kimono, watching, the position of your belt, and other adjustments of your costume, you place yourself in optimal situation to live the event that follows.

During the event, this ceremonial of the costume, facilitates the maintenance in your optimal concentration.

**Practice of the stimulating ceremonial ritual:**

o Choose a moment, when you are sure not to be disturbed. Consider this moment, as belonging to you completely.
o Take a shower, during which you begin your conditioning ceremonial for the practice. Then, put on clean clothes.
o Choose a place, which you designate as the privileged place of your practice. It can be a corner of your room, which you can later decorate, with for example a candle.
o Settle comfortably, relax and concentrate on the event that follows, with joy, and entire availability.

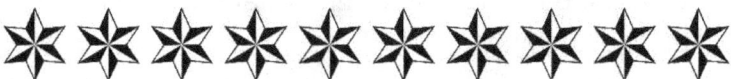

✳ ✳ ✳ ✳ ✳ ✳ ✳ ✳ ✳ ✳

**Practice of the still position :**

Succeeding in keeping the still position, requires practice, in order to know and to optimize, the position of your body, the necessary muscles to maintain the position, and the flexibility of your joints.

But do not worry, even if your muscles and flexibility are very weak. For the benefits are, as always, in the path that leads to the result, and not in an ideal result that will never be reached, but only approached. Now focus your attention on practicing, the perception of your feelings and on the perception of your progress.

o Perform the four stages of the stimulating ceremonial ritual, described on the previous page.

o The optimal academic position, for the practice of the stationary position, is the so-called lotus position. But this position is the privilege, of, many years of practice, or few particularly flexible people.
Just sit cross-legged.

o Place your hands on your knees, or join them in front of you, naturally. (There are several hand positions, you can study them if they interest you).

o Place your spine in a straight position. Stretch your column, by imagining a rope attached to the top of your skull pulling it you up.

o Tilt your chin slightly down to align the cervical vertebrae (your neck).

o Practice the respiratory balance that you now know:

- 3 seconds blocked breathing, at the end of three, more and more deep inspirations,

- 3 slow and long expirations,

- Then, a constant focus, on a comfortable regular breathing.

o Research, both relaxing your body, and maintaining a light tone of the muscles keeping you in this optimal position. Which, you will search to maintain, while looking for the silence of your body.

Feels no frustration or impatience when you feel the need to move, because on the contrary this need is part of your learning, and, you are moving to change for a more comfortable position.

After working, for some time, your comfort in this position, soon adds the work of the silence of your thought, for silences of body and thought are synergistic, and, one facilitates the other.

## 👀 Exercise 128 : OFF or Faded away

Here are two other techniques to fall asleep:

Today your body has moved a lot, he thought a lot and he felt many emotions.

Now that you've decided it's time to rest and sleep, here are two techniques that will help you fall asleep peacefully.

These two techniques are similar. You can try both and adopt the one that suits you best.

The first technique is to focus on parts of your body, starting from the feet and going up to the head, and imagine that you turn off this part.

The second technique is to make the same journey, but this time, imagining that the parts of your body disappear one after the other.

Thus, the feet are turned off, or faded away.

Then the ankles, calves, knees, thighs, pelvis, torso, arms, hands, shoulders, neck, face, brain and entire head.

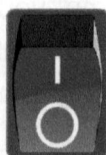

## ☺☺ Exercise 129 : The crackles

This exercise is placed, at the end of the manual, because its practice requires a thorough knowledge of sensations and relaxation of your body.
Also, because it marries very well to the practice of the Standstill position, especially in search of optimal position of the spine.

Now that you have better perceptions of your body, you will be able to more easily notice the moment when a crack occurs in your spine.
It happens, after you have felt an embarrassment and that you change position, to relieve this embarrassment.
This cracking corresponds to the release of one of the 142 joints, between your vertebrae, between the rib cages and the vertebrae, and between your pelvis and your spine. And it was the blockage of this joint that caused you the embarrassment. This blockage, more than a simple discomfort, can often be at the origin of future strong pains.

But now that you come to systematically notice these cracks, you will deepen your knowledge of the cracks, of the genes that preceded them, of the movements which have made it possible to unblock the joints, and the reliefs which have followed them.

This knowledge will enable you to unlock the nascent blockages before they cause acute pain and inflammation. You will gain physical, as well as mental, well-being. You will also gain efficiency in your actions which are not anymore disrupted by the discomfort.

**Interesting accessories to meditate:**

Meditation can be practiced without accessories, anywhere and at any time. That being said, some accessories are appropriate to facilitate the practice:

o **The place:**
If you can, use a room for meditation. Otherwise use a corner of room that is bright and well ventilated. You can decorate this corner of a room with a plant, a framed Mantra representation (eg Sri Yantra), crystals chosen for their beauty, the various vibrations of the colors and possibly to touch them.
Take care to always have water available to seize the opportunity to drink.

o **Incense:**
Its powerful perfumes cause strong states of consciousness.

o **The pyramids:**
the proportions of those of ancient Egypt have aesthetic virtues as well as vibratory virtues whose effects are measurable. To use those of small sizes in decoration, or to meditate under a large size.

o **The position of the tongue:**
glued to the palace is considered by some yogis as very important. You can linger to feel the sensations. And you can experience breathing exercises with the tongue glued to the palate.

## CONCLUSION OF THE CHAPTER ON MEDITATION:

Meditation is a technique that is as simple to practice as it is simple to breathe.

The only difficulties in meditation, are remembering to practice it, and remembering regularly, at least a few minutes, every day, to begin with.

Meditation brings us so many perceptible benefits, as well as others less perceptible, that we have a good time, and that we want to renew it.

The more you practice it, the more you get benefits, including the ones you've learned to feel.

If you practice meditation, a few minutes every day, for only a week, it is guaranteed that you will already feel new and very satisfactory sensations. It is not guaranteed that these new feelings of well-being, at the end of this first week, will automatically lead you to continue your daily integration of meditative and conscious experiences. Your intention, your choices, including the one to feel good, and your initiative of action will, as always, be necessary.

As they always do, the body sensations, will drive you to make mental discoveries.

Quickly, you will also perceive, becoming more effective in your actions.

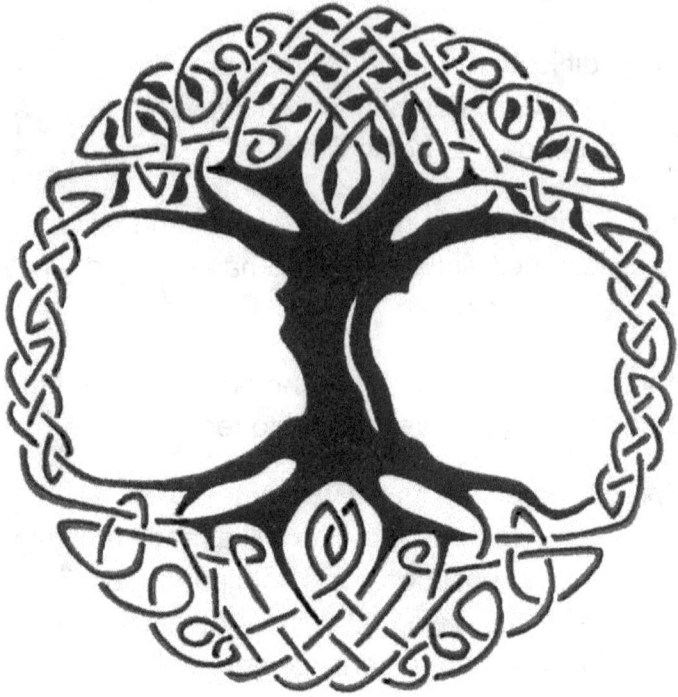

# CONCLUSION OF THE 101 GUIDES:

## CULTIVATE THE TREE OF HAPPINESS

Imagine that the human being is a fruit tree. Man, thus becomes a 'man-tree'.

To have a good harvest, beautiful fruit, and a blooming tree, with beautiful roots, a beautiful trunk, and branches receiving well the sun, our tree, we will take care of it, nourish it, caring for him, carving him.
And this is good, now, because it is the right time, to begin to care of trees.

First of all, let's think about the roots. They get our food from the soil. And they give us something to drink. They firmly anchor us in the ground, allowing us not to be torn away by the wind. Our roots have a vital symbiosis with the earth because in return they capture the excess of rain, enrich it with mineral salts drawn from the earth, and feed the ground water with pure and mineralized water. The man-tree will have as priority to ensure a solid anchorage in the ground. He will embrace his nurturing land. He will remember this symbiotic union.
As the man is a tree, mankind is a forest, he will remember that he is connected by his roots to all the trees of the forest. [40].

---

[40] The root length record is 622 km, 387 miles. By adding the lengths of the rootlets and the absorbent hairs, we arrive at the

Let us now, observe the trunk. Very important the trunk. It is like the energy column of the tree. Behind its bark is the nourishing sap enriched by the earth and by the leaves working with the sun light. It is important for a tree to reach its optimal life expectancy that the trunk is in good condition, that the bark is not injured preventing the sap flow. If the wound of the bark is too deep and cannot heal then the vermin progresses in the trunk and causes it to rot. Deep wounds can be clogged. The tree-man will remember that he is a column of energy in an energy field. He will remember that in his body circulates the energy of the earth and the sun, his feet on earth and his head in the sky. He will remember that it is good that the circulation is fluid in its column of energy.

Let us now look at the branches. In man-tree the branches are the thoughts. Good branches are the ones thinking positively about the function attributed to them. There are the mistress branches forming the framework of the tree. One of these thoughts is, thinking to live in the present moment, breathing well, drinking well, eating well, sleeping well, meditating, loving, relaxing, being active, being patient, being humble, being curious, forgiving, listening, accepting, laughing, studying, telling the truth. Among the smallest branches that bear fruit are the other guides in this manual. The bad branches, we will cut them, giving place to the good branches to manifest. In a simple and decided

---

network of a tree with a total length of tens of thousands of miles or kilometers.

manner, the man-tree will remove, one by one, these bad branches corresponding to negativity.

Then, there are the leaves, drawing, daily, the energy of the sun, subjected to the rains and the winds. The man-tree will remember the energy constantly within his reach, and unconditional happiness in spite of winds and tides. The falling leaves allow the tree to regenerate. The tree-man will remember that everything changes and that the losses turn into profits. It will rejoice in the abundance and optimum growth of its fruits. He will remember the pleasure of existing. Serene and happy, he will contemplate his verdant foliage, strongly immovable or dancing with the wind.

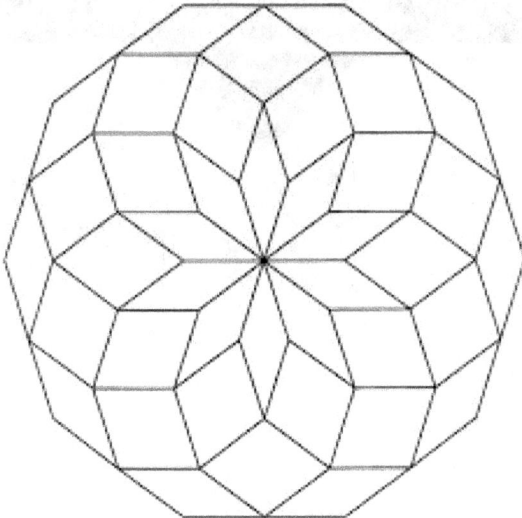

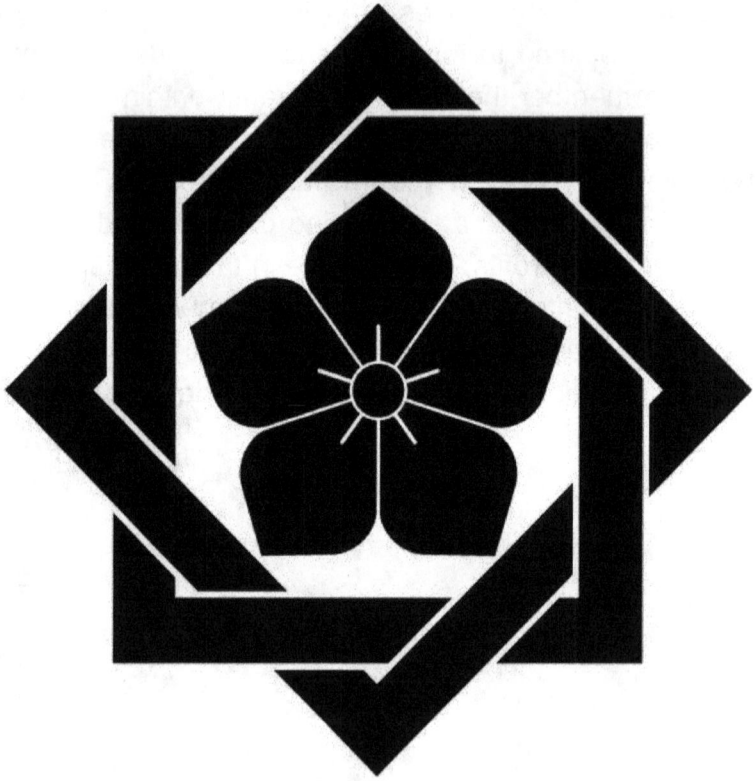

## 4. Afterword

That's it, the manual is finished. We had a great time together!

We got to know ourselves better. We have had new, and interactive, sensations of well-being, in our bodies: physical, energetic, mental, dynamic, magnetic, quantum, vibratory and cosmic.
You are happy when these bodies are aligned.
You can increase your ability to observe the origin of a possible imbalance. And,
You can instantly transform the discomfort into the happiness of being more efficient in this capacity of observation and in this rebalancing.

Guide    100:    Remembering, is the most important.
Exercise  04:    Conscious breathing is the key to happiness.

The rest of your construction of your happiness will happen smoothly, naturally and with joy.

Remember, Happiness is here and now.

Best regards, and wishing you a lot of happiness, building the new world.

Stéphane

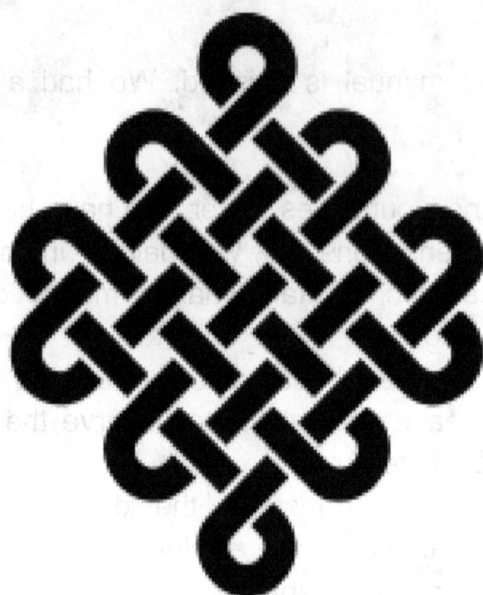

I invite you to join the Facebook page created for this Manual, where you can make a comment, share your experience, ask for a clarification, or give, friendly and without proselytism a contrary or concomitant opinion, and where, soon, will be presented videos, illustrating exercises.

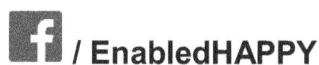

**f / EnabledHAPPY**

If the manual brought you happiness, made you stronger, and strengthened your participation in building a better world, thank you for sharing your enthusiasm. So, faster, more people become also, happier, stronger and more participative.

# 5. Poetry Collection

- 🌀 I have a dream
- 🌀 Universe's messages
- 🌀 Climate change
- 🌀 Here and now
- 🌀 Funky Tic Tic
- 🌀 Making plans
- 🌀 What's the value of my life ?
- 🌀 Clean up
- 🌀 It's for me
- 🌀 A hole my head
- 🌀 To be AND not to be
- 🌀 In the dead wood
- 🌀 What are you doing daddy ?
- 🌀 Bird
- 🌀 Corruption
- 🌀 M living in hell

- *Freedom*
- *Breath in*
- *Chocolate*
- *What a game play !*
- *Is that what you want ?*
- *I don't ask anymore*
- *Came back running*
- *Receive*
- *My tree*
- *M done*
- *Zen*
- *It's not my call*
- *A veil pulled out*
- *Lyli or Jimmy*
- *Communities*
- *Welcome on earth*

# I HAVE A DREAM

I HAVE A DREAM. Walking in the desert, no water, no
food no tree. Not even a scorpion to bit me
M not afraid to died. But it looks like m gone be
My thoughts became confused, ..., in lethargy
What? Is that a new mirage? Oh, my God! A real tree!
Clean water, clean energy, clean seeds, brothers, sisters,
Rainbow colors, timbers to make a house and a pit for
pee, as well as some intimacy, sweet sleep, sweet
dreams, morality, kids on wi-fi.
Taking everything as it comes and get along happy
Stop suffering, start now living. I HAVE A DREAM.
Sustainable poverty eradication, no more a utopia It even
proved to be the solution. The pyramid is now straight and
using cosmic energy. Let's have a mega party, then have
some intimacy. sweet sleep, sweet dreams, morality, kids
on WI-FI. Taking everything as it comes and get along
happy Stop suffering, start now living                    I
HAVE A DREAM, Love, loving, loveable, lovely
I HAVE A DREAM, Love, lover, lovesome, lovingly
I HAVE A DREAM, Love and loved, lovability
Sons and daughters, you're not going to die so soon
Please put pause on WI-FI. Rain is passing through the
roof. Risk losing dream and intimacy. Easy to fix we got
wi-fi. Sweet sleep, sweet dreams, morality, kids on wi-fi
Taking everything as it comes and get along happy

# UNIVERSE`S MESSAGES

A word. A scene. Advert on a bus.
Or coming from TV.
Answers without ambiguity,
Arriving so timely
Universe`s messages

I M 10.
Frightened and amazed by the event
Shall I forget about it?
What is that?
What is happening?

Now 15.
Many coincidences still coming
M I stupid or crazy?
What is that?
What is happening?

When adult. Neither crazy nor stupid, I know
Normal synchronicity
Messages.
Encouraging me to go.

# CLIMATE CHANGE

Ocean levels are rising.
Are you aware you'll have to swim?
And polar ices are melting.
Are you aware you'll have to think?

Climate changes.
I will always be next to you.
Climate changes.
My soul mate loved child and friends
Climate changes.

Are you aware you'll have to change?
To change your job, and what you eat.
Also, what you'll be wearing.
To change your roof, to change your place.
My sweet darling let me kiss you.

Climate changes.
I will always be next to you.
Climate changes.
My soul mate loved child and friends.
Climate changes.

Are you aware you'll have to change?
The tornadoes are twisting round.
Are you aware you'll have to change?
The villages are still flooded.
Whatever is I'll still love you.

Climate changes.
Thanks love for the new born baby.
Climate changes.
Our new house to be furnished.
Climate changes.

Are you aware you'll have to change?
Coping capacities decreased.
Are you aware you'll have to change?
Nationalisms to avoid.
I will always be next to you. Climate changes.

My son soon be getting married.  Climate changes.
I am granddad of a new born.    Climate changes.

Are you aware you'll have to change?
Poorest countries most affected.
Are you aware you'll have to help?
Those are your close neighbors.
Come on darling, let's go to dance.

Climate changes. Great joy to make a fuss of you
Climate changes. My duty to protect you
Climate changes. Are you aware you'll have to change?

Many things to reinvent.
Are you aware you'll have to change?
The world must be mobilized

My soul mate loved child and friends.
Climate changes.
This morning he lost his first tooth.
Climate changes.
The tooth fairy will bring a gift.
Climate changes

Climate changes. G-Eight, G-One, seventy-eight
Climate changes. Industrials, also traders.
Climate changes

Climate changes. Individuals and Consumers,
Climate changes. Associations, and the Schools
Climate changes.
Also, the Universities. Climate changes.
Also, the Organizations. Climate changes.
Please tell me, are you aware?
Climate changes. Climate changes.
General mobilization. Climate changes.
Survival is jeopardized. Climate changes

Climate changes. As from today we have to think. Climate
changes. To change our practices.
Climate changes.

Climate changes. Have better use of the resources
Climate changes. Discovering new ideas.
Climate changes.

Climate changes. Climate changes
Climate changes. Climate changes.

Climate changes. Climate changes.
Survival is jeopardized.
Climate changes.
General mobilization.
Climate changes

Climate changes. M confident we can do it
Climate changes.
Where I am having some doubts.
Climate changes.

Climate changes.
It's when we all going to start?

Climate changes.
Not to wait, not to be forced.
Climate changes

Climate changes.
Taking destiny seriously.
Climat changes.
Climat changes. Climat changes.

# HERE AND NOW

I was happy, and they told me.
To be happy you have to be. Rich and famous.
You have to have ... properties.
You have to have a job, a car a TV.
A beautiful partner. Great friends, long life, good health,
God and spirituality.
You have to do that at that time, wear that cloth, drink that
whisky.

I was happy, and they told me.
You'll be happy to have and be.

I 'have been craving to get there.
I found in it happiness. I found fear to lose it.
I also found happiness after loss.
Living in now, in reality. Cause m now free.
I can now find pleasure in all
Cause m now free ... in love
With this and that and contrary.

Cause m now free ... in love
Cause m now free ... in love
With this and that and contrary. Living in now, in reality.

# FUNKY TIC TIC

Ah ah ah ah, Lost my ethics
TIC TIC TIC TIC
Ah ah ah ah  Lost my ethics
HICK HICK   ICK HICK
Ah ah ah ah  Lost my ethics

Just found one here, ... mouse click,
CLICK CLICK CLICK CLICK CLICK CLICK

Ah ah ah ah  Lost my ethics
TIC TIC TIC TIC M removing, ..., sheep tick
TICK TICK TICK TICK TICK TICK
Delicious as, ..., joss stick

Ah ah ah ah  Realpolitik. Lost my ethics
TIC TIC TIC TIC  Ah ah ah ah Like amnestic
TIC TIC TIC TIC Ah ah ah ah  and not logic
TIC TIC TIC TIC Just found one here, ... Anecdotic

CLICK CLICK CLICK CLICK CLICK CLICK

Ah ah ah ah  Lost my ethics
TIC TIC TIC TIC
M removing, ..., sheep tick,
TICK TICK TICK TICK TICK TICK
Delicious as, ..., joss stick

# MAKING PLANS

MAKING PLANS, OK LET'S START
What will I do with all this wealth?
What will I do with the nuclear fusion?
What will I do with information' mass and pirates?
Will I participate to the knowledge revolution?
Will I control Artificial Intelligence?
Will I best use Super-High-Speed Internet?
How the best my quality life can be - interconnected?
Sure, I'll have best play with Nanotechnology,
and with Social-media literacy
What will I do, with, my long-life expectancy?
If I want it to happen, soon and in a good condition
What does it mean to me?
I maybe know already. What is the best I can do?
MAKING PLANS, AND LET IT GO
I want good food, water, health, tasks, a clean world, no
war, ... education, sciences and philosophies, good sport
and nutrition. Freedom of speech, gender balance,
ecosystems, vegetation, elephants, whales
and all what can be saved, multicultural, apiculture and all
what can be saved,
And many other things to say and invent.
What does it mean for me?
MAKING PLANS, AND LET IT GO
Open a link, watch a video, speak to your friend an' in a
forum. Go to a show. Make a blog, speak to your kid an'
in a forum. Read an article a book a comic, Under a tree,
under the sun. Focus on it, study on purpose,
communicate.

# WHAT IS THE VALUE OF MY LIFE?

AM I? AM I? AM I? AM I?          (x2)
Am I having the right?
What is the value of my life? Is it more than the ocean?
Is it more than the river, the forest, the soil?
Am I having the right to kill them all?
Throwing away the plastic bottle.
Throwing away the plastic bottle.
Soon one billion a day. I'll make of it an ocean.
Plastic balls green, blue, diamond.

Throwing away the plastic bottle.  (x4)

I want at any price maintain my comfort.
Throwing away the plastic bottle.
Has my life more value than the ocean?
I want to dive in the ocean.
Plastic balls green, blue, diamond.
The last sun ray, last green ray, then a deep grey.

AM I? AM I? AM I? AM I? AM I?
Am I having the right?
What is the value of my life?
Is it more than the ocean?
Is it more than the river, the forest, the soil?
Am I having the right to kill them all?
Throwing away the plastic bottle.

# IT'S FOR ME

| | |
|---|---|
| The moon isn'it there? | It's for me ! |
| The sun rising this morning, | It's for me ! |
| The good feeling, | It's for me ! |

| | |
|---|---|
| Beyond happiness | It's for me ! |
| The stone on the road | It's for me ! |
| Falling down to make me see | It's for me ! |
| Intention on what I see | Its' for me ! |
| The good feeling, pleasure to be. | It's for me ! |

M here and when I mean to be

I love myself and my journey

What a great fun to be with you.
I feel so good and energy

Beyond the fears
It's for me !
Waves of the ocean
It's for me !
Washing up all my worries
It's for me !
Washing up and set me free
It's for me !

# A HOLE IN MY HEAD

You are in a hole in my head.
Remains vague image of your face
You are in a hole in my head
I somehow remember our love
No remaining nagging recall
So much passion and suffering.
In the fire of our conjunction

Remains vague image of your face
I did remember my despair. Now not a single emotion.
I can remember our love.
And thanks to it we are here now

You are in a hole in my head
Remains vague image of your face
I even may have felt some hate. Certainly, now obliterated
I can remember our love.
And thanks to it we are here now

Free walking on the road again.
Hobbling along – Strolling about
This little stone in my boots.
How long m I going to keep it
But it's so easy to remove. Making easier the journey
You are in a hole in my head, Part of my personality
However, no more worry. At least no more one another.
I can remember our love.
And thanks to it we are here now

# CLEAN UP

Mother told me that.
Father showed me this.
My friend screwed me up.
I have been so greedy.
So much trouble!
Why did he win not me?
Why am I up side done
when thinking of him?

NO MORE!

The ocean waves clean up
the black spots on my memory

NO MORE!  NO MORE!
So much trouble
NO MORE!

I can now sing-song, laugh, smile, and dance.
I could see you again, and in all cases, I forgave me.
All the mistakes are made, to make it spicier.
Life is so fantastic, let it most time that can be
Let me hope to be alive the most to be,
acting the best in the fantastic seconds to be.
And I'll do the best I can,
telling-listening our fantasies.

I love mother
And father too
Even fucking friend
so greedy
No more trouble
Am I not crazy happy?
I do need no more your validation to be.
IN LOVE!
The ocean waves clean up
the black spots on my memory

CLEAN UP!  CLEAN UP!
So much trouble.  CLEAN UP!

I can now sing-song, laugh, smile, and dance.
I could see you again. And in any case, forgive me.
All the mistakes made to make it spicier.
Life is so fantastic let it most time be
Let me hope to be alive the most to be,
acting the best in the fantastic seconds to be.
And I'll do the best I can,
telling-listening our fantasies.

# TO BE AND NOT TO BE

It was not my choice.                    Was it?
I was just playing with your toys.      I did.
Helping you with your troubles.
Taking them into my heart.
Breaking your toys and finding mine.
Your fears are not mine,
neither yours betray, your ghosts and your bombs.
Let me answer to your question.
To be AND not to be, that is the answer.
Surfing the wave on the top on the down.
It is my choice.                     Is it?
I am playing with better toys.        Am I?
To be and not to be, that is the answer.
Relax. I know a lot of trouble around.
Relax. Then you'll find better toy.
They were all my choices.          They were.
Anyway, thank for your toys.         I played.
Do I need other troubles? I believe I`ll always do.
Breaking my toys and finding new.
Your fears are gone. M glad if you are happy,  cause I
am. Happiness will now stay here,
will stay here for a while, flying and crawling.
Surfing the wave of the day, the top the down.
It's my best choice.                It is.
Relax. Then you'll find better toy.
That is the answer. On the top, the down.
Today it's cold outside. Weather announced will get
better. Let's stay home for a while.
Relax. Then you'll find better toy.

# IN THE DEAD WOOD

In the dead wood there is the worm,
the carpenter and the banker.
In the dead wood, there is the earth, the seed,
sap from the tree, sun, rain, axe and ...
the wax of the cabinet-maker.
In the dead wood there are the scars,
of thousand arrows shot in my heart.
And ... our kiss at the feet of the oak.
My breath on your lips.
In the dead wood my breath on your lips, and the
woodpecker drumming
The travel of the bee, the flower, the bee keeper,
the honey, the wax, the businessman, the trader,
the transporter, you and me.
In the dead wood there is today, yesterday, last week,
next year and all around.
In the dead wood there are mushrooms,
an omelet, a glass of Beaujolais.
In the dead wood there is the shell,
the grain of sand and the black hole.
In the dead wood, furious ocean,
the boat, the fisherman, storm, wind, fear
and ... The helicopter rescue mission.
In the dead wood there are the waves,
repeated in the clock whirlpool.  And ... the photon, the
boson, the fermion. Back on my skin after a nice journey,
and the woodpecker drumming
In the dead wood there are mushrooms, an omelet, a
glass of Beaujolais.

# WHAT ARE YOU DOING DADDY?

Oh, daddy what are you doing?   And on who's name?
What is about me? What is my name?
Oh, daddy what are you doing?
Cold blood murder on way to jail
Sometime will be good to forgive
Sometime is also redemption. It can also be unity

What are you doing uncle?
Weapons trader?
Crazy scientist? Is that your name?
Uncle what are you doing?
Cold blood murder going to jail.

... We'll go over it. Finding the law, burst out laughing
and peaceful nap under the tree

You must be knowing dad. What is my name?
Is that the son of the dark' prince?
Tell you M going to change.
Maybe for Sleepy-Dopey-Happy?
Diamond on little earth band
that has survived, bloody idiot: → guitar

My name be love-happiness-passion

# BIRD

Bird, I like so much to see you flying,
Seeing you singing, hip hopping.
Bathing on the sun, Your red, orange, yellow,
green, blue, indigo, violet.

Sailing on the waves, symphony of joy.
Bon voyage, thanks making me feel joy and freedom.
M also now free singing, in full control,
on the spirals of my DNA.
This makes me feel I can also fly on infinite oneness
to love, return home and have time,
Safe surfing on what you say.
We are safe here. Our secret garden.
How beautiful this moonbeam reflecting on your face!
M surfing on the moon ray.

I know now. Bird, so much I like to see you flying,
Seeing you singing, hip hopping.
Bathing on the sun, Your red, orange, yellow,
green, blue, indigo, violet.
Bird, in the heart of the waves melting away,
Thanks for your singularity,
Dazzling generous sun, Your red, orange, yellow,
green, blue, indigo, violet.
Sailing on the waves, symphony of joy.
Bon voyage, thanks making me feel joy and freedom.

# CORRUPTION

Corruption! Accused. Rulers of this and this country.
You will know and admit. Corruption! Accused.
Billions of people enslaved.
Spoiled from their rights to food, water and electricity.

Corruption! Accused, Multiple false deals.
Bribes financing shame and criminality.

Corruption! Accused.
Flouted responsibilities.
Under the table the bill to pay.

So much cash, luxury. Billions diverted.
Comfort for everyone. But for a handful of dicks.
Corrupted bastards distorting the markets.
Distorting the logic, of a good well-earned bread.

Billions of people robbed. Fortune for a handful.
Dogs happy feeding their own fears to be caught.
Fine, you can shack corrupted.
Soon you'll have to pay.
Now you are surrounded. Justice on its way.
Criminals on your back. Accomplices and puppets.
Of your decadent show. Will also make you pay.

You think you are on your island, untouchable.

The volcano takes revenge, bury illusion.

No excuse, you knew, all return back to you.
However, you should have.
However, you could have.
An honest management. A sustained development.
An ideal of faire trade. Flourishing enterprises.
The reasons' benefits. Fair, shared, honest earning.
Cult of life not of market. I summon you to stop.
Your bullshit right away.
You have to start today.
First you correct your scale. It's old and distorted.
Rapidly you will see. Joy non-adulterer.
Functioning societies.
Blooming populations. School, health, arts, blossoming.
Fresh water, job for all, free and clean energy.
Fulfilling lives for One, for everyone.
Now the sun is rising, on a floral earth,
on the love of life.

# M LIVING IN HELL

M living in hell. What a strange idea !
My body hanging above the flames.
My flesh is crackling.
M burning. Burn, burn, burn, burn, burn.
The fire is burning. Burn, burn, burn, burn, burn.
The flames. Burning, burning, burning, burning, burning.

M consumed with jealousy. My regrets are molting.
Flashback of my defects. M living in hell.
What a strange idea !
My judgments carbonizing. My arrogance calcining.
M strolling on embers.

The fire surrounds my desires.
Reduced to ashes by my craving.
M not living but burning. M Burning in hell.
What a strange idea !

Giant fire of my recall. Burned out by my believes
Set in fire by my glances. M living in hell.
What a strange idea !

My lies branding me. Angers on the grill
Ardent Inaction. M burning. Burn, burn, burn, burn, burn.
The fire is burning. Burn, burn, burn, burn, burn.
The flames. Burning, burning, burning, burning, burning.
What a strange idea !

# FREEDOM

| | |
|---|---|
| My freedom, | What am I doing ? |
| My freedom, | What am I doing ? |
| My freedom, | What am I doing ? |

| | |
|---|---|
| Murdering you, | What am I doing ? |
| And raping you, | What am I doing ? |
| And swindling you, | What am I doing ? |
| And beating you, | What am I doing ? |
| Harassing you, | What am I doing ? |
| And judging you, | What am I doing ? |

However it shall be so nice !
To savor love and friendship,
Not having to pay after cheating,
And not for so long suffering,
After a short moment of pleasure

Again and again, starting from scratch.
Always having to give a tip.

| | |
|---|---|
| My freedom, | What am I doing ? |

| | |
|---|---|
| Suffocating, | What am I doing ? |
| Poisoning me, | What am I doing ? |
| And hating me, | What am I doing ? |
| And when moping, | What am I doing ? |
| Torturing me, | What am I doing ? |
| Remembering, | What am I doing ? |

What a karma m I making ?
Again, again, starting from scratch.
Always having to give a tip.

STOP !
However it shall be so nice !
Finding always new ideas,
To travel together the new path,
Each one finding satisfaction,
Together managing the challenges.

Again and again, starting from scratch.
Please enjoy the change as a tip.

| My freedom, | What am I doing ? |
| My freedom, | What am I doing ? |
| My freedom, | What am I doing ? |

| And hating you, | What am I doing ? |
| And stoning you, | What am I doing ? |
| And hurting you, | What am I doing ? |
| Also biting, | What am I doing ? |
| Locking you up, | What am I doing ? |
| Remembering, | What am I doing ? |

What a karma m I making ?
Again and again starting from scratch.
Always having to give a tip.  STOP !

However it shall be so nice !
Going with you for a walk,

Together tasting the silence,
enjoying singing laughing,
Understanding, helping, forgiving.

Again and again starting from scratch.
Please enjoy the change as a tip.

| | |
|---|---|
| My freedom, | What am I doing ? |
| My freedom, | What am I doing ? |
| My freedom, | What am I doing ? |

| | |
|---|---|
| Putting it right, | It's what m doing ! |
| Conscious breathing, | It's what m doing ! |
| Remembering, | It's what m doing ! |
| Best loving you, | It's what m doing ! |
| Listening you, | It's what m doing ! |
| Making you laugh, | It's what m doing ! |

Again and again, starting from scratch.

# BREATHE IN

Breathe out ! Enjoy living.          Breathe in !
With entire body.                    Breathe out !
In every cell.                       Breathe in !
Feel air flowing.                    Breathe in !
You have a thought.                  Breathe out !
That's normal let it go.             Breathe in !
Just a single focus.                 Breathe out !
It's just about air flow.            Breathe in !
Very often we get so stacked,
thinking about a past event,
thinking about my future plans.
But, breathe, only present can be.
Breathe, Breathe, Breathe, and be present.
Breathe in !  And your intuition is growing.
Breathe in !  At last you find the solution.
End to the turning obsession.        Breathe in !
See the serenity growing. Become alive not asphyxia.
Now see you mind is opening.
You're alive not navel gazing.       Breathe in !
Find new meaning to your life.       Breathe in !
And be present.                      Breathe in !
At each moment.          Breathe in !  Everywhere.
In every cell Max oxygen.            Breathe in !
Pain and sadness are dissipated.     Breathe in !
Present is life and energy.          Breath out !
Enjoy living.                        Breath in !
With entire body.                    Breath out !
In every cell

# WHAT A GAME PLAY

So many truths,      what a game play
Multi-dimension Universe
So many truths,      what a game play

There, over there. Here, and here also.
And that, and that also.
This solution, and this one two.
Multi-Universe expanding in all directions.
M choosing mine.
Thanks my mistakes for better play
Thanks my success for better play
Feeling good is my pathway
I trust in Love, love, love. Love, love, love

There, over there. Here, and here also.
And that, and that also.
This solution, and this one two.
One way for me and the best play
Son of the stars. Just emotions
Thanks my mistakes for better play
Thanks my success for better play
Always happy on the new day.
I trust in Love, love, love. Love, love, love

# CHOCOLATE

Sometimes I would prefer, not have to take a decision,
Never ending eating cake. Never creating delusions.

CHOCOLATE!   … Its for my mouth not my body.
CHOCOLATE!      Even for my mind only.
Can't even be sharing you now.
I want you more, infinity.
Celebrating each piece of yours,
and never feeling guilty.
I always want you to be with me.

Sometimes I would prefer, not have to take a decision,
never ending eating cake, never creating delusion.

CHOCOLATE! I can't find the peace,
until I'll finished the box.

CHOCOLATE! I like how you treat me.
I want you, more and more and more.
Not ending at any cost.
No matters when. No Where. No Who.

CHOCOLATE!      I wish you'll be with me eternally.

Sometimes I would prefer, not have to take a decision,
never ending eating cake, never creating delusion.

CHOCOLATE!   … Now I could give you my life!
CHOCOLATE! My life is now only my mind not my body.

My desire of you back and forth. I could cry like a baby.
Melting in my mouth, blowing my mind.
Chocolate, only you and I, and now.
No time, no space, no energy.

Sometimes I would prefer, not have to take a decision,
never ending eating cake, never creating delusion.

CHOCOLATE! I want the time to freeze now,
at the moment you are melting.
CHOCOLATE! I like how you treat me.
Thanks you, more and more and more
I know you're here somewhere.
Also enjoying ecstasy. CHOCOLATE!
Thanks sharing with me your heaven.

I LOVE YOU CHOCOLATE!

# IS THAT WHAT YOU WANT

Choice between joy and misery.
Stop all these wars. Is that what you want ?
Barbed wires and walls. Is that what you want ?
At a cross-road for humanity.
Between peace and despair.
Could be starvation or the end.
Between fresh air and nausea.
Between knowing and ignore.
At a cross-road for humanity. Is that what you want ?
Between devil and deep blue sea.
Is that what you want ?
Or being the one with good feeling.
Between solar and equinox.
Between the love and the fear.
At a cross-road for humanity. Between legal illegality.
Between loyal and spoiled child.
Between love and premature.
Merry-go-round and stillborn.
At a cross-road for humanity. Is that what you want ?
Between devil and deep blue sea.
Is that what you want ?
Or being the one with good feeling.
Stop all these wars. Barbed wires and walls.
Is that what you want ?
There is one day you shall stop.

# I DON'T ASK ANYMORE

One could ask the question.
Life is really simple. Healthy food, Breathing and love.
Loving ourselves for what you do.
This is best that you could do, all around will just enfold.

Healthy heart and big cleaning.
Healthy wave cleaning my grief.
Oxygen is pure energy.

In my energy field,   m getting strong and loved.
In your energy field, m coming in if you're smiling.

Other models are deep falling.
Healthy wave of love energy.
Arrivederci my dear toxins.
Good food is good energy.
The sun did rise this morning.
The rain had fed all the chicks.

In my energy field, m getting strong and loved.
In your energy field, m coming in if you're smiling.
Breathing deeply, not asphyxia.
Healthy breath and Healthy body.
So long so long my carbonic.

# CAME BACK RUNNING

My intuition came back running.
Feeling my thoughts and all their journeys.
Feeling peaceful on immensity.
Feeling motivated and free.
Feeling loved and loving me.

Loving souls and infinity, in absolute and in quantity.
M so happy to meet with you, and to agree on fraternity.

In this deal we are both happy,
in absolute and in quantity.
Feeling peaceful on singularity.
Feeling relax on individuality.

My intuition came back running.
Feeling my thoughts and all their journeys.
Feeling peaceful on immensity.
Feeling motivated and free.
Feeling loved and loving me.

Colors, sounds, originality. Your energy your company.
M so happy to meet with you, and to agree on fraternity.

In this deal we are both happy in absolute and in quantity.
Feeling peaceful on singularity.
Feeling relax on individuality.

# MY TREE

My tree
You're alive with the rain
You're alive with the earth
With the sun and also the wind

My tree. I can't live without you
Your beauty is marvel
Nice nap under your shade
After you leave m muted

The juices from all your fruits
When sweet or when bitter
Each time m enchanted
The curves of your body
Swinging in the wind
Your shine and your colors

I can't live without you
Believe I promise you, to knowing loving you
And also protect you
Can't stop smelling flowers. Can't stop painting colors
Can't stop watching you dance

My tree
Please don't leave me

# RECEIVE

Life is simple.
Give it to me. Give it to me. Give it to me, now.
As easy as, add one to one.
Give it to me. Give it to me. Give it to me, now.

One thing for all. A simple rule.
Give it to me, Give it to me. Give it to me, now.
To receive. First is to give.

Give it to me. Give it to me. Give it to me, now.
Give it to me. Give it to me. Give it to me, now.

Looking for love give now love.     .
Give it to me. Give it to me. Give it to me, now.
Lets share it now.  One earth-one love.

Wish some money?
Give he'll comes back.
Give it to me. Give it to me.
Give it to me, now.
Success is guaranteed.
Rich and happy.

Searching friendship?
First give yours out.
Give it to me. Give it to me.
Give it to me, now.
To receive.
First is to give.

Wanting respect?
Give out first yours.
Give it to me. Give it to me.
Give it to me, now.
Then enjoy,
the recognition.

The people listening to you.
First is to learn, how to listen.
Give it to me. Give it to me.
Give it to me, now.
Give it to me, now.

It is working for everything .
Give it to me. Give it to me.
Give it to me, now.
To receive First is to give.
Give it to me. Give it to me.
Give it to me, now.

# IT'S NOT MY CALL

| | |
|---|---|
| Your war, | IT'S NOT MY CALL. |
| Your vice, | IT'S NOT MY CALL. |

I don't want to speak with you.
Somehow, I may become interested.
But definitely I know.
You're compromising my journey.
By the corrupted way you are walking.
Get up !      Other tune your inspiration.
Get up !      Slightly more of some compassion.
Get out !     I do not need validation.
Neither your boots, critics nor oppression.
I've all to be happy, leave me alone.

| | |
|---|---|
| Your war | IT'S NOT MY CALL. |
| Your vice | IT'S NOT MY CALL. |

I have my story, my war, my compassion.
Get out !     I do not need validation.
Neither your boots, critics nor oppression.
I've fine tune dreams, freedom, passions.

| | |
|---|---|
| Your war, | IT'S NOT MY CALL. |
| Your vice, | IT'S NOT MY CALL. |
| Your stress, | IT'S NOT MY CALL. |
| Your air, | IT'S ALSO MINE. |
| Freedom, | NO COMPROMISE. |

I've fine tune dreams, pleasures, passions.

# M DONE

M done, m done, m done. The pain gone away, m done.
Found good vib, m done. Energy optimized for now,
 m done. Happy what I do, m done
Loving me, m done. Loving you, m done.
Suffering, m done. CHOCOLATE!
The best i can do so far Loving me, Loving you,
Keep going on the miracle of live
What you are doing hurting me no more, ...
or still some time, but shortly. Loving me, Loving you.
I visited paradise. Looks good to me.
will stay here for a while. CHOCOLATE!
Thanks so much. It was nice to meeting you, suffering
It brought me here. I'll visit you sometime but shortly
Will stay more on my good vib
reconnect with nature, with you, I, All
Looking, feeling your colors. Keeping going
Feeling good. Knowing what I don't want
allowed me to know what I do. Loving me, Loving you,
Learning from your words. Learning from mine
Loving me, Loving you,
Learning from my mistakes. Learning from yours
Loving me, Loving you.
Learning from your keys, finding new
Loving me, Loving you, Happy what I do, m done
Now it`s the best I can do. Keep going, going, going
No more stress, m done.
Feeling good easy life, m done. Happy what I do,
m done. Happy of what I've done, I'll do
Now it`s the best I can do

# ZEN

You and I, no distinction. Like a cable-knit sweater.
You and I, here and there. All a single energy.
One life, one world, one being.
Singularity in All. All in singularity.
Zen!
Whatever the event is. It's neither good nor bad.
Just matter of perception.
Can be strange, but it's all good.
Aren't galaxies turning? Don't be such an arrogant !
You're much more than accident.
Who, what, when this is happening,
Equal to understanding.
Zen! Source of happiness,
All is to be found inner. There is the outer and more.
It's my choice and it's my life.
JUST! Managing my response.
STOP! Bad reaction on the event.
JUST! Managing my response.
Is event good or bad? It is neither of them.
JUST! Managing my response.
M free facing the event. Golden pearl in each event.
Who, what, when is happening,
Is exactly for my need. ZEN! Positive energy.
Joy coming from my spirit. Neither things nor the events.
Grief coming from my spirit. Neither things nor the events.
Zen!

# LILI OR JIMMY

Lili  iiiii        Love you always on one pathway
Jimmy  iiiii    Wish you the best the other way
Always my love follows your day.
Love my new born, blessed parent's days
Lili  iiiii        Kids are pure love on any way
Jimmy  iiiii    Love you always on one pathway
Flying with stars an other day. Lili  iiiii    What a great fun
the other day. Growing around on lover play
Jimmy  iiiii    You got so high on your pathway
M on mine too the other day. Feeling the sun going this
Way. Lili  iiiii        Like you new house and its pathway
Will walk in through on the planned day.
Nice to know you are happy every Way
Jimmy  iiiii    What a great fun the other day
Lili  iiiii        All going there the other day
Jimmy  iiiii    Always my love follow your Way.
Somewhere a life all in one day
M now loving me more, what can I say
Lili  iiiii        Love you always on single way
Jimmy  iiiii    You do the same on one pathway
All this is done on any day. Lili  iiiii        Love you now
more this is my day. Love you always on one pathway
Jimmy  iiiii    You got so high on your pathway
M on mine two the other day.
Feeling the sun going the way
Lili  iiiii        Like you new house and its pathway
Will walk in through on the planned day.
Nice to know you are happy every day
Jimmy  iiiii    What a great fun the other day

# A VEIL PULLED OUT

Today walking on the beach
I telepathy chatted with a Heron.
I discovered later during our conversation,
He was the angelic delegate of the nature.
We were standing at marveling,
The nature's beauty displayed.
The swarming of life all around at low tide,
The blue-green algae,
The seagulls triangular flight,
Merging with the white of the waves,
The silvery gleam of the anchovy,
Savored by my brother the Heron,
And by his valiant little bird friend,
Fast running between his legs.

Our conversation became sorrow,
As we mourned man-made massacre of nature.

Then we became ecstatic,
As my friend received from Universe,
The right given to nature,
To furthermore unveil to humanity
Its marvelous beauty.

From now enjoy my friends,
This unprecedented unveiled beauty.

After I continued on the beach,
Collecting corals and shells.
Each and every time amazed, by fabulous treasures.
And by their flowery demonstration of being.

In one of the multiple caves of these precious gems,
I found keyed one of these plastic refill lead of pencil,
Fine moreover,
looking like a lighthouse in middle of the cliff,
Enabling the vessels to not run aground,

Like a sign of our violation of nature,
And telling me to compose for you these words.

# WELCOME ON EARTH

Argentina, Brunei, Namibia, Paraguay,
Turkey, Madagascar, Nepal, Cape Verde,
Switzerland, Tunisia, Armenia, Brazil,
Algeria, Suriname, Germany, UK,

Afghanistan, Benin, Nigeria, Panama,
Thailand, Martinique, Norway, Cayman Islands,
Swaziland, Andorra, Burundi, Russia,
Indonesia, Angola, Malawi, Bhutan,

Azerbaijan, Bahrain, Cambodia, Gibraltar,
Vietnam, Coco Islands, Burma, United-States,
Singapore, Senegal, Netherlands, Maldives,
Bermuda, Ethiopia, Botswana, Guinea,

Antarctica, Chile, Portugal, DRC,
Cuba, Eritrea, China, Jamaica,
Canada, Ecuador, Palestine, Seychelles
Malaysia, Colombia, Djibouti, France,

Guatemala, Fiji, Kazakhstan, Bolivia,
Denmark, El Salvador, Egypt, Nicaragua,
Italy, Israel, Bangladesh, Finland,
Grenada, Guadeloupe,     Guernsey, Hong Kong,

South Africa, Greenland, Hungary, Macau,
India, Sierra Leone, Iceland, Ivory Coast,
Australia, Monaco, Lesotho, Japan,
Sri Lanka, Kyrgyzstan, Liberia, Gabon,

Costa Rica, Sweden, Mozambique, Peru,
Taiwan, Venezuela, Mali, Mauritania,
Slovenia, Philippines, Lebanon, Togo,
Lithuania, Bahamas, Samoa, Ireland.

# COMMUNITIES

Slowly take off your shell. A sign of friendship
Slowly take off your shell. Make a step aside.
Slowly take off your shell. You are welcome, pleasure.
Slowly take off your shell.
The air is fresh and pure outside.
Please be my guest. Thank you so much.
So kind of you. Have a nice day.

Evening community. Compound Community
Gathering at the park. Around a game, a play.
Or around a project. Meeting of art lovers.
Or sharing a hobby. Passionate gathering.
Or praying together. Or meditating.

I go party tonight. I 'have plans for the weekends.
Saturday skating rink. Sunday will be movie.
A walk in nature. You will stay for dinner.
I will send it by mail. I'll join the photos two.
Here is the address. You'll find this on the web.

Global community. Village community
Corp'rate Associations. Students at the school.
College and faculty. Groups of volunteers.
Helping groups, charities.
Communities in need. Communities for fun.
Chatting and smiling.

# 6. Appendix

## ❷ Human Rights

Universal Declaration of Human Rights (1948)

Article I : All human beings are born free and equal in dignity and rights. They are endowed with reason and conscience and should act towards one another in a spirit of brotherhood.

Article 2 : Everyone is entitled to all the rights and freedoms set forth in this Declaration, without distinction of any kind, such as race, colour, sex, language, religion, political or other opinion, national or social origin, property, birth or other status.

Furthermore, no distinction shall be made on the basis of the political, jurisdictional or international status of the country or territory to which a person belongs, whether it be independent, trust, non-self-governing or under any other limitation of sovereignty.

Article 3 : Everyone has the right to life, liberty and security of person.

Article 4 : No one shall be held in slavery or servitude; slavery and the slave trade shall be prohibited in all their forms.

Article 5 : No one shall be subjected to torture or to cruel, inhuman or degrading treatment or punishment.

Article 6 : Everyone has the right to recognition everywhere as a person before the law.

Article 7 : All are equal before the law and are entitled without any discrimination to equal protection of the law. All are entitled to equal protection against any discrimination in violation of this Declaration and against any incitement to such discrimination.

Article 8 : Everyone has the right to an effective remedy by the competent national tribunals for acts violating the fundamental rights granted him by the constitution or by law.

Article 9 : No one shall be subjected to arbitrary arrest, detention or exile.

Article 10 : Everyone is entitled in full equality to a fair and public hearing by an independent and impartial tribunal, in the determination of his rights and obligations and of any criminal charge against him.

Article 11 :    1. Everyone charged with a penal offence has the right to be presumed innocent until proved guilty according to law in a public trial at which he has had all the guarantees necessary for his defense

2. No one shall be held guilty of any penal offence on account of any act or omission which did not constitute a penal offence, under national or international law, at the time when it was committed. Nor shall a heavier penalty be imposed than the one that was applicable at the time the penal offence was committed.

Article 12 : No one shall be subjected to arbitrary interference with his privacy, family, home or correspondence, nor to attacks upon his honor and reputation. Everyone has the right to the protection of the law against such interference or attacks.

Article 13 : 1. Everyone has the right to freedom of movement and residence within the borders of each State.

2. Everyone has the right to leave any country, including his own, and to return to his country.

Article 14 : 1. Everyone has the right to seek and to enjoy in other countries asylum from persecution.

2. This right may not be invoked in the case of prosecutions genuinely arising from non-political crimes or from acts contrary to the purposes and principles of the United Nations.

Article 15: 1. Everyone has the right to a nationality.

2. No one shall be arbitrarily deprived of his nationality nor denied the right to change his nationality.

Article 16 : 1. Men and women of full age, without any limitation due to race, nationality or religion, have the right to marry and to found a family. They are entitled to equal rights as to marriage, during marriage and at its dissolution.

2. Marriage shall be entered into only with the free and full consent of the intending spouses.

3. The family is the natural and fundamental group unit of society and is entitled to protection by society and the State.

Article 17 : 1. Everyone has the right to own property alone as well as in association with others.

2. No one shall be arbitrarily deprived of his property.

Article 18: Everyone has the right to freedom of thought, conscience and religion; this right includes freedom to change his religion or belief, and freedom, either alone or in community with others and in public or private, to manifest his religion or belief in teaching, practice, worship and observance.

Article 19 : Everyone has the right to freedom of opinion and expression; this right includes freedom to hold opinions without interference and to seek, receive and impart information and ideas through any media and regardless of frontiers.

Article 20 : 1. Everyone has the right to freedom of peaceful assembly and association.

2. No one may be compelled to belong to an association.

Article 21 : 1. Everyone has the right to take part in the government of his country, directly or through freely chosen representatives.

2. Everyone has the right to equal access to public service in his country.

3. The will of the people shall be the basis of the authority of government; this will shall be expressed in periodic and genuine elections which shall be by universal and equal suffrage and shall be held by secret vote or by equivalent free voting procedures.

Article 22 : Everyone, as a member of society, has the right to social security and is entitled to realization, through national effort and international co-operation and in accordance with the organization and resources of each State, of the economic, social and cultural rights indispensable for his dignity and the free development of his personality.

Article 23 : 1. Everyone has the right to work, to free choice of employment, to just and favorable conditions of work and to protection against unemployment.

2. Everyone, without any discrimination, has the right to equal pay for equal work.

3. Everyone who works has the right to just and favorable remuneration ensuring for himself and his family an existence worthy of human dignity, and supplemented, if necessary, by other means of social protection.

4. Everyone has the right to form and to join trade unions for the protection of his interests.

Article 24 : Everyone has the right to rest and leisure, including reasonable limitation of working hours and periodic holidays with pay.

Article 25 : 1. Everyone has the right to a standard of living adequate for the health and well-being of himself and of his family, including food, clothing, housing and medical care and necessary social services, and the right to security in the event of unemployment, sickness, disability, widowhood, old age or other lack of livelihood in circumstances beyond his control.

2. Motherhood and childhood are entitled to special care and assistance. All children, whether born in or out of wedlock, shall enjoy the same social protection.

Article 26 : 1. Everyone has the right to education. Education shall be free, at least in the elementary and fundamental stages. Elementary education shall be compulsory. Technique and professional education shall be made generally available and higher education shall be equally accessible to all on the basis of merit.

2. Education shall be directed to the full development of the human personality and to the strengthening of respect for human rights and fundamental freedoms. It shall promote understanding, tolerance and friendship among all nations, racial or religious groups, and shall further the activities of the United Nations for the maintenance of peace.

3. Parents have a prior right to choose the kind of education that shall be given to their children.

Article 27 : 1. Everyone has the right freely to participate in the cultural life of the community, to enjoy the arts and to share in scientific advancement and its benefits.

2. Everyone has the right to the protection of the moral and material interests resulting from any scientific, literary or artistic production of which he is the author.

Article 28 : Everyone is entitled to a social and international order in which the rights and freedoms set forth in this Declaration can be fully realized.

Article 29 : 1. Everyone has duties to the community in which alone the free and full development of his personality is possible.

2. In the exercise of his rights and freedoms, everyone shall be subject only to such limitations as are determined by law solely for the purpose of securing due recognition and respect for the rights and freedoms of others and of meeting the just requirements of morality, public order and the general welfare in a democratic society.

3. These rights and freedoms may in no case be exercised contrary to the purposes and principles of the United Nations.

Article 30 : Nothing in this Declaration may be interpreted as implying for any State, group or person any right to engage in any activity or to perform any act aimed at the destruction of any of the rights and freedoms set forth herein.

## 7. Table of contents

www.ingramcontent.com/pod-product-compliance
Lightning Source LLC
Chambersburg PA
CBHW071726270326
41928CB00013B/2581